# Health Wars

# Health Wars

## On the Global Front Lines of Modern Medicine

Richard Horton

NEW YORK REVIEW BOOKS

nyrb

*New York*

THIS IS A NEW YORK REVIEW BOOK

PUBLISHED BY THE NEW YORK REVIEW OF BOOKS

HEALTH WARS: ON THE GLOBAL FRONT LINES
OF MODERN MEDICINE

by Richard Horton



This edition published in 2003
in the United States of America by
The New York Review of Books
1755 Broadway
New York, NY 10019
www.nybooks.com

The illustration on page xxiv appears courtesy of
Erich Lessing/Art Resource, New York

Library of Congress Cataloging-in-Publication Data

Horton, Richard C.
Health wars: on the global front lines of modern medicine /
Richard Horton.
p. ; cm.
Chiefly articles originally published in the New York review of books.
ISBN 1-59017-024-5 (hardcover : alk. paper)

1. Medicine—Miscellanea. 2. Medical care—Miscellanea.
3. Social medicine—Miscellanea.
[DNLM: 1. Medicine—trends—Popular Works. 2. Physician–Patient Relations—Popular
Works. WB 130 H823h 2003] I. Title.
R708.H785 2003
610—dc21

2003007252

ISBN 1-59017-024-5

Printed in the United States of America on acid-free paper.

June 2003

1 3 5 7 9 10 8 6 4 2

*for Ingrid and Isobel*

# Contents

# Preface

THE FIRST JOB I took after I qualified as a doctor in 1986 was "house officer" (an intern, in US parlance) for a surgeon who specialized in stapling the stomachs of very large people. My main responsibilities were taking histories from new patients, doing scut work for the rest of the surgical team (such as ordering take-out dinners when we were on call), and accepting the blame when things went wrong. My boss was an impatient man—he was an obsessive squash player—and he insisted that I stand in the operating room all day watching him cut and sew. That meant I had little time for pleasant conversation with new patients. One morning, the ward was chaotic with nurses ushering out barely sutured but nevertheless grateful patients while squeezing in, as best they could, a new cohort of the hopeful sick. I had eight names on the day's operating list, so my encounters with each of them amounted to hardly more than "Hello, are you the person with a right inguinal hernia? Good, then sign here." I was halfway down my list when I arrived at the bedside of a man in his sixties. I went through a brief and routine lecture about the dos and don'ts of the ward. He looked at me rather vaguely. I pushed the consent form in front of him—again he looked at me uncomprehendingly. My heart sank. All doctors will recognize this feeling. I raised my voice a little, asking him again to sign the consent form *please*. He mumbled something back to me, but I did not understand him. My eyes projected irritation. And then he picked up a pad of paper and a pen and wrote, "I am deaf." I will go to the grave remembering (and deserving to remember) the cruel discourtesy I inflicted on this man.

But I shall also remember this. On a Saturday afternoon at a busy teaching hospital in Birmingham, England, I was the medical resident on call for the weekend. I carried the pager, which, if it went off, would alert me that a patient had collapsed somewhere close by with a suspected cardiac arrest. It did go off that afternoon, around three o'clock, and a crackling voice reported that a man had arrested in the hospital's swimming pool. I ran with the house officer, who was on call with me, to the pool, across a road and pushing a rickety cardiac arrest trolley, all the time trying to hold on to the defibrillator as we went. When we finally reached the pool area we saw that the man, who was in his fifties, had been pulled out of the water and was lying unconscious at the poolside. He was pulseless, had stopped breathing, and his heart was flatlining on the cardiac monitor. We bagged air into his lungs and shocked his chest several times with escalating voltages of electricity. At last, a weak pulse started and he began taking shallow breaths. He had a rough course over the next day or so. But he recovered and went on to have specialized diagnostic studies which showed that the electrical impulse of his heart followed an abnormal path on its journey through the cardiac muscle. Surgery rectified the problem completely, as surgery so often does. His wife was a receptionist at the hospital. She baked me a lovely cake.

Medicine is inevitably about death as well as life. And death makes its mark on all doctors, whatever defenses they (say they) might develop or deploy. Doctors are not unique witnesses of death. If we are fortunate, we will all have the privilege of being with those we love most when their last breath leaves their body. The difference for doctors, perhaps, is not only that they experience death more often, but also that the circumstances of the deaths they experience are frequently more extreme—the consequences of violence or trauma, the multiple lines hastily inserted into arteries and veins in the emergency room, tubes pushed down the trachea or esophagus, and, of course, blood. We do not do death very well in Western cultures. Even in an age that celebrates its lack of respect for tradition, the details of how a person dies remain taboo, presumably because they bring us face-to-face with how we ourselves might die. Our inquiries stumble and our interest falters, and we will go to almost any lengths to avoid such a confrontation until the day when we have no choice in the matter.

One death still haunts me because of its silent ferocity. I had admitted a man in his seventies to the hospital one evening with a history of bleeding from what seemed to be his stomach. He had vomited a little blood earlier in the day. His blood pressure was low and so we put him to bed. His condition was monitored regularly by the nursing staff. Later in the evening, a nurse called me to say that he had vomited a small amount of what looked like fresh blood. I walked to the ward, drew the curtains around the man's bed, and sat down beside him to examine his heart and lungs. He seemed unconcerned by his episode of sickness and was more bothered by the fact that I had been troubled. I put up another bag of fluid to run through his intravenous line, but as I was about to leave he began to retch. A little blood oozed out between his lips, which I collected into a bowl. The ooze then became a trickle, which soon became a steady stream. A constant flow of blood was now coming out of his mouth—faster and faster and in ever-increasing quantities. He began to panic because he could not catch his breath. I leaned him forward trying to speak calmly to reassure him, but at the same time beginning to panic myself. Would the bleeding stop on its own? If not, how would I stop it? The situation was rapidly spinning out of my control. I squeezed the bag of fluid hard into his vein, and I called the nurse to ask her to find a more senior doctor. Meanwhile, blood was now gushing from the man's mouth all over himself, the bedclothes, and me. For what seemed like several minutes I was alone with him on the bed behind the curtains as he bled determinedly to death. When the blood finally did stop flowing, I sat there with my arms around a warm corpse. His skin was white and his eyes stared forward into the pool of blood lying before him. He had watched himself die and he had seen and felt my complete inability to do anything to help him. This scene comes into my mind most days, even now some fifteen years later. It was not a violent death in the ordinary sense of the word. There was no external sign of injury. I found out later that the large blood vessel carrying blood from his heart—the aorta—had fused with his esophagus. When the aorta finally ruptured into his esophagus, as it sometimes does, his heart simply emptied all the circulating blood into his mouth and stomach. He had no chance of surviving once the rupture took place, but he knew nothing of this as he watched the blood accumulate in front of him. What must his last thoughts have been?

These are the sort of personal stories that all doctors can tell. And we do tell sanitized and satirized versions of them to one another—all the time. When I have occasionally ventured to repeat them to non-doctors, there might be a horrid fascination, but rarely does a serious discussion follow. It is all just too intimate. We prefer to see medicine as a series of impersonal scientific discoveries or, if we must attach disease to real human beings, as successes ranging from the routine to the extraordinary. Sometimes the story of a terrible mistake is disclosed, and then we express outrage because we do not have the language or experience to discuss medicine as it truly is. We can only talk of medicine as it is not—bloodless, aseptic, and somehow divorced from our own understanding of humanity.

This volume of essays tries to take some of what I see as the most interesting and important issues in contemporary medicine and to spend time reflecting on their implications not only for health and disease but also for our wider culture. After traversing so many subjects, it may seem that medicine is an irredeemably fractured discipline, divided into a multiplicity of specialties with competing interests. In some respects, this is true. But there remains a unifying idea binding together all parts of medicine: the notion of the dignity of an individual incapacitated by illness. I find dignity a tremendously powerful and inspiring concept, yet it is one that is outside the mainstream of medical and cultural discussion about disease and the purpose of healing. If I had to single out one argument in this book that is more important than any other it would be that a successful future for medicine depends on recovering the notion of human dignity and making its restoration the conscious objective of every practicing physician. This is the subject of the final chapter.

I also see medicine as an immensely important cultural force in society, one that is largely underrecognized, even dismissed, by the contemporary authorities of our culture. In an otherwise excellent analysis of the erosion of news values in America, two distinguished editors of *The Washington Post*, Leonard Downie Jr. and Robert G. Kaiser, argue that

> government, political, foreign, and other news of importance to peoples' civic lives was largely supplanted [in the late twentieth century] by crime, weather, health, consumer, investor, entertainment, and other news believed to be of more interest to viewers and readers in their personal lives.[1]

Downie and Kaiser see this focus on health as a means "to attract and entertain audiences to sell advertising and make money." I understand this argument and have felt the force of it myself. In the late 1990s I wrote a weekly column for a British Sunday newspaper, *The Observer*, about medicine. This paper is a serious broadsheet, but the supplement in which my column appeared was devoted to lifestyle (it was called *Life*) and it was packed with advertising. I was regularly sent press releases and product announcements describing new beauty treatments or cosmetics. Medicine, to the editors of that newspaper, meant the surface appearances of health—beauty and cosmetics—and nothing too shocking for its Sunday readers. The only column I wrote that was spiked was an attack on monthly women's and men's magazines for their near-exclusive focus on health as a commodity of narcissism. The piece was something of a rant and the editor was right to turn it down. Yet health is so much more than tanned skin and toned musculature. The forces that surround medicine are some of the most potent and political of our times.

Issues such as the global burden of disease, the threat of infection, war, HIV/AIDS, the epidemic of cancer, bioterrorism, the implications of the human genome, genetically modified organisms, vaccination, surgery, and euthanasia help to define modern global societies in ways that conventional political, economic, and social forces barely touch upon. These threats are shaping the opening decade of a new century and are likely to influence human history well beyond that. They are events that are usually the concern of a closed professional discipline, but they are also matters that all citizens should be informed about and have a say in. Doctors, with a few notable exceptions, have not done especially well at taking their subject to the public and debating it with those they tend and treat.

Take tobacco. This multibillion dollar industry kills about five million people each year.[2] The figure is rising annually—there were one million more deaths attributable to tobacco in 2000 than in 1990, with most of the increase coming from developing countries where aggressive advertising campaigns are finding new and younger markets for would-be smokers. Evidence shows that the tobacco industry and its lobbyists have sought to thwart legal efforts to protect the public's health from a proven addictive drug.[3] In 2003, the US Justice Department filed court documents claiming that these practices required a payment of $289 billion in reparations to American taxpayers.

Worse, governments have tried to derail the world's first ever global health treaty—the Framework Convention on Tobacco Control. The US embassy in Saudi Arabia wrote to the Saudi Ministry of Foreign Affairs in 2003, immediately before the final negotiating session on the framework convention. The US government was seeking to weaken this treaty by countering public health arguments with the concerns of trade ministries. In a letter to President Bush, Representative Henry Waxman pointed out that the US government's position was even more pro-tobacco than that of Philip Morris! Fortunately, the World Health Organization (WHO) won agreement for its groundbreaking treaty in March 2003. The legal conditions have now been created to use taxes, product labeling, and advertising restrictions to limit the consumption of tobacco products.

Or look at the pharmaceutical industry. The US market for prescription drugs is around $130 billion (£7 billion in the UK). Many valuable medicines have been designed and brought to market successfully by drug manufacturers. But the pharmaceutical industry is, above all, and in the words of Professor John Abraham from the UK Centre for Research in Health and Medicine, "a political player." He argues that

> the present drug regulatory systems are insufficiently robust in their political relations with the pharmaceutical industry, because they prevent proper public accountability, are highly vulnerable to industrial capture, and permit the industry's scientific experts to have extensive conflicts of interest while providing their expert advice.[4]

Two former editors of the *New England Journal of Medicine*, one of the world's leading medical research journals, have claimed that "the consequences of continuing to allow an essential industry to put profits above public interest are simply too grave."[5] The public responsibilities of the tobacco and pharmaceutical industries are civic issues of our time.

The shape of modern global society is also being molded by disease. The most tangible example is the effect of HIV/AIDS in Africa. A devastating mix of biology and behavior has produced an epidemic that threatens to destroy the future of a continent. The disease is eliminating working adults and young children. In 2001, 700,000 children became infected with HIV in Africa; 500,000 children died. Life expectancy is expected to fall in countries such as South Africa, Zimbabwe, and Botswana from sixty years of age in 1990 to thirty by 2010. The economic impact of these huge and rapid shifts in population structure will accelerate an already measurable decline into poverty. When families are threatened by the loss of their main income-earner, children are taken out of school and put to work. Education then collapses along with the economy. Orphanhood, once only the result of short-term episodes of war or famine, is now a long-term challenge that neither the international political nor humanitarian communities have a response to. By 2001, over 12 million African children had lost their mother or both parents to HIV/AIDS. That figure is expected to double by 2010, representing one in ten children.[6] The lack of concerted global action to stop the 16,000 new HIV infections estimated to take place each day has been called a crime against humanity by leading international AIDS experts.[7]

The evolution of human settlements is further fertile ground for those pathologies that are a product of our short-term success as a species. The creation of urban centers seems to be linked to the emergence of asthma,[8] a disease almost undetectable in rural communities. And Salim Yusuf, a leading researcher into cardiovascular disease, claims that it is urbanization, with its associated increase in consumption of high-calorie foods, fragmenting social structures, diminished physical activity, and greater tobacco use, that is driving new waves of heart disease across the developing world.[9]

The present news—and so the public—agenda in medicine is driven mostly by events, whether these are new discoveries reported in scientific journals or epidemics of new diseases, such as a deadly outbreak of severe acute respiratory syndrome (SARS), which prompted the World Health Organization to issue a global alert on March 15, 2003, and to coordinate international efforts to identify and treat this puzzling illness.[10] But the slow news of disease also deserves front-page coverage, since the existing standards of news reporting hide issues of not only health but also public policy importance.

One example of this hidden news is China. While the March 2003 National People's Congress focused on the transfer of power from the septuagenarian old guard of Zhu Rongji as prime minister and Jiang Zemin as state president to Wen Jiabao and Hu Jintao (both aged sixty), respectively, China was facing several largely unreported public health disasters. Suicide is now China's fifth-most-common cause of death, and it is the leading cause of death among young adults. Unlike elsewhere in the world, the suicide rate is far higher among women, especially those women living in rural areas—the number of women committing suicide outweighs the number of men by three to one. Why is this? Most theories point to the low status of women in Chinese society, the absence of legal or religious prohibitions against suicide, weak social-support networks in rural areas, the ready availability of pesticides in the homes of most families, and a lack of medical staff to treat episodes of attempted suicide.[11]

Sexually transmitted diseases are recognized to be another growing problem in China—a "hidden epidemic," according to one recent report.[12] The reemergence of prostitution in an era of aggressive capitalist-style economic reform, after the virtual eradication of commercial sex work under Mao, is the likely explanation for this new health crisis. Almost one in ten Chinese men report visits to prostitutes in the preceding year, and over 90 percent describe irregular use of condoms.

Given the sheer size of China's population—1.3 billion people out of a global total of 6.1 billion—its blood supply could have important effects on the global community. Traditional cultural beliefs in China, according to Hua Shan and colleagues working in China and the US,[13] encourage citizens to view loss of blood as harmful to health and as a betrayal of their family forebears. Volunteer donors are therefore in short supply, producing a sometimes coercive employer-driven market in blood. The risk of infection from hepatitis B and C and HIV remains. Shan concludes his analysis by arguing that

> Improvement of blood safety in China is of global importance. As the world becomes an increasingly interconnected community, the spread of infectious diseases in one part of the world can pose a serious threat to the rest of the world. Therefore, control of existing infectious diseases and surveillance for new diseases in China have the potential to benefit the entire global community.

And yet China is largely ignored by news reporters—and so by the wider Western public. SARS is likely to erase such indifference. This mysterious and fatal lung disease caught Chinese officials by surprise. In March 2003, the government banned WHO scientists from visiting Guangdong Province, which borders Hong Kong and where the SARS outbreak was concentrated. China claimed that after a brief epidemic (the number of cases was first reported to be 305), the disease had burned itself out. But by the end of March, the government realized that SARS was a far bigger problem than it had initially thought. WHO experts were allowed into the country to conduct their own independent investigation. China's demands for privacy could no longer be sustained in the face of thousands of infections worldwide.

China's authoritarian overmanagement of information was strongly criticized by WHO and others. After decades of fear about threats to the country's political stability, the government found being in the global media spotlight hard to tolerate. Zhang Wenkang, China's minister for health, rejected WHO's travel warning about Hong Kong and Guangdong. Poor surveillance systems made following the epidemic difficult, and WHO's efforts were hampered when its team was shut out of military hospitals. Government officials continued to claim, despite evidence to the contrary, that SARS was under control. But by mid-April, the disease had infected two thousand people. The country's reputation for "socialism with Chinese characteristics"—that is, rapid economic liberalization—so carefully crafted by its leaders was being badly damaged. Eventually, Hu Jintao and Wen Jiabao admitted that the public health emergency was "grave" and "too dreadful to contemplate." The May Day holiday was canceled. Zhang Wenkang was sacked. China was beginning to enter the global information as well as trade communities, for the first time in its history.

A further area of neglect is child health. Western culture has spawned sometimes violent protests about animal rights. And yet very few people take to the streets, call public meetings, or write to newspapers about the 11 million children under five years of age who die each year, half of whose lives could easily be saved if the correct measures were put in place.[14] These measures do not require high-tech solutions. Two million children die from diarrheal disease every year. Solution? Clean water, good sanitation systems, and oral rehydration therapy. About two million children die from pneumonia. Solution? Breast-feeding and access to cheap antibiotics. Another million die from malaria. Solution? Insecticide-treated bed nets and, again, cheap drugs. Seven hundred thousand children die from measles. Solution? A very effective vaccine. In the Western world, the challenge of child health is diametrically opposite to that facing the developing world. Whereas over 60 percent of childhood deaths in developing countries are linked directly to undernutrition, in the rich world it is obesity that is the foremost public health crisis among children—a crisis, it must be said, fueled by an advertising-driven sugar-sweetened soft-drinks industry aiming specifically to attract children through promotions linked to games, toys, films, and clothing.[15]

Why are these issues—deemed "soft news" by Downie, Kaiser, and other supposedly high-brow commentators on our culture—not center stage in today's political debates? Partly because health and disease are interpreted as matters of lifestyle and not—as they are—profoundly existential, public policy, and geopolitical concerns. But the marginalization of medicine also owes a great deal to sclerotic establishment attitudes in journalism and public affairs, which have failed to adapt to changing forces within society. Perhaps most fundamental of all, the inattention to medicine that does the public such a disservice is due to a straightforward lack of knowledge among the opinion-forming political and journalistic elite about why disease matters beyond the confines of the clinic or hospital.

Doctors have not helped this cause. Their public disputes have usually focused on their threatened professional rights, eroded financial status, or declining political influence. The substance of what they do has been carefully protected, until recently, from public scrutiny. But science is now demanding that doctors step further into the arena of public debate. As Craig Venter, a co-discoverer of the sequence of the human genome, pursues the elusive and possibly crazy goal of creating life (albeit bacterial life) from nothing more than a bag of chemicals,[16] and as animal cloning reveals that genetic technologies can bring diseases forward in time (Dolly the sheep developed premature arthritis and died from a progressive lung disease usually found in older sheep), doctors will not only need to interpret the implications of these developments for a concerned public but also help shape opinion about the place of these technologies in modern society. They have done little of either so far.

Doctors are also well placed to influence public debates about the evolution of research into human disease. A good example is the announcement in 2003 by Bill Gates that his foundation is donating $200 million to pinpoint critical research questions about the major causes of disease and disability in the world today. But which questions? Gates has put together a panel of scientists, led by Harold Varmus, the Nobel Prize winner and former director of the National Institutes of Health, to devise ten questions, the answers to which "would save the most lives." Gates wants the panel to take a global view, shifting the emphasis of research away from richer nations. At present only 10 percent of research money is spent on the diseases that cause 90 percent of the health burden in the world today. The public too has a part to play in deciding what questions matter most to them, and doctors, together with scientists, have a valuable role in stirring this debate. So far, they have been silent.

I wanted to call this book "Wretched Arguments at the Sick-Bed,"[17] in homage to my hero, Pliny the Elder (AD 23–79), who leveled many correctly trenchant criticisms against doctors and the medicine of his day. Wiser publishing heads prevailed. But that is nevertheless what this book is about. Wretched arguments about human disease, debates that I passionately believe are central to an understanding of our most personal worlds as well as global society. The best that I can hope for, if you read any part of this book, is that you will strongly take issue with me.

* * *

The rule in writing medical research papers is that one should ask permission before acknowledging another person. The idea is, of course, that the person being thanked may not want to be associated with the work in question—the embarrassment may simply be too great. One final—perhaps *the*—joy in writing this truly last paragraph (even though it comes near the beginning) is that I can thank whomever

I wish, and they may be mystified, angry, upset—or just plain embarrassed. The influence of others on a person's work does not conform to a linear relationship, in which the greater their physical presence, the greater the force they exert on your life. The very briefest encounter may have the most profound effect. I have included people who have been materially decisive to this book—decisive in the most personally conceivable sense—two of whom, sadly, I have never met: my birth parents. Thank you, then, to (alphabetically) Robert Beaglehole, Barbara Beddow, Anne Bowler, Iain Chalmers, Ron Cockitt, Peter Cooles, Robin Fox, Hopelyn Goodwin, Clarice Horton, Ken Horton, Martin Kendall, Ann Löfgren, Stephen Lock, Steve Logan, Faith McLellan, Maren Meinhardt, Bob Michel, Karl Miller, Jane Padfield, Eldryd Parry, Duncan Payne, Albert Pearson, Drummond Rennie, Ken Rothman, Ken Schulz, Tom Sherwood, Richard Smith, Jan Vandenbroucke, Pierre Vinken, Mary Waltham, David Wolfe, and all my colleagues at *The Lancet* who constantly remind me why medicine is such an engaging and enjoyable world to be part of. But particular thanks go to two people. Robert Silvers was the person who took a chance and gave me my first opportunity to write for *The New York Review of Books*. I doubt that there could be any better training for a hopeful writer than being edited by Bob. Michael Shae has been my unflagging editor for this book. His gentle but firm encouragement has meant that I only missed my deadline by one year, instead of several. His questions exposed many unsupportable assumptions throughout these chapters, and anything that makes sense in what follows is in no small part thanks to Michael's forensic reading. Only I bear responsibility for the errors and imperfect arguments that follow.

—Richard Horton
April 25, 2003

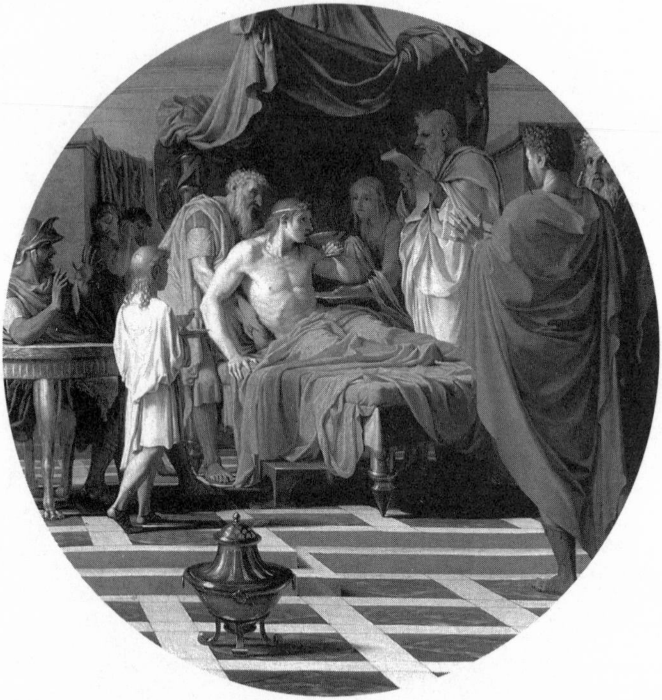

Eustache Le Sueur: *Alexander and His Doctor*, circa 1648–1649

# INTRODUCTION:
# THE DIS-EASES OF MEDICINE

> There are three factors in the practice of medicine: the disease, the patient, and the physician. The physician is the servant of science, and the patient must do what he can to fight the disease with the assistance of the physician.
>
> —Hippocrates, *The Epidemics*, Book I

A PALE AND half-naked Alexander lifts the cup to his lips, his mouth open and ready to drink. Unmistakably, the King is ill. He requires the support of an elderly attendant and a clutch of servants who stand fussily around him and stare. Alexander's eyes are fixed on an old man, dressed in white robes, who towers above him reading a letter, although the word "reading" does not quite do justice to the old man's expression of shock. His mouth is open too, and he has pulled the letter close to his face, eyebrows raised, brow furrowed, and cheeks flushed. His embarrassment, shading into fear, is striking, and seems also to have caused extreme discomfort among those waiting nearby. At the foot of Alexander's grandly canopied bed, a man wearing a red toga is holding out his hand in exclamation. A companion turns to him in wide-eyed surprise. To Alexander's right is a soldier, possibly a bodyguard, also horrified at the prospect of his general's hasty swallow. To the rear a woman clasps her hands together in sorrow, unable to look at the scene before her, while the man next to her, eyes shut, casts his head down in fatalistic sadness. The whole scene evokes a sense of profound dread. Will Alexander's imminent sips cost him his life?

The drama of Eustache Le Sueur's seventeenth-century painting *Alexander and His Doctor*[1] is high—and unresolved. The details of the story must be sought in Le Sueur's source, Plutarch's *Age of Alexander*.[2] According to the famous chronicler, Alexander was an impulsive young man "prone to outbursts of choleric rage," yet he was intrigued by the art of healing. Aristotle had kindled in him not only an interest in the theory of medicine but also "the habit of tending his friends when they were sick and prescribing for them various courses of treatment or diet." Alexander inherited his kingdom in 336 BC when he was only twenty years old, and wars marked much of his time as monarch. In 333 BC, while engaged in a standoff against Darius, the king of Persia, he fell ill, either through the sheer exhaustion of this latest military campaign across Asia or, Plutarch suggests, less honorably by catching a chill while bathing in icy river waters.

Alexander's doctors had written their patient off. They were frightened of Macedonian vengeance should their treatments fail, as they surely would. Only one of them—Philip—thought it his duty to intervene. Plutarch continues:

> And so he prepared a medicine and persuaded [Alexander] to drink it without fear, since he was so eager to regain his strength for the campaign. Meanwhile Parmenio had sent Alexander a letter from the camp warning him to beware of Philip, since Darius, he said, had promised him large sums of money and even the hand of his daughter if he would kill Alexander. Alexander read the letter and put it under his pillow without showing it to any of his friends. Then at the appointed hour, when Philip entered the room with the king's companions

> carrying the medicine in a cup, Alexander handed him the letter and took the draught from him cheerfully and without the least sign of misgiving. It was an astonishing scene, and one well worthy of the stage—the one man reading the letter and the other drinking the physic, and then each gazing into the face of the other, although not with the same expression. The king's serene and open smile clearly displayed his friendly feelings towards Philip and his trust in him, while Philip was filled with surprise and alarm at the accusation, at one moment lifting his hands to heaven and protesting his innocence before the gods, and the next falling upon his knees by the bed and imploring Alexander to take courage and follow his advice.

Thanks to Alexander's sorely tested trust, he lived—and so did Philip.[3]

Trust remains the pivot of any successful relationship between doctor and patient. By virtue of their ready access to many means of harm as well as healing, physicians—and even more those surgeons who wield a scalpel—have considerable power over their patients. As a result, early medical commentators understood the importance of emphasizing the doctor's benevolence. In the Western medical tradition, Hippocratic writers made this principle famous in their oath: "I will use my power to help the sick to the best of my ability and judgment; I will abstain from harming or wronging any man by it."[4] The Hippocratic Oath goes on to state that doctors will not exploit patients when making house calls, will not "indulge in sexual contacts with the bodies of women or men," and will maintain patient confidentiality. From Hippocrates to the present day, trust has been the foundation of medical practice. Alfred T. Tauber, a dual professor of medicine and philosophy at Boston University, summed up his views about a "new medical ethic"—in his words, "ethics as *the* priority for a philosophy of medicine"—by calling on the unashamedly old-fashioned values of empathy and trust.[5]

All of this helps to explain why it is so terrifying when the trust between doctor and patient is breached. In the UK's *Medical Register* for 2000, there is the following bare entry:

> **Shipman,** Harold Fredrick 23 Jul 1970, 05 Aug 1971
> 15 Roe Cross Green Mottram Hyde Cheshire
> SK14 6LP
> MB ChB 1970 Leeds 1470473 m

That same year, the UK General Medical Council issued another notice:

> **Shipman, Harold Frederick** [sic] ***Registration number 1470473*** As required by section 34 (1) of the Medical Act 1983, the Medical Register represents the Principal List of the register of medical practitioners as at 1 January in the year of publication. Dr. Shipman was on the Principal List on 1 January 2000 and his name is therefore included in Part 4 of the Medical Register 2000.
>
> On 11 March 2000 Dr. Shipman's name was erased from the Principal List following a decision taken by the Professional Conduct Committee on 11 February 2000. The erasure was in accordance with section 36 (1) of the Medical Act.

Shipman's name was erased because he had been proven to be a serial killer, the worst in the history of English law—and medicine. On September 7, 1998, Shipman was arrested by the Greater Manchester police when he forged the will of one of his patients and after colleagues raised concerns about excessive numbers of deaths among those under his care. In January 2000, he was convicted of murdering fifteen patients. A year later, Richard Baker, a respected academic physician interested in the quality of clinical practice, and Liam

Donaldson, the UK's chief medical officer, published a report setting out the scope of Shipman's crimes.[6]

After examining Shipman's death certificates, Baker concluded that 236 "excess deaths" had occurred either at the homes of his patients or on his private premises. From Baker's calculations, he could not be absolutely sure of this number. In estimating the degree of uncertainty, he found that the figure could have been as high as 277. When Baker compared the total number of death certificates issued by Shipman with similar figures for doctors practicing nearby, he found 297 excess deaths, with the degree of uncertainty indicating a maximum of 345.

The most grisly aspect of this investigation was the pattern of murders. Shipman liked to kill in the early afternoon, after a good lunch. He preferred to attack older women in their own homes; claim that they had died of strokes, heart attacks, or simply old age; and more often than not would report that they had died within a half-hour of his arrival, beginning with a dramatic faint or collapse. A typical note on a cremation form read: "Saw patient at home, diagnosis made, arranged admission ambulance, patient dead when went back, all within 10 mins." Shipman frequently chose a lethal dose of heroin as his weapon. As far as anyone could tell, the motivation was neither money nor sex. A former heroin addict himself, Shipman simply seemed addicted to murder. He reveled in his power to end life. And many of his living patients reacted with incredulity—for Shipman was famous for his wonderful bedside manner.

The shock of this unprecedented betrayal of trust reverberated through newspaper reports for several days after Baker's findings were published on January 5, 2000. *The Times* led its front page with "Shipman killed up to 265," and its editorial called him the "British Mengele." On January 6, *The Sun* exclaimed, "Death Doc 'killed 345,'" "Monster Shipman did one murder a month for last 25 years." *The Mirror* noted, "Doctor Death: 297 victims." *The Daily Express* shouted, "For God's Sake, just tell us the truth," and also plumped for 297 as the definitive number of those killed. *The Independent* focused the wider blame on medicine's dismal complacency: "The career of Dr. Shipman strengthens the case for medical accountability." By January 7, news coverage had given way to feature articles about Shipman's frugal life in prison. The church bells in his hometown rang out 215 times in July 2002 for each of his finally confirmed victims.

Harold Shipman was an exceptional case of the doctor as murderer, but harm caused by doctors is not exceptional. Medical error has only become a respectable subject for study during the past decade. The landmark investigation was the Harvard Medical Practice Study,[7] which grew out of concerns about malpractice litigation: legal scrutiny of medical practice was not an effective means of solving problems of poor-quality care. And yet there were no empirical data about the extent of iatrogenic illness—illness caused by medical treatment itself. By randomly reviewing hospital records from over 30,000 patients in New York State in 1984, the Harvard researchers found "a substantial amount of injury to patients from medical management," with many injuries being the result of substandard care. Over a quarter of those occasions when the course of surgery went badly wrong were due to negligence, and one in six led to permanent disability or death. Increasing age was an especially important indicator of risk. When the investigators looked at the causes of adverse events they found that almost half were linked to surgical operations and 58 percent were caused by "errors in management." The most common adverse events were harmful drug reactions, wound infections, and technical complications, such as stitches coming undone.

Ten years later, in 2000, the US Institute of Medicine published a report that not only added its imprimatur to these figures but also called for a radical overhaul in the way error was dealt with by a largely complacent medical community.[8] The report concluded that, based on extrapolations of figures such as those obtained from New

York, between 44,000 and 98,000 Americans "die each year as a result of medical errors." The authors of the report wrote that more people died in a given year as a result of medical errors than from traffic accidents (43,458), breast cancer (42,297), or AIDS (16,516). These errors are "costly in terms of loss of trust," and yet "silence surrounds this issue."

The Institute of Medicine recommended that a Center for Patient Safety be established to set goals for safety and to gather information about errors[9]; that a mandatory national reporting system for adverse events be created; that legal protection be given to these data so that fear of litigation is removed for those reporting errors; and that safety once again be made a more explicit goal of clinical care. The official response to the report was as quick as it was unexpected. President Clinton immediately ordered a feasibility study to determine how the Institute of Medicine's recommendations might be implemented. Some critics claimed that the institute's findings were exaggerated,[10] but the authors of the original Harvard study fiercely disagreed.[11] The one point all protagonists seemed to agree on was that medical error was now rightly at the center of discussions about health care. It was as if Hippocrates' dictum—"I warmly commend the physician who makes small mistakes; infallibility is rarely to be seen"[12]—could at last be uttered in public without fear of prosecution or shame.

The Institute of Medicine's report stands as a watershed in Western medicine. For the first time in the profession's history, doctors were being asked to face up to their own limitations. And yet we still know remarkably little about how errors take place or might be prevented. For example, Atul A. Gawande and his colleagues at Harvard were some of the first to review surgical adverse events among 15,000 patients admitted to Colorado and Utah hospitals in 1992.[13] They searched for and classified preventable incidents, which were defined as "related to an operation or a surgeon's non-operative care or occurring within 30 days after an operation." Procedures that went wrong most often included appendectomy, Caesarean section, gall bladder removal, coronary bypass surgery, hysterectomy, hip replacement, and resection of the prostate—all common operations. The patients on whom mistakes were made were often young (their average age was thirty-nine). The overall annual incidence of unexplained surgical complications was 1.9 percent. This figure translated into over 11,000 adverse events across the two states in 1992. Over half were preventable and one in twenty led to death. These numbers provided good reason for alarm.

The details of these investigations are illuminating, and perhaps contrary to our expectations of medicine today. The most frequent complications stemmed from the way surgeons actually used their instruments, together with wound infections and bleeding (both one in ten of all incidents). The 100 percent preventable complications of surgery were diagnostic mistakes or delay and inappropriate therapy, each accounting for just 2 percent of adverse events. But there were opportunities for substantial prevention of at least a quarter of all errors.

Not surprisingly, certain types of operations carried more risk than others. Repair of an abdominal aortic aneurysm—a dangerous and life-threatening condition—was associated with a one in five risk of a surgical adverse event; a gall bladder removal carried only a one in twenty risk. Again, exact reasons for these differences remain unknown; the likely explanations relate to the complexity of the operation and the overall health of the patient. These findings also indicate that a distinction should be made between human errors (that is, practical inexperience) and system errors. Gawande includes within system errors variables such as a low number of procedures completed in the hospital (inexperience), lack of the best available technical support, poor communication between health professionals, time of day, and low staff numbers.

If Gawande is correct, how might the "system" of medicine discover which doctors are a problem, who might become a problem, or simply how errors occur in the first place? These human factors have been studied by one unusually inquisitive cardiac surgeon, Marc R. de Leval. He reviewed over two hundred operations involving complex arterial surgery in newborn children.[14] Human factors were measured among all surgeons who conducted these rare arterial switch procedures. As a group, the death rate was 7 percent but near misses totaled a far more worrying 18 percent. The risk factors for these near misses included not only uncontrollable variables, such as uncommon anatomical patterns encountered by the surgeon, but also controllable human errors—both major and minor. Major human errors were potentially life-endangering, and ranged from difficulties for the anesthetist to technical errors by the surgeon. In this group, thirty-eight patients suffered one major error that was successfully compensated for in thirty-three cases. If the major error was left uncompensated for, it became an important predictor of a poor outcome. Minor errors were failures that, taken alone, had negligible consequences. But minor errors were multiplicative in their effect—what mattered was the accumulated number, and the fewer, the better.

A slew of studies has followed these early forays. In 2003 alone, reports appeared showing that adverse events are common after patients are discharged from the hospital and that many of them are easily preventable. At least a fifth of American hand surgeons reported operating on the wrong hand at some point in their careers. And drug errors seemed to be especially frequent; both in hospitals and in primary care.

The study of a doctor's fallibility is new to medicine. It is a significant challenge to the philosophy underpinning traditional clinical research, which deals with populations of patients and assumes that the quality of medical care provided by doctors is a constant that can be disregarded. But clinical investigators need to study people, not merely populations, the detailed activities of medical teams and not only groups of patients. Five propositions about this new approach to medicine follow:

1. Research on error is producing huge and unpredictable changes in medical culture. Instead of a preoccupation with blame—a doctor's personal failure—emphasis is moving toward understanding the complexity of modern medicine and the impossibility of assigning mistakes to individuals alone. The notion of critical weaknesses in the situations in which doctors work—mistakes simply waiting to happen—is gaining ground. However, the expanding awareness of these weaknesses is likely to undermine the confidence the public has in medicine as a profession and as a science.
2. Factors that are commonly ignored—for example, resources, time, the role of the managers of medicine—may be more important than the actions of any one individual doctor in causing medical errors. These causes are hard to pin down and they are resisted by practitioners (for obvious reasons). Emphasizing the complexity of the culture that fosters error also seems like a profession trying to hide the truth of its own failure. But the failures—professional, practical, and managerial—are even worse than we first thought.
3. Analyses of errors and their causes—a shift from the quick indictment of an individual to thoughtful inquiry about the whole health care apparatus—will eventually become the new norm. Yet it is still true to say that research into a doctor's inherent capacity for error is desperately neglected.
4. Part of the reason for professional resistance to independent external scrutiny of medical practice is that doctors are taught to feel an exclusive personal responsibility for what they do. Although a sense of personal responsibility is right and proper, its counterpart—the shared responsibility among an entire health

care team—is rarely emphasized in either medical school (medical students are not routinely mixed with nurses, physiotherapists, clinical laboratory scientists, or other members of the teams they will subsequently work in) or in clinical practice (by which time this professional elitism is firmly entrenched).

5. Present-day health care systems, focused as they are on cost containment and fear of litigation, cannot hope to create the conditions necessary to encourage disclosure and discussion of error.[15] Indeed, as errors do gradually come to light, the public may lose confidence in doctors as well as the system of medicine they practice. And doctors may feel even more isolated in an ever more critical civic culture that demands unattainable standards of perfection.

These propositions invite us to reevaluate the state medicine is in—for diseases, doctors, and their patients. It seems time to stop taking health care—and the science of medicine on which this care is based—for granted.

Our understanding of disease depends upon our understanding of the human body. Galen's theories of disease, for example, were based on the belief that animal bodies are composed of hot, cold, wet, and dry elements.[16] In Book I of his *Mixtures*, Galen weighs the evidence for and consequences of mixing these four elements. One school of thought believed in the existence of only wet-cold and hot-dry mixtures, while another school held that wet-hot and dry-cold were also valid combinations. Galen lays out the arguments for and against each point of view and he criticizes them both roundly for missing the most obvious point—namely, that "they have completely left out of the account the well-balanced mixture, which is actually superior to all those mentioned above, in both excellence and potential." After long reflection, and to our modern eyes rather bizarrely, Galen comes to the conclusion that there are nine types of mixture that make up the human body: one well-balanced; four ill-balanced in a simple way (too wet, dry, cold, or hot); and four ill-balanced in a more complex manner (hot and wet, hot and dry, cold and wet, and cold and dry). He classifies the human body's tissues according to these mixtures.

This is all nonsense. Yet the basic principle of understanding disease in terms of the interaction among the elements that compose the human body has lasted well into the third millennium of the Western medical tradition. Although contemporary medical histories bestow glory on Andreas Vesalius for his anatomical studies in the sixteenth century and William Harvey for discovering the circulation of the blood in the seventeenth century, the full force of the mechanistic attitude toward the human body was only realized in René Descartes's *Treatise on Man*,[17] published posthumously in 1662. Descartes opens his inquiry by claiming that the body is "just a statue or a machine made of earth." We see artificial fountains, mills, and clocks, all made by us, and the machine that is the human body is similarly constructed, only this time "made by God." Descartes is not interested in anatomy. Instead, his purpose is to explain the movements of the human body. In his descriptions of the stomach, lungs, heart, eye, ear, and brain, the mechanical nature of human functions is repeatedly emphasized, usually by compelling analogy. In the nervous system,

> the nerves of the machine that I am describing can indeed be compared to the pipes in the mechanical parts of these fountains. Its muscles and tendons to various other engines and springs which serve to work these mechanical parts, its animal spirits to the water that drives them, the heart with the source of the water, and the brain's cavities with the apertures.

The church organ proved to be another useful metaphor:

> You can think of our machine's heart and arteries, which push the animal spirits into the cavities of the brain, as being like the bellows of an organ, which push air into the wind chests, and of external objects, which displace certain nerves, causing spirits from the brain cavities to enter certain pores, as being like the fingers of the organist, which press certain keys and cause the wind to pass from the wind chests into certain pipes.

Sometimes, Descartes stretches his readers' credulity beyond reason. He argues the case for "animal spirits" that are carried with the blood and nourish the brain. These animal spirits flow from the brain into nerves and then into muscles. But the logic of his theory presents an insoluble problem:

> Animal spirits are able to cause movements in all bodily parts in which the nerves terminate, even though anatomists have failed to find any that are visible in parts such as the eye, the heart, the liver, the gall bladder, the spleen, and so on.

Still, these mechanistic theories were, Descartes claimed, an essential foundation for the practice of a rational medicine. The doctor can cure disease, prevent illness, even slow the aging process. But to do so, he must "know the nature of our body, not attributing to the soul functions which depend only on the body and on the disposition of its organs."

Cartesian doctrines reached their apogee in Germany two hundred years later. In twenty lectures delivered at the Pathological Institute of Berlin between February and April 1858, Rudolf Virchow inaugurated the new discipline of cellular pathology.[18] His intentions did not lack ambition. Virchow wished "to furnish a clear and connected explanation of those facts upon which, according to my ideas, the theory of life must now be based, and out of which also the science of pathology has now to be constructed." The great idea that Virchow delivered was cell theory. By looking at the collections of cells that made up tissues—the science of histology—he could classify systematically both the normal and the abnormal. No matter how a disease was conceived, everything led back to the cell:

> The chief point in this application of histology to pathology is to obtain a recognition of the fact, that the cell is really the ultimate morphological element in which there is any manifestation of life, and that we must not transfer the start of real action to any point beyond the cell.

Virchow's cellular approach had a profound effect on his attitude toward disease:

> I consider it necessary to trace pathological facts to their origin in known histological elements;...I am not satisfied with talking about an action of the vessels, or an action of the nerves.... I consider it necessary to bestow attention upon the great number of minute parts which really constitute the chief mass of the substance of the body, as well as upon the vessels and nerves.

Until very recently, this cellular view of disease remained the dominant organizing principle of Western medicine. Despite enormous scientific progress in understanding the mechanisms and treatment of disease, most pathology textbooks still begin with discussions of cell structure and function. Virchow's legacy seemed untouchable.

But the study of human genes now threatens to throw Virchow into the shadows of medical history. New origins of "pathological facts" beyond the cell have at last been discovered, and a new pathology is slowly being assembled. Laboratory techniques called microarrays now enable pathologists to answer questions about which genes are switched on or off in tissues—normal and diseased—at particular times. A microarray is made up of tiny pieces of human tissue taken from a larger sample. As many as a thousand different specimens can be analyzed simultaneously for their gene content, or for the products of those genes, which indicate gene activation in the tissue under study. They may be single-stranded RNA molecules transcribed directly from DNA itself (messenger RNA) or they may be proteins created from the messenger RNA code. By studying thousands of activated genes in tissue samples, the pathologist can begin to make more accurate diagnoses, offer more precise prognoses, investigate how genes might drive cancer growth, and discover whether treatments can be specifically targeted to particular patterns of gene expression within diseased tissue.

I report these shifts in thinking from cell to gene not in any triumphalist salute to modern genetics, but rather as a tentative pointer to a significant break with past understanding. What will follow for medicine cannot hope to entirely erase fear or uncertainty in the face of illness. But little by little, medicine should get more precise, and new questions will be asked that will take it closer to the wellspring of disease.

One example of how our perception of disease might change concerns breast cancer. Traditional approaches to breast cancer commonly divide the disease into two types—carcinoma in situ and invasive carcinoma. A carcinoma is a malignant growth of cells derived from epithelium, one of the four tissue types found in the human body (the other three being nerve, muscle, and connective tissue). Carcinoma in situ accounts for no more than a third of all breast cancers and, by definition, does not invade surrounding tissues. It is more frequently diagnosed today because of mammographic screening. There are many types of carcinoma in situ—ductal, lobular, solid, cribriform, comedocarcinoma, papillary, and micropapillary—all quaintly named according to their appearance under the microscope. Invasive carcinoma is also classified by its microscopic appearance.

The outlook for a woman diagnosed with breast cancer depends on the "stage" of her disease. Staging categorizes the tumor in terms of its size, its degree of invasion into surrounding tissue, and its spread to nearby lymph nodes. Other factors are also known. One of the most important is estrogen receptor status. Well over half of all breast cancers have receptors for estrogen, a female sex hormone, on their surface. A receptor is a protein that usually sits on the cell surface, binds another substance to itself, and then switches on a cascade of chemical reactions within the cell. Nobody knows why estrogen receptors are there. But they are, and their presence or absence affects the prognosis of a woman with breast cancer. Drugs such as tamoxifen, which binds to and blocks the breast cancer estrogen receptor, substantially improve a woman's chance of surviving the disease.

This mixture of histology, staging, and receptor status underlies modern breast cancer medicine. But it is frustratingly crude and descriptive —arbitrary tumor sizes are set for determining the stage of the cancer, for example. None of these various measures links treatment or outcome to the biological mechanisms producing the disease. We remain a long way from Descartes's mechanical vision of human function.

If specimens of breast cancer tissue are embedded into microarrays, distinctive patterns of gene expression are seen.[19] These "molecular portraits" provide telling insights into the genetic diversity of breast cancer. By looking at clusters of genes and their expression, one can identify families of breast cancer subtypes, which both confirm and refute present thinking about the disease. For example, gene clusters within breast cancer tissue are often closely associated with a particular cell type—genetics giving a final encore to Virchow. Two broad groups of gene expression in breast cancer are apparent. These two groups largely reflect the distinction between estrogen-receptor-positive and estrogen-receptor-negative cancers. But within the estrogen-receptor-negative group, two distinct and previously unknown genetic subtypes seem to exist. One is called basal-like, since the genes expressed are similar to those expressed by a particular type of epithelial cell. Another is labeled Erb-B2 positive, since the genes expressed are associated with overexpression of the Erb-B2 oncogene. So although gene expression microarray studies can help to confirm or refute our existing understanding of a disease (estrogen-receptor-positive or -negative tumors, for example), they also uncover what could be entirely new diseases, with possibly different clinical outcomes or treatments (for instance, Erb-B2).

Gene expression studies also reveal new information about the outlook for women diagnosed with breast cancer. Marc Van de Vijver and colleagues from the Netherlands have found a poor-prognosis genetic signature that correlates with survival and risk of cancerous spread beyond the breast.[19] This genetic predictor was better than existing techniques based on clinical examination or histology. Similar studies have been completed on prostate, colon, kidney, and liver cancer, and they will be a major theme of medical research during the next decade.

This mechanistic method of inquiry has proved extraordinarily successful in medicine. If one takes the example of the commonest cause of death in the developed world—ischemic heart disease, which includes angina pectoris and acute myocardial infarction (heart attack)—the advantages of the Cartesian attitude are shown to their fullest degree. William Osler, in his 1892 treatise *The Principles and Practice of Medicine*, devotes just four pages of his thick book to angina pectoris, which was then deemed a "rare" disorder. Osler summarizes the state of nineteenth-century knowledge concerning the causes of angina. But he begins by cautioning, "The nature of the affection is doubtful." He then discusses three competing theories. First, that angina is "a neuralgia of the cardiac nerves," by which he means that the pain of an attack originates in and follows the path of nerves to and from the heart. Osler is skeptical of this idea, since anginal pain is "unlike any neuralgic affection." His second theory is that angina might be a "cramp of heart-muscle itself." But if so, surely such a total cramp of the heart would cause death in almost all cases, which it clearly does not. Third, and even more unlikely, angina could follow "great stretching and tension of the nerves in the muscular substance" of the heart—an idea for which there was not one shred of evidence.

A century later, we know a great deal about the pathology of angina and acute myocardial infarction, from the gross anatomical changes that take place in the wall of a coronary artery—the microanatomy of the advanced cholesterol plaque—to the molecular mechanisms by which these damaged walls attract blood clots that aggregate and eventually cause the typical cardiac symptoms of crushing chest pain, nausea, breathlessness, and sweating. The subject of ischemic heart disease occupies over fifty pages of the 1996 edition of the *Oxford Textbook of Medicine*. And where Osler recommended little more than "a quiet life," supplemented by the occasional dose of nitroglycerin, as a treatment, the authors of modern medical treatises have a vast pharmacopeia to choose from. In addition to drugs, there are now balloons to blow open closed blood vessels, metal stents to stop them from closing again, and surgical procedures that insert pebble-sized electrical-assist devices to help the heart do its job, as well as now almost routine cardiac transplantation.

Today, comprehending a disease weaves together phenotypic (symptoms and signs), pathologic (cellular damage), and genetic descriptions,[20] but there is still something missing: an explanation of just what it is that disease does to us as whole human beings. Descartes has no answer to this question (other than what must presumably be in the mind of God), nor do Virchow, Osler, or modern scientists. It is neither a wholly mechanistic nor a wholly metaphysical question. Yet it remains for many patients a deeply important one: What is this disease doing to me? Doctors tend to recoil from these more holistic matters. In asking the question, I am not seeking an ultimate final meaning of human disease, a teleology of illness, so to speak. Instead, I am trying to find a way to make sense of what it is that disease does to us, not only as human bodies but also as human beings. It is a question of ontology as much as it is one of pathology.

One writer who struggled with this larger conception of disease was Georges Canguilhem (1904–1995). He trained to become a doctor in the 1930s after a lengthy period as a teacher and as the editor of the journal *Libres Propos*. He was a committed pacifist—one story has it that he purposely failed an examination for officer training by dropping a rifle on the foot of his examiner. Nevertheless, he joined the French Resistance and threw himself into writing anti-fascist polemics. As a doctoral student in Strasbourg (he fled the Vichy regime in 1940), Canguilhem wrote a thesis entitled *The Normal and the Pathological*. It is one of the few works of philosophy that deals directly with concepts of disease and health, together with the contrasts between pathology and so-called normal physiology. Completed in 1943 and first published in 1966, it is not taught to English-speaking medical students and it is rarely read by doctors.[21]

Canguilhem's interest is the evolution of medical knowledge. He contrasts two ways of looking at the history of medicine. One involves the chronological documentation of factual progress while the other seeks to identify the far more obscure development of concepts. Canguilhem emphasized the priority of concepts over facts because of their explanatory power and practical value. He studied how ideas developed, matured, and superseded one another, and argued that on each accepted conceptual framework hung an ideology of scientific belief. For example, the notion that an infectious pathogen causes a disease drives a program (a scientific ideology) to treat that disease by eliminating the pathogen or preventing its transmission from one person to another.

Given that the study of concepts is a powerful means of studying how physicians acquire practical knowledge, what methodology does Canguilhem use to discover the links between concepts and care? His method is fundamentally historical but with a twentieth-century twist. Canguilhem fuses philosophy ("the questioning of received solutions") with history in his evaluation of conceptual progress in medicine. The history of medicine becomes a branch of epistemology. According to Canguilhem, "The history of science is not only science's memory but also epistemology's laboratory." The history of medicine is no longer some arcane and literal discussion about scientific progress but a vital debate about the evolution of scientific ideologies.

Canguilhem developed this philosophical outlook to understand how medicine establishes norms of human function. The concepts of normality and the norm are at the heart of his work. He saw the history of medicine as a continual conflict between descriptive (the act of producing evidence free of values) and normative (the interpretation of evidence according to a set of values) forces. The application of experimental methods to medicine led to a laboratory and animal-based research approach that rejected purely descriptive traditions. The quest to acquire meaningful data led medical scientists to develop quantitative methods for interpreting results in terms of averages (the true meaning of norm). Advocates of this mathematical attitude aimed to replace the intuitive judgments of physicians with sound statistical reasoning.

The intellectual conflict between experimental medicine and armchair reflection, however, is not so easily resolved. Canguilhem argued forcefully that experimental medicine is inextricably intertwined with rational conceptualization (even when made from the armchair). Data led researchers to formulate theories that are themselves validated or falsified in the light of further experimental data. Empiricism and rationalism are not opposing methods; they are interdependent processes that make up the science and practice of medicine.

Canguilhem went on to confront the then-prevailing view that disease was mainly a quantitative variation from the normal. By drawing on the writings of Auguste Comte, François Broussais, Claude Bernard, and René Leriche, Canguilhem showed how this difference of degree had become the standard model of disease by the end of the nineteenth century. This view remains dominant today. Disease differed from health only according to the intensity of the phenomenon in question. If one had thyroid disease, for example, the clinical outcome was either *hyper*thyroidism or *hypo*thyroidism—that is, too much or too little thyroid function. The same was true for diabetes (glucose), Cushing's disease (cortisol), and menopause (estrogen).

An alternative view was that sickness differed qualitatively from health. Canguilhem put it this way: "To be sick means that a man really lives another life, even in the biological sense of the word." This philosopher-doctor might sound rather pretentious to modern scientists. But his point is, I think, telling, and I admire his refusal to be conciliatory toward a reductive history of medical science:

> It is completely illegitimate to maintain that the pathological state is really and simply a greater or lesser variation of the physiological state.... Normal and pathological have no meaning on a scale where the biological object is reduced to colloidal equilibria and ionized solutions.

So what is disease if it is not to be reduced to its most fundamental mechanical elements? Canguilhem argued that disease is a natural part of life, but that it is different from what we consider normal because "it tolerates no deviation from the conditions in which it is valid." In other words, although disease is "a positive, innovative experience in the living being... a new dimension of life," it severely narrows the livable environment. "Disease is characterized by the fact that it is a reduction in the margin of tolerance for the environment's inconstancies." Disease reduces our freedom to maneuver. It limits our ability to adapt to challenges posed by the environment. We are unable to create new norms for new settings. Disease, then, is not defined at some point along a spectrum of biological variation. Instead, disease should be defined by the functional meaning of any disturbance for the whole person. For Canguilhem, health "means being able to fall sick and recover"; "to be sick is to be unable to tolerate change."

This attitude—that disease offered a new but narrow dimension to life—is radically different from Virchow's cellular pathology and today's genetic redrawing of old boundaries, and it remains a refreshing perspective half a century after its first publication. In a medical school curriculum designed to cram facts into students, reading *The Normal and the Pathological* would perform a valuable function. The book would encourage doctors-in-training to do something rarely asked of them—namely, to think about the relation between the patients they see and the diseases those patients suffer from and live with.

The future path for the science of disease is an ever more precise description of gene malfunction, as well as efforts to solve the complex riddles of how proteins interact with one another to cause cell and tissue failure. Yet the reality is that this necessary and important project will come to mean less and less to those very people responsible for listening to patients and translating what they hear into some plan of care. Doctors are not laboratory scientists. Their knowledge of molecules is limited—and rightly so, since they have to retain more than enough facts about the practical aspects of diseases and their treatments. The detail of how those diseases come to be is, for the most part, an unnecessary burden.

But as an understanding of disease becomes more distant from practitioners, how will they conceive the pathologies presented to them? How will the doctor connect those pathologies to the lives of those who possess them? Canguilhem's views hold the potential to rejuvenate a presently arid territory of understanding for the physician. Nevertheless, Canguilhem was a realist in his philosophizing. His analysis was original and valuable. But he knew that his abstract intellectualism would be greeted with skepticism by his former medical colleagues. In reflecting on how ordinary doctors might view his arguments, Canguilhem concludes that

> It is perfectly understandable, then, that physicians are not interested in a concept which seems to them to be too vulgar or too metaphysical. What interests them is diagnosis and cure.

The challenge for present-day medicine is to debate how Canguilhem's humanistic pathology has a very real part to play in the care of patients.

The most important event in the English medical calendar is the Harveian Oration, an hour-long homily that takes place at the Royal College of Physicians in London in October each year. Indentured in 1656 by William Harvey, the most revered experimentalist in the history of Western medicine, it is an opportunity for a distinguished physician to speak to his or her colleagues. The purpose of the lecture, according to Harvey's initial description, was to celebrate "a general feast... for all the Fellows" of the college. The lecture is, in addition, for "the honour of the profession to continue mutual love and affection amongst themselves." The lecturer is commonly a knight or a lord of the medical aristocracy, someone officially recognized by royal patronage as an honored and honorable representative of the profession.

The millennial oration was delivered by Lord Turnberg, a past president of the college, a respected academic physician, and a gifted university administrator. His lecture was entitled, "Science, Society, and the Perplexed Physician."[22] The evening of his speech was extraordinary in every respect. Here was a man who could usually be found either ambling peacefully through the corridors of the college or relaxing in the leather armchairs of the Athenaeum. But on this day of supposed celebration, Lord Turnberg chose to turn an anxious eye inward, to the problems facing doctors themselves. He began by speaking of his "beleagured colleagues" in England and around the world. He sensed that his profession had "lost control" of itself, and he asked —imploringly—"Who will need physicians?" He hoped to offer reassurance that "physicians will continue to have roles to play." But his encouragement sounded strangely hesitant, even hollow.

Lord Turnberg set out to diagnose what was going wrong for doctors. The first problem lay with the science of medicine. As the human genome began to assert its presence in clinical practice, how would doctors adjust, not only to this highly technical new knowledge but also to a shift in the balance of information power, thanks to the Internet, toward the patient? A second difficulty facing the profession was that patients were no longer the passive and happy recipients of a doctor-driven medicine. Patients now criticized, complained, and sued. As public expectations of medicine grew, failure was no longer acceptable—and somebody, often the doctor, had to be blamed. The marble plinth of respect from which the physician presided over medicine was thus being eroded. Turnberg argued that these cultural evolutions meant that the public needed an even stronger medicine—more, not fewer, physicians, and ones who could analyze and interpret information, offer choices to patients, and make decisions together with them. Added to this typically doctoring role, they should also be recommitting themselves to the old-fashioned but neglected values of empathy and compassion. And doctors should become passionate advocates for science too.

Turnberg was responding to serious loss of confidence among his fellow practitioners. An Anglo-American consensus on this precipitous state of insecurity had been building for several years. Jerome P. Kassirer, a past editor of America's most influential medical journal, the *New England Journal of Medicine*, has written of doctors' discontent and dismay with current medical practice.[23] He too identified loss of control as a cause of frustration, together with threats to physicians' independence and integrity, escalating administrative burdens, and the improper commercialization of medicine. The business ethic was replacing the Hippocratic ethic. Doctors were selling out, moving on, and giving up. Meanwhile, Richard Smith, the editor of the *British Medical Journal*, asked, "Why Are Doctors So Unhappy?"[24] They are overworked and undersupported, he concluded. They feel that they are fighting the system of health care rather than working harmoniously within it. Doctors and their leaders seemed surprised by this turn of events. They could not understand why patients were dissatisfied, why governments were interfering with their professional autonomy, or why medicine now served the interests of money rather than the values passed on lovingly from one generation to another for two thousand years. Yet they should not be surprised. The fracturing of the profession is a predictable and irreversible trend of our time.

In *Death of the Guilds*, his study of professions in the twentieth century, Elliot A. Krause shows how the tensions inside and outside professional classes have become so strained as to be no longer sustainable.[25] His model of professional power has four dimensions—association, workplace, market, and state. Professional associations first formed as a means of organizing their members' work. They set their own standards of training, practice, and governance. They also controlled the workplace—the space where work was done and the way in which that work was done. The control the association had over its members' work gave it a monopoly over the professional skill being provided—its accumulated knowledge and its application in the marketplace. Invariably, it suited the state to acquiesce in this monopoly. The profession then sought to retain its influence when threatened by another provider. For much of the past century, the medical profession has succeeded in protecting its power. It did so by setting out a unique professional code of conduct and by obtaining the legal right to license new members. Those who encroached on this sanctified professional territory were labeled as quacks or frauds.

But today each of these four pillars of the professional edifice is cracking under the weight of mounting dissatisfaction. In no country is there now a single association that includes all doctors. Separate associations exist for surgeons, physicians, psychiatrists, obstetricians, and so on. Within these tribes, subassociations have formed—cardiologists, neurologists, gastroenterologists, and oncologists. Training is thereby fragmented, governance splintered. Professional success has become a source of professional weakness. Unity has been lost, interests clash, and conflict is fostered. The workplace is no longer under an exclusive professional jurisdiction. Nonmedical managers are common, and business governs hospitals and clinics as much as medicine once did. The market within which orthodox medicine is offered is now open to alternatives—complementary medicine being a catch-all phrase for widely differing approaches to health and disease, from chiropractic (respectable) to iridology (not at all). And finally the state, once content to leave medicine to its own self-governance, can no longer risk doing so. The greater transparency of medicine—and of medical errors—has forced governments to intervene and hold doctors accountable in more explicit (and punitive) ways than ever before.

Professions are changing, and their power is declining. Doctor discontent is one result. There is no clear view as to how this upheaval will turn out. We are in an era of transition, perhaps of similar importance to the era in which scientific Greek medicine was created or enlightened seventeenth-century Western medicine was formed. The likelihood is that the state and the consumer will take a more active part in medicine. This political and civic involvement is already apparent in most Western health care systems. A majority of doctors do not know how to respond to these changes, but two trends have emerged to counter the prevailing threats. The first aims to recover a past that seems to have been lost, while the second has aggressively laid out a new medical rationalism, one that wants to reinvest power within the hands of the doctor, and the doctor alone.

David Weatherall, a former Regius professor of medicine at the University of Oxford, began *Science and the Quiet Art*, his 1995 inquiry into medicine,[26] with the question "Why does modern medicine seem to have lost its way?" He revisits the widely held perception that the personal art of medicine has given way to an impersonal high-technology mutant. Worse still, "There is a widespread belief that many of the qualities of good doctoring have been lost in our efforts to understand diseases rather than the problems of sick people."

Weatherall sees no contradiction between the science and the practice of medicine. While fascinated by the prospects for medical science, he reasserts the old and traditional value of treating patients as people, not diseases. He closes his investigation by returning to "the love of our patients." He is scornful of those who believe that doctors are less compassionate today than, say, thirty years ago, when the paternalism of the postwar era imbued all aspects of medicine. Thankfully, that time is past. But he accepts that the present mechanistic view we have of disease can appear dehumanizing. Weatherall advocates an attitude that reclaims the art of medicine, by which he does not mean a naive sentimentality toward the sick patient. Instead, he wants doctors to study and embrace the biological, social, and personal complexity of illness:

> Apart from clinical and pastoral skills, good doctoring requires an ability to cut through many of the unexplained manifestations of disease, to appreciate what is important and what can be disregarded, and when to get to the core of the problem, knowing when scientific explanation has failed and simple kindness and empiricism must take over.

Weatherall calls this "the real art of clinical practice." Bernard Lown, a respected American cardiologist, has called it the "lost art of healing."[27] Allen B. Barbour, a professor of clinical medicine at Stanford University, has written a treatise on the notion of "person-centered care."[28] He recalled that in his medical practice, "I learned that if I didn't know the person I didn't really understand the illness." Without that understanding, "it was less likely that the patient would become well."

Various epithets have been attached to this style of medicine—

biopsychosocial, humanistic, personal. None is altogether satisfactory, although "personal medicine"[29] perhaps comes closest to the ideal of fusing a sometimes brutish scientific medicine with a rather softer person-centered care. Although attractive, this idea has a rather wistful feel to it. Writing about the art of medicine has a backward-looking appeal. It fails to deal seriously with contemporary issues in medicine, to provide a coherent foundation for reinterpreting medicine in a new era of science, and to help doctors understand the justification for and problems within medical practice today.

The second major trend initiated by doctors is evidence-based medicine. The goal of these new rationalists is to make maximum use of the best available research evidence for clinical practice. It seems odd, hardly believable even, to think that doctors have spent years practicing non-evidence-based medicine. And yet it is largely true that acquired experience and remembered anecdote have counted more for many doctors than the knowledge gained from, for example, clinical trials. Such complacency about getting research evidence into clinical practice is no longer acceptable. Governments have embraced evidence-based medicine as a means to stop unproven (and expensive) treatments from becoming entrenched in routine care.

The home of evidence-based medicine is McMaster University in Hamilton, Ontario, and its principal proponent has been David L. Sackett, a charismatic man whose writings are treated with almost sacred significance by his followers. Evidence-based medicine is a movement that aims to quell what its more extreme supporters see as two malevolent attitudes in medicine. One is that the favored basic science for medicine is done in the laboratory. Respectable medical researchers point themselves toward the bench, not the bedside. Sackett and his colleagues want to replace this laboratory-oriented preeminence with a new basic science for medicine that deals with whole people and entire populations—clinical epidemiology. The other attitude concerns the power of and respect for the clinical professor, awarded by virtue of his or her long experience. Proponents of evidence-based medicine wish to set experience in its proper place and thus to democratize practice. The most junior medical student is free to know more medicine than the most experienced professor simply because the student has taken the time to study the best evidence rather than rely on the prejudices of a hazy and lazy memory.

Evidence-based medicine is not without controversy. Unsurprisingly, many within the senior professoriate of medicine rather resent the discomfort brought about by skeptical students or junior colleagues. But Sackett and his entourage provide compelling arguments in favor of rigorous evidence-based practice: valid information is obviously essential for effective patient care; traditional sources of information—out-of-date textbooks, biased expert opinions, and ineffective didactic tuition—are often useless; and while clinical skills may improve over time, scientific knowledge usually withers surprisingly fast.[30] Evidence-based medicine also aims to supplant the traditional apprenticeship model of medical learning. As Henrik R. Wulff, a Danish medical philosopher, and Peter C. Gotzsche, a clinical epidemiologist, argue: "The apprentice learns to imitate the decisions of the master but he does not learn to assess the basis for the decisions."[31] Learning how to criticize provides that missing element.

Advocates of evidence-based medicine wish to provide doctors with a theoretical and practical foundation for making clinical decisions. It takes an uncommon mix—usually untaught at medical school—of statistics, epidemiology, ethics, and history to make those decisions. If one looks at evidence-based medicine as part of our earlier discussion of a theory of professions, one can see how it might help to resecure medicine within the framework of association (a new group of professionals with specialized knowledge), workplace (a new science of practical bedside medicine), market (new and better skills on offer to patients), and state (renewed commitment by government to medicine on quality-of-care and cost-containment grounds). Evidence-based medicine may provide the best road to future professional security. In that sense, it would be profoundly reactionary, emphasizing a rigid hierarchy between the doctor who knows and patient who gratefully receives.

The language of medicine discloses small clues about how we doctors perceive our patients. And there is no doubt that doctors do see those who consult them as *their* patients. In some sense, doctors possess the sick. They belong to us. Patients give themselves—sometimes freely, sometimes not, in settings of extreme emergency—to doctors at certain moments in their lives: moments when they feel the need for advice, or when they feel incomplete, imperfect, damaged, or disabled—that is, in a general and intuitively well-understood way, when they are ill. The doctor–patient relationship then slips into one of master and servant, a contract of service and ownership. There are unstated terms and conditions to this contract—trust and duty, for patient and doctor, respectively, for example. But many doctors nevertheless retain—indeed, firmly believe in—an attitude of benevolent possession. It is *their* patients who define what it is to call oneself a member of a profession.

Why do doctors use words that suggest this need for appropriation? The simple answer is that the language we commonly use is a vestige of tradition, from a time when paternalism was seen as a virtue —the skill of a good bedside manner, when doctors were expected to act with the kindness and care of a father. That kindly version of a doctor's work is now seen in more oppressive terms: the doctor as an authority figure who imposes rules and regimens on those who are dependent upon him. The very word "patient" reinforces this accusation of paternalism. "Patient" is derived from the Latin word for suffering. Today it means a person receiving medical treatment. Note the passivity—receiving, not taking. The word "patient" is an adjective as well as a noun. Here again, the impression left is of a person wholly dependent on (and grateful for) the actions of another—a person who expects to wait for something to be done.

But this easy answer to the question of appropriation—one driven by the social conception of doctor as technician—does not capture a more subtle explanation. For the experiences of patients serve as the warrant for professional action: "I do what I do, and I am justified in doing what I do, because my patients have this particular set of problems." This epistemological rather than social interpretation is important for understanding how doctoring truly works. A few examples should help to make this point clearer.

The relationship between doctor and patient is reduced and reified by medical research. If one picks up a medical journal, any of several thousand published each year, the patient has metamorphosed into a subject. Some examples in one such journal by my side: "fifty-six subjects were referred for diagnostic assessment"; "the subjects sat comfortably with their carers"; "thirteen subjects were lost to follow-up." Patients who consent to take part in medical research are *subjected* to the manipulations of the investigator. No doctor or scientist uses the phrase "guinea pig" about a human being taking part in research. The reality is worse than this demeaning cipher: a patient has been transformed into a subject who, in turn, is little more than an event to be counted, a person whose identity has become a number. Research is an indispensable tool not only for the doctor to improve medical practice but also for the patient to receive the benefits of specialist attention that a research study brings. Yet the notion of subjects helps investigators to set a distinctive tone when they write up and discuss their work, an orientation of the mind that aims to force the vicissitudes of medicine into the shape of an exact science and that strips the sick of their unique circumstances.

One of the most egregious episodes of exploitation and abuse of patients in medical research involved *The Lancet* shortly after I joined the journal as an assistant editor in 1990. The study concerned a selection of complementary medical treatments offered at the Bristol Cancer Help Centre in England. Publication of this profoundly flawed study in *The Lancet* on September 8, 1990,[32] was immensely damaging to the reputations of the two cancer charities in the UK, the Cancer Research Campaign and the Imperial Cancer Research Fund, which had supported the investigation. One of the principal scientists involved in the study, Professor Tim McElwain, committed suicide two months after publication of his *Lancet* report. But it was the effects on the women who attended the center and took part in the study that have had the most significant influence on British medicine. Their experience is extreme, but emblematic of what can go wrong when an overly zealous attitude to medical research is mixed with a totalizing ideology of what modern medicine is—and what it is not.

The Bristol Cancer Help Centre first opened in 1979, and set out to provide complementary treatments for patients with cancer. Part of the regimen in Bristol involved a vegetarian diet, together with other activities aiming not only to improve the quality of life for cancer sufferers but also to encourage a positive attitude toward the disease. The center received a great deal of favorable media attention. Prince Charles lent royal support to its work. But many cancer specialists were openly skeptical, even hostile, about the services offered in Bristol. And with this strongly negative view in the forefront of their minds, a group of researchers began a study of the efficacy of the Bristol project in 1986. The work was planned to be a collaboration between those running the center, its patients, and such senior medical scientists as Dr. (later Sir) Walter Bodmer, Professor Ian (later Lord) McColl, and Professor McElwain.

The protocol for the study is interesting in light of the subsequent controversy. First, this plan emphasized that the center's regimen was "complementary to orthodox medical treatment rather than competitive with it." In the final published report, however, the Bristol regimen was called "alternative," an entirely different and more divisive statement about the care being offered to women with breast cancer. Second, the protocol stressed that the best way to investigate a new treatment is by means of a randomized controlled trial. The research team chose a different study method, one they knew to contain "problems and potential biases." Third, the protocol stated that the outcomes of women with breast cancer attending the center were to be compared with women who did not attend the center. In doing so, women at Bristol would be "matched" (compared directly) "on the main factors which influence prognosis." This plan was never implemented, and the omission turned out to be the fatal flaw in the published report. Finally, the protocol noted that before publication not only would staff and patients at the Bristol Cancer Help Centre have the opportunity to comment on the paper but so would the scientific experts—Bodmer, McColl, and McElwain. None of these experts, and sadly none of *The Lancet*'s editors (including myself), discovered the fatal flaw.

The study purported to show that women receiving complementary medical care had a substantially—three times—worse survival rate than those not attending the center. This result was devastating for the women and it needed to be reported cautiously to allow careful reflection about what the findings meant to all those who had taken part in the study. But the *Lancet* paper was leaked to the press, by whom no one quite knows, in early September 1990. A September 2 report in a British Sunday newspaper was headlined "Blow to Cancer Hopes." The report opened:

> Cancer patients who use alternative therapies as well as orthodox treatments die sooner than those who use orthodox treatments only, according to new research.

This message became the central theme of press reports throughout the week. The report was finally published on the following

Friday. In it the authors of the research paper speculated on why they found that women attending Bristol fared worse than women who did not:

> While it is possible that BCHC attendees may, in some subtle way, have worse disease than our control series, the possibility that some aspect of the BCHC regimen is responsible for their decreased survival must be faced.

The cancer establishment felt vindicated. They now had evidence to prove that this version of alternative medicine was not only useless but also poisoned its recipients. McElwain was the most vigorous opponent of the Bristol center and other complementary medicine practitioners. He commented that "other alternative practitioners should have the courage to submit their work to this type of stringent assessment."

The hoopla did not last long. In the very next issue of *The Lancet*, Dr. Tim Sheard from the Bristol Cancer Help Centre raised the possibility of differences between the "cases" (women who attended Bristol) and "controls" (women who did not). For example, were there differences in the severity of the tumors between women in these groups? The study report alluded to, but extraordinarily did not explore, this possibility.

Professional and press disquiet mounted when it was realized that some of the women in the Bristol group had only attended the clinic for one day. How could one day's exposure to a variety of relaxation techniques, counseling, and a vegetarian diet triple the risk of subsequent relapse from breast cancer? The result made no sense. The final blow to the study's integrity was delivered by three respected epidemiologists at the London School of Hygiene and Tropical Medicine. In a letter published in *The Lancet* on November 11, 1990, Richard Hayes and his colleagues pointed to several important inconsistencies in the paper. They supported the assertion that cases and controls were not comparable. Indeed, Bristol women were considerably sicker. It was hardly surprising that their outcomes were worse.

In that same issue, Claire Chilvers, the senior scientist involved in the research, published a reanalysis of her team's data, this time taking account of the more severe disease among Bristol women. In a total about-face, she wrote, "It is much more likely that the differences could be explained by increased severity of disease in BCHC attendees." She offered regret for the misimpressions created by the earlier report. There has rarely been such a hasty retreat by a group of distinguished scientists in the history of medicine.

Walter Bodmer, by then promoted to director of research for the Imperial Cancer Research Fund, delivered his own words of explanation. Critics of the *Lancet* paper were asking how the ICRF could have funded and endorsed the publication of such an erroneous piece of work. Bodmer added his voice to the view that women attending Bristol had more serious disease. (A pity he had not said so earlier, before the study was published.) As time went by, the ICRF's position shifted still further. In a statement drafted by its director of clinical research, Professor Nicholas Wright, in May 1991, the ICRF concluded, "It is not possible to interpret the nature of the difference between women attending the Bristol center and those who do not." In short, a major sponsor of the study had concluded that the research was meaningless.

A further aspect to this tragedy reflected even more poorly on doctors and their institutions. The research paper had been rushed into print with only cursory, and certainly no statistical, peer review. The reason for this incautious speed was the imminent broadcast of two television programs reporting the results of the Bristol research. In a statement made in March 1992, the then editor of *The Lancet*, Robin Fox, noted, "I greatly regret that *The Lancet*, along with those who designed, analyzed, and funded the study, failed to spot these defects earlier." For the journal, the first lesson learned was that we needed to substantially strengthen our peer-review procedures. This we did. The second lesson was not to dance to the tune of other news media—to do so reflected a greater concern for our own interests (the risk of being scooped) than the interests of those on whose shoulders rested the research we were reporting.

Worse still, the news leak led the investigators to hold a press conference before publication of the study, enabling them to criticize the center and its practices without the public having full access to the study to form its own opinion. McElwain took the lead again. He said that his advice to women wishing to attend the center would now be "that for some unknown reasons women who go to Bristol relapse sooner and die earlier." He committed suicide fifteen days after publication of the letter by Claire Chilvers. He was fifty-three years old.

What good came out of this desperate episode? In January 1991, twenty-three women came together to form the Bristol Survey Support Group. The intention of this group was, in the words of a foreword to *Fighting Spirit*,[33] a collection of stories by women who took part in the Bristol research, "to challenge the results of a study in which they had taken part." The feelings of these women were best summed up by Isla Bourke and Heather Goodare in a letter to *The Lancet* a year after the Chilvers amendment:

> The release of the purported results of the study before *The Lancet* article was published left us angry, frustrated, and betrayed. That anger and a sense of having been used as pawns in a game have continued for many of us because the research team has never apologised. Nothing short of complete retraction can make amends for the psychological damage caused by the [*Lancet*] report and the research-workers' lack of interest in us, the individual human beings whose records they misused.[34]

A public apology to these women from the original scientists who completed the work has still not been forthcoming. Bourke and Goodare together produced their own scientific critique of the *Lancet* paper, one more thorough than any provided by the sponsoring charities, the investigators, or even *The Lancet*'s editors. They entitled their report "The Bristol Research—The Patient's Perspective," and it systematically dissected inconsistencies in the study's design, data collection, and statistical analyses. When reviewing the chaotic events surrounding publication of this research, the Bristol women summed up their reactions:

> They were talking about *us*! We knew *from our own experience* that their figures must have been at fault, that there must have been some hideous mistake. We knew that Bristol could not possibly have harmed us in any way. But at that time we could not know (without doing our own research) exactly how faulty these figures were.... The patients themselves are no longer objects of study but active participants in the debate. It cannot proceed without their goodwill, which most unfortunately has been forfeited.... In our view, the [research] team have been looking down the wrong end of the telescope. They have been focusing on relapse and death, while we think it is more interesting to focus on survival and life. Five years on, some of us *have* survived, from pre- and postmenopausal age-groups, with excellent quality of life. It would have been interesting to discover how we have done this, and we would have appreciated some encouragement and support from medical researchers in our fight for life, rather than slings and arrows.

The culmination of this work was *Fighting Spirit*. Goodare described the Bristol Survey Support Group's challenge to the scientists who had so badly let them down as "a milestone in medical history." And so it was. The eleven testimonies of women who went to Bristol at last allowed them "to speak for themselves," having been earlier silenced by the publication of the *Lancet* paper. Goodare criticized the doctors who had labeled the Bristol women as somehow different from other women with breast cancer—women, perhaps, with fighting spirit. She wrote that she was "tired of scientists making unscientific assumptions and hazarding guesses about us." *Fighting Spirit* aimed to extract the women from the straitjacket of scientific debate. The validity of medical research depends on counting numbers of people, together with the events, usually deaths, that befall them. But instead of assembling research papers, tables, graphs, and letters to learned journals, *Fighting Spirit* recounts stories of lives that display enormous differences. What is written here cannot fit the pattern of a research protocol, a study questionnaire, or a scientific report.

Even now, I feel some resistance to the words in the last paragraph. The conditioning of a career in medicine is hard to put to one side. *The Lancet* publishes research papers that conform to a highly formal structure. A dull title designed to keep the result of the study secret. A summary next, distilling the important features of the research. Then comes what journal editors call IMRAD—a brief introduction, the researchers' methods, their results, and, finally, a discussion about what they have found. Every research paper in every medical journal conforms to this style, or a very close version of it. There is no room for the patient here. Indeed, to add the patient's story would be seen as a violation of scientific etiquette. Somehow, it would be unseemly, detracting from the scientists' intention of conveying experimental purity and precision. The best a patient might get is a brief note of thanks at the end of the paper, in far smaller type than the rest of the text. Goodare asks for "the patient's own authentic voice to be heard." Only recently has this call been partly heeded.[35]

What was breached in the study of women attending the Bristol Cancer Help Centre? To say their trust was damaged is correct but hardly sufficient. Trust is a hard concept to nail down. In ordinary language, most of us probably think of trust as an expectation that someone will do what is required of him or her. That expectation may be explicit—for example, a prescription for a drug which, on presentation to a pharmacist, will be exchanged for a bottle of pills—or it may be implicit. If I visit my doctor, I do not expect the first ten minutes of the consultation to involve a series of promises—that she will do me no harm, that she will keep what I tell her confidential, or that she will offer me the best care she can. Those unstated expectations are assumed. They are part of the trust I invest in her as my doctor.

Trust may operate at an institutional as well as a personal level. Does the system of health care that I am taking part in—Western, Chinese, alternative—deserve my trust or confidence? What are the grounds for this trust? And can I rely on the competence of the staff—nurse, primary care physician, specialist, surgeon—responsible for delivering my care? Trust thus begins where my knowledge and control end. And that step beyond the information within a patient's grasp involves a risk. Modern society would collapse without a large measure of trust in all that we do—crossing the street, taking a bus, riding in a cab, eating in a restaurant. Trust lies at the heart of all our interactions with one another. If this trust is violated—the car runs us down, the bus crashes, the cab loses its way, the food puts us in the hospital—we feel various degrees of betrayal. And so it is with our doctor.

As the basis for medical care—and the existence of medical error—has become more explicit, so our trust in trust has been challenged. The nature of trust in medicine is changing rapidly. Patients ask more questions of their doctors than they once did; many want to know the evidence on which the doctor is basing clinical judgments and decisions; some will even bring their own evidence to the consultation, taken most often from the Internet. Many doctors have been unable to keep pace with this trend. Some feel uncomfortable with a new-found assertiveness among their patients. This is not what their teachers at medical school said medicine would be like. Doctors are frequently unprepared to meet these new expectations.

The fundamental change between past and present medicine is access to information. There used to be a steep information inequality between doctor and patient. No longer. As more people understand the risks as well as the benefits of modern medicine, we increasingly desire more information before we are willing to rely on trust to see us through. This need to be transparent about what doctors know (and what they do not), to engage in a consultation on closer to equal terms with patients, has changed the way medicine is practiced. Patients now want to know how good their surgeons are compared with other surgeons. Before we consent to the knife, we want to know the likely complications and how successful the surgeon will be at avoiding them.

Some doctors see these social changes as unpleasant incursions on their historic authority and clinical freedom. Many more, I suspect, simply feel that this devaluation in trust somehow reflects a sad decline in the respect in which the doctor is held. I am sure this is part of the explanation for the prevalence of doctor discontent. But for the patient, the erosion of trust is liberating. If doctors see these shifts as damaging, they miss the point about how and why medicine is changing. Trust is simply more qualified now. The patient still relies on the doctor to prescribe the drug, the surgeon to cut open the abdomen and remove the tumor, the obstetrician to deliver a baby in distress. What has changed is that trust is now more circumscribed to a specific technical skill. And before we allow that technical skill to be given free rein on our bodies, we want certain specific qualities of trust to be fulfilled. Together, these qualities constitute a working definition of trust in medicine. Trust requires:

- *belief*, in the person providing care;
- *confidence*, in the theory or system of medicine being offered

by this person;
- *dependence*, on the competence of those working in that system; and
- *transcendence*, from feelings of fear created by ignorance.

The importance of these qualities will vary according to individual patients, and will depend on the setting. If I am involved in a traffic accident, I want immediate medical care—and my trust is less qualified, if I am sensible, than if I am seeking advice about occasional headaches.

Trust, so central to the patient's experience, has become a subject for much sociological reflection.[36] Anthony Giddens, in *The Consequences of Modernity*, has written a powerful study of trust as a critical component of modern globalized culture.[37] Although not explicitly concerned with medicine, his analysis provides an important perspective on trust in patient–doctor encounters. In his book, Giddens charts the rise of information as a force in modern social life. He places great weight on a process of globalization called disembedding. By disembedding, he means the lifting of particular social relations out of their immediate local contexts and their application across large expanses of space and time. One important type of disembedding mechanism is that of expert systems. Successful disembedding depends on the trust we place on these expert systems.

Medicine is a good example of an expert system. It is a discipline that lays down expectations of doctors for patients—largely because of their specialist knowledge and widely agreed-upon professional codes—independent of space and time. Western medicine is disembedded from local contexts and operates at a global level. For example, evidence acquired from research conducted in New York is equally relevant in London, Paris, and Rome. Trust plays its part by stabilizing this global expert system because for the patient there can never be full access to the same information base of experience and evidence as the physician has. How does the patient in London know that she can rely on evidence generated in Chicago about the safety of a drug? The expert system works because patients invest trust in it. But these expert systems also need reembedding back into local contexts. Patients see doctors in real time, not in some abstract global ether. Reembedding takes place, according to Giddens, through facework and faceless commitments. Facework commitments are, as the phrase implies, concerned with person-to-person trust, or, in Giddens's rather forbidding description, "in circumstances of co-presence." These are the verbal and nonverbal cues that set us at ease (or not) with the doctor we are face-to-face with.

Faceless commitments concern trust in abstract systems. This type of trust is more difficult to secure. It depends on a meeting ground—Giddens writes of "access points"—between individuals and the abstract system. Hospitals are one such access point for the expert system of medicine. And, increasingly, medical journals are another, as they become sources of information for public as well as professional use (half of those who access *The Lancet*'s Web site for information, for example, are not health professionals). Giddens observes that these access points not only help to strengthen trust but also act as points of vulnerability between the public and the expert system. If the doctor repeatedly fails the patient, or if the information source is persistently wrong, a patient's trust in the system, as well as in the individual doctor or information source, may well be damaged. Thus, the opposite of trust is, for Giddens, not simply mistrust, but "persistent existential anxiety." As we come to place ever-greater trust in abstract systems—science, technology, supranational governments, international agencies—the importance of this anxiety increases.

Today, these systems are not only more widely distributed but also the trust demanded by them is intensified. The risks are greater, and so are the costs if the system fails. Think of bovine spongiform encephalopathy and new-variant Creutzfeldt-Jakob disease. A change in farming practice introduced a new kind of disease into the human food chain. Thousands of people who had put their trust in the food they were eating were infected.

Expert systems like medicine are more complex than in the past. For the patient, modern risk environments—such as the hospital—are likely to induce profound anxiety. Awareness of risk is greater, and the public is also more aware of the limitations of expert systems. To be sure, patients will develop adaptations to these risk cultures. Giddens identifies four general adaptive variations that we will all recognize from our own experience of friends and colleagues: pragmatic acceptance (the stoic), eternal hope (the optimist), world-weariness (the pessimist), and radical engagement (the idealist). But whatever we try to do, we cannot escape the "institutionalization of doubt."

In my view, doctors are wrong to lament loss of trust. Less trust is a good thing, for it suggests a greater transparency regarding the reality of medical practice. The present difficulty is not the loss of trust, or the challenges to doctors' traditional authority. It is that we are in a phase of uncertain transition. Information is all around us, but it is hopelessly disorganized. There are huge gaps in the information available to patients and there is no agreed-upon means of judging the quality of that information.[38] Patients may be ready to give up part of their trust in doctors but at present they have little to replace that trust with. The predicament for the patient today is acute.

Have doctors now become the chief threat to the public's health? Ivan Illich certainly thought so, and his 1975 book *Medical Nemesis*[39] has become a key document in the case against modern Western systems of medicine, and a reference point for writers wishing to report on today's state of medical science and practice. Most of these commentators, myself included, still feel the enormous originality of Illich's influence,[40] but few seem to take his arguments seriously. Born in 1926, Illich studied theology, philosophy, and history in Europe before moving to America in 1951. He then turned his inquiries to institutions and industrialization. Illich is variously regarded as a religious eccentric, an obsessive maverick, and a fascinating crank. He wrote books on education, technology, work, transport, energy, literacy, book learning, and pain. (He died of disfiguring cancer in December 2002.) Like many other controversialists, Illich is more cited than read, but this combination of neglect and dismissal means that much of value in his critique is ignored.

If one does accept Illich's invitation to debate his proposition that "the medical establishment has become a major threat to health," one begins to see how his analysis prefigures much of what has preoccupied doctors during the past decade or so. Time has seen many of his predictions come true. Illich opens *Medical Nemesis* with a challenge: modern medicine has not been designed to treat epidemics of disease; rather, modern medicine is itself an epidemic, and a virulent one at that. Like any pestilence, it must be defeated. According to Illich, progress in medical science has done little except expand the disease burden associated with medical interventions. Contemporary medicine and its product, iatrogenic disease, are little more than man-made misery. To talk of doctors' effectiveness is therefore to indulge in myth. Western medicines, according to Illich, "redefine, but do not reduce morbidity." Treatments commonly lack evidence to support their widespread use. Doctor-inflicted injuries are now being recognized as a major source of illness in their own right. Patients are becoming overdependent on their physicians, and on the drugs they prescribe. Doctors are less concerned with the sick than they are with sickness. Their hospitals are nothing more than museums of disease. It is within these specimen houses that patients become "cases" to be studied and discussed as objects of scientific curiosity. An overindustrialized economy has created an overmedicalized society. And, paradoxically, while the corpus of medicine continues to grow, so inequalities in health services between rich and poor widen still further. Doctors now "perform as priests, magicians and agents of the political establishment." In other words,

> *Medical Nemesis* is more than all clinical iatrogeneses put together, more than the sum of malpractice, negligence, professional callousness, political maladministration, medically decreed disability and all the consequences of medical trial and error. It is the expropriation of man's coping ability by a maintenance service which keeps him geared up at the service of the industrial system.

Illich predicted that hospital-based medicine was approaching a crisis. Problems of too few medical staff and lack of resources in the face of rising consumer demand, difficulties in accessing services wherever and whenever required, and the sheer management complexity involved in the bureaucracy surrounding modern health care systems were all indicative of flaws in the way rich societies dealt with disease. He argued that those few treatments that did more good than harm were generally cheap and easy to administer, and did not require the professional monopolies of physicians. Illich wanted to see a deprofessionalization of medicine. Doctors should not be accrediting one another. Their work should not be reviewed by peers but rather by "informed clients." Professional power should be limited and medical interventions reduced to a minimum. For Illich,

> Deprofessionalisation of medicine means the unmasking of the myth according to which technical progress demands an increase in the specialisation of labour, increasingly arcane manipulations, and increasing dependence of people on the right of access to impersonal institutions rather than on trust in each other.

Medicine has changed a great deal since Illich wrote his prescription for the future. First, a consumer movement that reaches far beyond medicine has challenged what was once the protected order of almost all professional elites. Transparency, accountability, and governance are now common words in our civic vocabulary where, a generation ago, they were unheard of. Second, a renewed public health movement has pushed preventive medicine into a position of prime importance within health care. Screening services for breast and cervical cancer are two obvious examples. The HIV/AIDS epidemic has encouraged a public discussion of sexual behavior that even activists in the liberal climate of the 1960s would have found astonishing. Who could have imagined, for example, that fisting and rimming would become acceptable dinner-table conversation or subjects for academic research?[41] Third, the means of acquiring new clinical knowledge has undergone a revolution in both the size of the enterprise and its qualitative nature since 1975. Thanks largely to the project of sequencing the human genome, biomedicine has become the new Big Science after physics. But instead of medicine relying on inferences from laboratory research for its treatments, the clinical trial has become the foundation for judging the efficacy of any new intervention, be it drug, device, or any other tool for patient management. The rise of the clinical trial is the single most important change in research and clinical practice since Virchow's cell theory finally consigned the four humors to the annals of anachronism. Therefore, medicine has changed in ways that would have both pleased and displeased Illich. He would have applauded consumer activism, but likely regretted the overall strengthening of medicine as a discipline.

Still, the present state of medicine accords with at least a part of his profoundly negative assessment, even if the looming implosion predicted by Illich has failed to materialize. Diseases and their molecular mechanisms have become the preoccupation of a new cadre of doctors more focused on the intellectual challenges of pathology than on the ordinary needs of patient care. Indeed, doctors are presently rewarded —in salary, rank, and honor—more for their contributions to research than for their devotion to the bedside. The mechanistic preoccupations of medicine have driven a wedge between the doctor and the patient since fundamental clinical skills that physically connect patient with doctor are no longer valued as they once were. Too often I have heard it said to a talented young physician thinking of his future career, "Anyone can be a good doctor, but you are too bright for that." Clinical practice is endured only as the route to a life in the far more challenging climes of research. Doctors, meanwhile, have seen their professional status eroded and their public trust threatened. They are discontented and unsure how to reclaim past respect and authority. The patient, although theoretically a beneficiary of today's vast expenditures on medical research and the altered balance of power in the relationship with the doctor, has yet to acquire the means—organized and valid information—to take advantage of this gradual democratization of medical practice.

However, I part company with Illich in his final conclusion. I do not see the essential problem in modern medicine as one of professional monopoly and self-interest. To be sure, there are difficulties to be faced. A medical monopoly has bred institutional complacency and fostered a clinical culture that has systematically hidden the real uncertainties underlying a doctor's decision-making. Much of medicine operates on the principle of best guess. The central challenge for contemporary medicine is epistemological.[42] Putting this challenge as a single question, it is this: How can the patient and the doctor share ways of knowing about disease that enable each to fulfill their expectations of one another? I readily admit that this formulation has little of the iconoclastic emotion of Illich, but then, I do not want to sweep away modern medicine. I hope I can show, however, that this question matters. For example, there is a great deal of evidence proving that stopping smoking, tackling obesity, reducing high blood pressure and high cholesterol levels, and controlling diabetes can prevent serious heart disease. There are dozens of effective drugs available to manage these conditions, yet doctors are making little progress in treating them. For example, a comparison of patients in Europe between 1995–1996 and 1999–2000 revealed that smoking prevalence had increased from

19.4 percent to 20.8 percent, that obesity had increased from 25.3 percent to 32.8 percent, and that diabetes had increased from 18.0 percent to 21.9 percent.[43] The prevalence of high blood pressure fell only slightly (from 55.4 percent to 53.9 percent), although rates of high cholesterol fell substantially (86.2 percent to 58.8 percent). The scientists who completed this survey concluded that their results were "a call to action" for doctors across Europe to come to grips with these preventable risk factors of heart disease.

These findings prove that even when a huge amount of original and conclusive scientific evidence is available, its impact on clinical practice can be almost nil. It is not clear where the blame for this failure lies—with researchers, specialists, primary care physicians, their public health counterparts, or governments that are at least partly responsible for public education. Perhaps it is your fault for not heeding the advice being given to you. In truth, it is everybody's failure. But it *is* a failure of modern medicine. And since the patient–doctor encounter is the one place where high blood pressure, high cholesterol, diabetes, and obesity can be properly addressed, it is within this encounter that the failure is more striking.

We might get closer to finding the cause of this failure if we see how medicine has come to be equated exclusively, and quite inaccurately, with science. Each medical student is introduced to an idea called "clinical method." This means understanding a patient's main reason for visiting the doctor by taking a detailed medical history, completing a thorough physical examination, making a diagnostic assessment, and designing and implementing a care plan for the patient. These clinical skills have traditionally been revered in medical training, and in some schools they still are. But at a time when the patient's history is seen as unreliable, and where touch, the tapping finger, and the stethoscope are all judged insensitive by comparison with the latest computer imaging techniques, the reputation of clinical method has been seriously damaged.

Far superior, so it is said, is the scientific method, whose aim is to secure reliable knowledge. By applying the unbiased rules of this scientific method, the vagaries of human judgment and its attendant errors can be eliminated. What are these rules? When discussing a treatment, they include basing our decisions on research conforming to a preplanned protocol, on results from large numbers of patients (several thousand), on random allocation of those patients to treatment or placebo, on masking these patients from the investigator so that an objective assessment of treatment efficacy can be made, and on measuring "hard" outcomes, such as death. How different these rules are from the reality of daily practice. Here one cannot plan a consultation in advance; the doctor must deal with a unique patient, not the average of several thousand; the doctor must help determine the patient's care, not randomly allocate it to one of multiple possibilities; masking the doctor would destroy what was left of the patient–doctor relationship; and death, one presumes, is to be avoided.

What medicine has achieved is the creation of a powerful means to acquire evidence, but at the cost of frequently devaluing the evidence gathered during the patient's encounter with a doctor. The rules of scientific method render that "anecdotal" evidence inadmissible when making assessments of treatment efficacy. To make matters worse, although a body of evidence may have been accumulated in the way I have described about the value of a drug for a particular disease, researchers provide almost no assistance for the doctor to judge whether that evidence is applicable to the individual patient. In short, there are two epistemological gaps. The first is between the rules of scientific method and the reality of clinical practice; the second is between the acquisition and the application of evidence secured according to those rules.

A backlash to this view may be emerging. A group of American cardiologists recently found that old-fashioned clinical method—watching the pulsation of a vein in the neck and listening for an abnormal heart sound with a stethoscope—is a "clinically meaningful" way to judge the outlook for patients with heart disease.[44] These specialists wrote about the "overall decline in cardiac auscultatory skills in physicians," and they urged doctors "to refine their skills in physical examination." Is clinical method about to undergo a renaissance?

Let me now break my earlier question down—that is, how can the patient and doctor share ways of knowing about disease that enable each to fulfill their expectations of one another—to its constituent parts so as to show how all that I have discussed so far makes an answer elusive. I place the patient alongside the doctor in a one-to-one relationship of shared understanding because it is this relationship that remains, whatever the technology introduced into medicine, the indissoluble core of clinical practice. The patient's predicament must still be confronted in an encounter with somebody who is called "doctor." Very little time in modern medical curricula is devoted to the clinical consultation, and an even smaller fraction of resources is expended to study this process. The consultation is not taken seriously; it is too low-tech to command the interest of most medical scientists. But the patient–doctor encounter is worthy of reflection. For example, the physician's case history begins with the patient's name, age, ethnicity, sex, marital status, and main occupation. This sequence is taught as the standard format for any communication between one doctor and another. It is a universal means of summing up the essential personal and demographic features of the patient. Next comes the "presenting complaint," the reason why the patient is consulting the doctor.

The word "complaint" suggests an expression of dissatisfaction, a lament even, indicating an emotional cause for visiting the doctor. Lament implies sorrow, regret, disappointment, grief. There is a dis-ease in the person before any proof of disease. The doctor thus conceives the patient on first meeting as possessing a psychological rather than merely a physical motivation for seeking an appointment. From the moment the clinical encounter begins, a division is made between mind and body. The patient is not merely categorized as a pathological diagnosis. There is a mental expression of whatever biological process is evolving, an expression that precipitates the need for a medical opinion. The doctor, therefore, begins the encounter with a humanistic appraisal of the person rather than a scientific evaluation of the case.

When these clinical consultations are studied, the findings can be revealing. John Skelton and F. D. Richard Hobbs applied techniques of computer concordancing to the language used by forty doctors in almost four hundred separate consultations, in order to study patterns of use of words and phrases in conversations.[45] Skelton and Hobbs were especially interested in how doctors used jargon, how they exercised authority, and the ways in which language was used to modify the perceived threat of the presenting complaint. In this sample of doctors working in Birmingham, England, jargon was mostly absent from their encounters with patients. They seemed to know that obscure technical descriptions should be avoided. However, patients often used language in ways that suggested perceived social inferiority in their relationships with doctors. Instead of a direct request, for example, it was common for patients to begin their question with the phrase "I was wondering." Finally, and perhaps most interestingly of all, they found that doctors commonly used language to diminish threats and allay anxieties felt by patients; they repeatedly offered reassurance to quell patients' worries.

The consultation is a shared exchange of evidence. From the patient, a history of the presenting illness given to the doctor; from the doctor, an examination of the patient's body, a discussion of what may be wrong, and the options for dealing with the symptoms in question. Within this exchange, however, there are tensions. Doctors are now encouraged to pay less and less attention to the patient's story. The reason is that patients are, so doctors are constantly told, unreliable and biased in what they report. A woman may describe a history of chest pain that raises the suspicion of a heart attack. But only by measuring the activity of a chemical in her blood will the doctor know whether her heart muscle has been truly damaged.[46] A man with HIV infection may feel perfectly well, but an accurate assessment of his HIV disease can only be made by measuring the viral load present in his bloodstream. There are many more examples where the patient's testimony is set aside in favor of an "objective" test result.

The reasons why doctors now rely less on what the patient says and more on tests that the doctor believes he can judge independently of the patient are twofold. First, these tests are measuring a variable at a particular point in time and place in the progress of the disease. The results of such tests help the doctor to gauge how much hold the disease has over the body, a hold that the patient is unable to sense accurately by himself. Second, as treatments become increasingly complex and carry greater risks—a drug's adverse effects, the dangers of a general anesthetic or an inexperienced surgeon—more precise means are sought to determine when to intervene, or, more important, when not to intervene. Medicine has moved from the qualitative—the subjective history of the patient—to the quantitative. The experiences and feelings of the patient are of marginal importance in making judgments about what treatments to offer. The patient is an obstacle in the consultation rather than a source of critical information. The patient may be offered a treatment (or not) quite at odds with how he or she feels. In addition, the rhetoric of evidence-based medicine creates the impression that medical science has reached a Newtonian age of certainty. The patient can expect precision, and the doctor, if he embraces the rigors of evidence, can deliver on that expectation. The expectations of doctor and patient are hopelessly unrealistic, of course, and both parties to the clinical encounter will frequently be let down by events. Despite treatment for high blood pressure, the patient may suffer a stroke. Despite drug therapy for high cholesterol, the patient may still have a heart attack. Despite surgery for cancer, the disease may still recur.

My plea, therefore, is for humility to become the binding force between experience and evidence. Today, experience is regarded as something of a sin to be repented for—it is at best an old-fashioned way to practice, at worst, dangerous. In our new quantitative worldview of medicine, experience is out because it cannot be measured, packaged, examined, manipulated, or tested experimentally or statistically. Experience exists only in the mind. In hierarchies of valid evidence, experience sits at the bottom, the weak associate of scientifically acquired evidence.

Yet any doctor will report that he or she possesses a body of practical knowledge that was not taught at medical school. This practical knowledge may be expressed in the way one can "feel" the needle as it penetrates the thick tissues between vertebrae when doing a lumbar puncture. It may be the way a pattern of symptoms triggers a memory of an idea that is not immediately obvious from the history. Or it may be the way a surgeon touches an organ that sparks an impression of its state of health or disease. These sensations, vague as they are, are an important part of the epistemology of medicine. And when they are ignored, the consequences can be severe. When I was a student, a woman in her twenties came to our medical clinic with ill-defined abdominal pain and a story that suggested she had lost weight. The doctor who saw her judged that she had an eating disorder and required no active intervention. The primary care physician sent the woman to the clinic again a few weeks later—vomiting had now been added to her symptoms of pain and weight loss. The same doctor took this turn of events as an indication of a bulimic pattern to her eating disorder. The patient was again returned home. A month later she returned at night with an obstructed bowel. The pancreatic cancer that had been slowly growing was now so large that it was blocking her colon. True, this kind of tumor is rare in a young woman. But a more experienced doctor would almost certainly have looked at this woman's symptoms in a different way. A second visit, an added symptom, the vomiting—nothing definitive, but a pattern that should have triggered a sixth sense.

We are now in the realm of intuition as a means of securing knowledge. Intuition is about as unscientific as one can get in writing about reliable evidence. But in medicine, as in many practical disciplines, intuition is a powerful tool in the right hands. It also has a respectable (if now forgotten) past, one that deserves to be recovered. In his *Essay Concerning Human Understanding*, John Locke begins his classification of degrees of knowledge by reflecting on the intuitive faculty of the human mind:

> For if we will reflect on our own ways of thinking, we shall find, that sometimes the mind perceives the agreement or disagreement of two ideas immediately by themselves, without the intervention of any other: and this, I think, we may call *intuitive knowledge*. For in this, the mind is at no pains of proving or examining, but perceives the truth, as the eye doth light, only by being directed toward it. [IV.ii.1]

For Locke, "this kind of knowledge is the clearest, and most certain, that human frailty is capable of," for "there is no use of the discursive faculty, *no need of reasoning*" [IV.xvii.14]. In medicine today, doctors are rarely interested in studying how intuition influences practice, how their accumulated experience affects their clinical decisions. And so, in its pursuit of molecular certainty, the Academy of Medicine is becoming ever more separated from the realities of practice and the experiences of patients.

This defense of experience naturally brings me to a second defense: the defense of the consultation. The global nature of medicine—research done in the US is applicable in the UK—tends to disembed evidence from the ordinary experience of the clinical consultation. The fact that we privilege desituated evidence over situated experience means that the messy social issues of family, income, occupation, class, gender, or leisure and how they influence the interpretation or application of that evidence receive little attention from today's professors of medicine. The fears a patient might have, her values and beliefs, are matters that are not, perhaps cannot, be included in gathering global evidence. Doctors are not prepared, for example, for the patient who, perhaps because of a religious conviction, refuses treatment. Or the patient who will try anything, no matter what the risk. These examples are extremes. The doctor is rarely tutored in how to respect and balance a patient's preferences with what the evidence is pressing him to do.

Inevitably, one returns to the consultation as the source of mutually agreed-upon ways of knowing, ways to understand dis-ease as well as disease. As Kathryn Montgomery Hunter has argued:

> Narrative shapes clinical judgment. In medical practice, the vast body of knowledge about human biology is applied to the patient analogically through narratives of the experience of comparable instances.... The construction of the case history is an integral part of medical thinking, essential to clinical education and to making decisions about the care of an individual patient.[47]

My final defense concerns the nature of this judgment. Again, the rather qualitative and individual thinking implied by a word like "judgment" seems to militate against the guideline culture now pervasive in medicine. Literally thousands of guidelines exist, exhorting doctors to practice medicine in one particular way for each particular disease. The goal is a worthy one—namely, to ensure the best possible practice. But the fact that these clear and authoritative guidelines float freely above the less organized world of practice makes them formidably resistant to implementation. They are often of poor quality.[48] And guidelines seem to make little difference to clinical practice.[49] Doctors, recognizing the gap between their personal experience and the prescribed evidence, tend to ignore the latter. Guidelines represent rationality taken to ridiculous lengths. Medicine is not reducible to lawlike rules. We are not dealing with planetary orbits or gravitational fields. The challenge for doctors is far trickier. It is to make the best use of the pluralism of available evidence—from experimentation and experience—to fashion a new knowledge shared by both doctor and patient. We are searching for an interpretive medicine, not an evidence-based medicine.

John Dewey tried to devise a theory of judgment that throws some useful light on the difficulties facing medicine.[50] For Dewey, judgment was inextricably related to inference, and both concepts depended on there being uncertainty. The conditions that are present for a judgment to be made include a controversy or choice between various options, "sifting the facts," and a decision. Dewey cautions that "information does not guarantee good judgment." The person making the judgment has to decide what information matters in reaching a decision, what those selected data mean, and what "aspects of the situation" will shape the interpretation of these data:

> To be a good judge is to have a sense of the relative indicative or signifying values of the various features of the perplexing situation; to know what to let go as of no account; what to eliminate as irrelevant; what to retain as conducive to outcome; what to emphasize as a clue to the difficulty. This power in ordinary matters we call *knack*, *tact*, *cleverness*; in more important affairs, *insight*, *discernment*. In part it is instinctive or inborn; but it also represents the funded outcome of long familiarity with like operations in the past.... Long brooding over conditions, intimate contact associated with keen interest, thorough absorption in a multiplicity of allied experiences, tend to bring

> about those judgments because they are based on intelligent selection and estimation, with the solution of a problem as the controlling standard. Possession of this capacity makes the difference between the artist and the intellectual bungler.

I am not arguing that we should accept the truth of all our judgments, or that experience inherently carries more validity in reaching a judgment than quantitative evidence. I am simply claiming that we should take experience more seriously as a source of useful information contributing to a judgment. If we do, we can begin to clarify its weaknesses as well as its strengths. For example, Amos Tversky and Daniel Kahneman have laid out ways in which judgments are made and the biases that can result from each approach.[51] Judgments are made according to a limited set of principles, such as how representative one's situation may be, how the present situation matches one's remembered experience, and how one adjusts a point of view depending on the point one started at. Thus, in judging whether to give drug x to a particular patient, I might compare this patient with those enrolled in a clinical trial for which a result is known. I might compare this patient with one I have treated before. Or I might simply make an educated guess that, given all I know about the patient, the drug, and the logical interaction between the two, the treatment will be beneficial, or not. Each of these methods of judging has its own particular cognitive biases that lead to predictable errors.

This interpretive rather than evidential approach to the consultation, to experience, and to judgment has implications for all three aspects of medicine—doctor, patient, and disease—that Hippocratic writers identified long ago. The goal for the doctor is to collaborate with the patient to identify what a disease means to that person's way of life. The doctor will trust the qualitative evidence that the patient gives up in the consultation and find ways to reembed abstract quantitative evidence back into that same consultation. This reciprocity between patient and doctor, centering on their understanding of the reason for the consultation, is one likely way to rebuild trust between the doctor and the patient. The key is participation by doctor and patient in constructing a framework of understanding within their relationship rather than simply seeing it as an exchange of services, usually for money.

In parallel with these changes, medical research is best put in the service of practice, thus reversing the present tendency to put practice in the service of research. The patient as subject needs to disappear, with the doctor entering as a participant in the research as much as the patient. Any therapeutic strategy can only be applied through that encounter, whether it be in the clinic, at the bedside, or in the operating room. The doctor cannot exclude himself from the acquisition of knowledge. The fact that he has largely tried to do so explains much of the present frustration among patients *and* doctors with modern medicine and its methods. The clinical encounter is both social and physical; understanding the consultation and improving on it therefore require the efforts of social scientists, anthropologists, historians, psychologists, and philosophers, as well as laboratory scientists and clinical trialists.

The forces currently operating in medicine are all aligned to undermine the patient–doctor encounter, to render it harmful to both the patient (who may not see any relation between mental or physical feelings and the diagnosis or treatment) and the doctor (who cannot rely on either the patient's story or research evidence). Using Giddens's term, medicine is increasingly disembedded from its human reality. Here is a schism in medical practice that is at the heart of the present challenge to medicine. The solution is to discover a way to reconnect doctor to patient through a bridge of common understanding and shared ways of knowing about disease. We need nothing less than a new philosophy of medical knowledge.

There are signs that medicine might have the capacity to adapt to these new forces. Let me give just three recent examples to counter tentatively some of the propositions I have so far set out. First, the idea that doctors cannot rely on what patients tell them. When parents of children who had suffered from cancer were interviewed, about half reported disputes with their doctors.[52] These disagreements centered around the special knowledge parents had—they had detected subtle changes in behavior, together with nonspecific symptoms and signs—about their own children. Parents felt that their doctors dismissed their concerns, in some cases delaying a diagnosis of cancer. These cues were not well-defined symptoms, they would not appear in textbooks, and doctors would not recognize them as diagnostic for cancer. But for parents, "not wanting to play," "nightmares," "becoming very quiet," and "loss of boisterousness" all indicated that something was wrong. Here is empirical evidence to encourage doctors not only to listen to what patients have to say but to believe it.

Second, the idea that the dynamics of the clinical consultation have little impact on understanding the patient's concerns. Studies of the doctor–patient encounter are now beginning to be reported. For example, a routine question that doctors are all taught to ask concerns whether there has been a family history of illness.[53] When this question was probed in the specific context of heart disease, there was a wide and surprising variation in understanding of "family history." Whether one judged oneself to have a family history of heart disease depended on the number of close relatives affected, their age, sex, social class, and type of relation. Moreover, interviewees often made judgments that they were not personally at risk despite the evidence of their family history. A question that seems straightforward to doctors may be fraught with ambiguities for patients. After centuries of assuming that doctors and patients are speaking the same language, at last we are coming to accept, even to study, the gulf of understanding that exists at the heart of this supremely important relationship.

Third, the idea that the context of the consultation is meaningless and that what matters is the application of quantitative research evidence to the patient's illness. When all available research studies are examined carefully,[54] context is clearly important. If patients' expectations are enhanced by providing information about the illness or its treatment, the outcome for that illness can be substantially improved. Management of patient–doctor relationships can affect the disease process. The situation in which care is offered is therefore a powerful therapeutic tool. Warm, friendly, and reassuring relationships make a difference.

Given these moderately encouraging developments, how might we begin a more substantial reconciliation between the science and practice of medicine? The rather large problem that remains is summed up in this tiny phrase: the false dichotomy between practice and science. Practice implies all that goes on at the bedside; science suggests a more objectively derived collection of evidence from experiments either in the clinic or the laboratory. Inevitably, each new piece of research evidence prompts a debate about its relevance to practice. Medicine thus divides into two very different communities—the producers and consumers of research—and these two groups sometimes seem barely able to tolerate one another.

The responsibility for resolving this division rests mostly with doctors on the front line of care. The skill that they need most of all is the ability to reason successfully. Reasoning first and foremost involves thinking critically about a particular clinical proposition: Does this patient who has suffered a stroke require speech therapy? Why are these parents fearful of allowing their child to undergo vaccination? Is it necessary to wire up a woman who has gone into labor with an electronic monitor? When I add up all the pieces of information before me, what should I do? Physicians are poorly trained to answer these sort of questions. They are not taught how to make clinical decisions—a practical grammar for medicine, if you like. Medical teaching is didactic and crammed, emphasizing patterns of symptoms and signs and how to respond to those patterns, instead of encouraging a fresh critical approach to each new patient. The process of questioning our claims and assumptions in clinical decision-making is fundamentally one of criticism and interpretation, and it stands in opposition to evidence-based medicine. Relying on evidence alone forces doctors to stop too soon in their clinical reasoning. So what can one do to help doctors do better? It is not only a matter of reorientating the education and training of doctors.

There is one aspect to medicine that we have too easily given up on—time. Time allows for the full range of information to be collected, weighed, reviewed, analyzed, refined, and finally agreed on. Medicine desperately needs to create a better temporal space for the patient and doctor to work in. My final hypothesis is that doctors who practice in a time-rich environment provide better care—and more carefully thought through and shared decisions—than doctors who do not. The one "treatment" that doctors can, but rarely do, offer a patient is their time. One could design a clinical trial to test this theory. Patients with chronic diseases could take part in a study in which they are randomized to receive care either in a time-poor setting (the current standard) or in a time-rich setting. The benefit, if there truly was one, could easily be measured. It is true that science has provided doctors with powerful, although sometimes dangerous, tools to alleviate symptoms of diseases and to challenge disease. But the evolution of doctor as diagnostician to doctor as technician has, for many different reasons, taken time away from the patient's encounter with his physician. It is time for time, and the judgment that it permits, to be taken more seriously. This change is necessary if medicine is to retain its place as society's chief source of healing. It is by no means certain that it will do so.

# ADVANCING THREATS

# I

## INFECTION: THE GLOBAL THREAT

> If disease is an expression of individual life under unfavorable conditions, then epidemics must be indicators of mass disturbances in mass life.
>
> —Rudolf Virchow

BEGIN WITH A thought experiment: What might it take to produce a virus with the potential to eliminate *Homo sapiens*? For a start, it should be one that we are unfamiliar with; our physical naiveté insures only perfunctory resistance to virulent infection. To preserve the element of surprise, the virus must cross to humans from another species. Airborne transmission would encourage such a leap: a cough or simply sharing a breath, especially if only a tiny amount of virus were needed to establish a human foothold. Once inside us, the virus must multiply with extraordinary rapidity, producing catastrophic and irreversible damage to all major organs: liver, heart, lungs, brain, kidneys, and gut. During this phase of fertile proliferation, subtle but significant changes to its structure (mutations) would enable the virus to evade any rearguard attempt by our immune system to reestablish control. To give the virus the ultimate upper hand, we should possess neither drug nor vaccine to challenge the infection. Finally, we should be denied the means to restrain viral spread, an easy condition to fulfill if one is ignorant of where it normally (and peacefully) resides.[1]

If this wish list of virulence sounds improbable, Richard Preston will quickly extinguish your skepticism, even if SARS leaves you unimpressed. With almost unseemly relish, he described in *The Hot Zone*[2] the dramatic emergence from Africa of two viruses—Marburg and Ebola—that fit our "perfect" virus rather too well. For instance,

> Ebola... triggers a creeping, spotty necrosis that spreads through all the internal organs. The liver bulges up and turns yellow, begins to liquefy, and then it cracks apart.... The kidneys become jammed with blood clots and dead cells, and cease functioning. As the kidneys fail, the blood becomes toxic with urine. The spleen turns into a single huge, hard blood clot the size of a baseball. The intestines may fill up completely with blood. The lining of the gut dies and sloughs off into the bowels and is defecated along with large amounts of blood.

The strain of Ebola found in Sudan, and first discovered in 1976, is twice as lethal as Marburg, killing half of those it infects. The Zaire strain of Ebola is nearly twice as lethal as its Sudanese counterpart. In *The Coming Plague: Newly Emerging Diseases in a World Out of Balance*, Laurie Garrett recounts the details of these discoveries.[3] In the Yambuku Mission Hospital in northern Zaire, Belgian nuns gave out injections of antimalarial drugs with unsterilized needles. Thirteen days after Mabola Lokela, a schoolteacher recently returned from vacation, received such an injection, he became the first known fatality from Ebola Zaire. Eighteen members of his family and friends perished soon after. The virus proceeded to spread through the hospital and surrounding villages. Thirty-eight of the Yambuku staff died, including all of the missionary nurses. A single needle at Yambuku had magnified this chance tragedy into a devastating epidemic.

The first Western physician to be notified of this public health emergency by Zaire's minister of health was Dr. William Close (whose daughter is the actress Glenn Close). He immediately informed the US Centers for Disease Control (CDC) in Atlanta. Samples of blood and tissue from the Ebola victims were distributed to laboratories throughout the world for analysis. At the University of Anvers in Antwerp, a youthful Peter Piot (who is presently director of the Joint United Nations Program on HIV/AIDS[4]) and his colleagues discovered an unknown virus in the Yambuku samples. With not unnoticed irony, the microscopic image of the virus assumed the appearance of a "?".

A small team of virologists, including Piot, was sent to Zaire to investigate. They found that villagers had soon recognized the highly contagious nature of Ebola. Families had been quarantined, the dead had been buried far away from villages, and strict roadblocks had been placed between settlements. The international team of scientists visited 34,000 families in more than five hundred villages. Of 358 confirmed episodes of infection, there were 325 deaths. Yet despite intense study, the origin of Ebola remained a mystery. Where was it hiding? Most likely in a nonhuman host, perhaps a spider, a bat, or a monkey. But as a World Health Organization report later noted, "As in the case of Marburg virus, the source of Ebola virus is completely unknown beyond the simple fact that it is African in origin."

Certainly these events were alarming, but they were also remote. To most people living in the Northern Hemisphere, the risks that these new viruses posed seemed distant. But an unknown strain of Ebola turned up in Reston, Virginia, a few miles outside Washington, D.C., in 1989. One hundred crab-eating monkeys had arrived at the Reston Primate Quarantine Unit from the coastal forests of the Philippines on October 4. Two monkeys were dead on arrival and a further score died during the next few days. Such evidence of the unpredictable and far-flung meanderings of Ebola caused panic.

The laboratory's veterinarian suspected a common monkey virus, but soon, and contrary to all expectations, the illness spread to the unit's non-Philippine monkeys. Samples of monkey tissue were sent at once to the US Army Medical Research Institute of Infectious Diseases for examination. When Thomas Geisbert looked into his microscope, he saw the telltale ?-like virus. To the horror of the American team, their tests proved positive for Ebola Zaire. The investigation at Reston quickly moved from an intriguing diagnostic treasure hunt to a potentially volatile political crisis. The quarantine unit was a hot zone containing an organism classified as "biosafety level four": one for which neither cure nor vaccine existed. Ebola Zaire was now only a few yards away from the Beltway. While the military was being alerted, more Reston monkeys were dying far away from the Philippine shipment, strongly suggesting airborne spread. The biocontainment mission began.[5]

At this point one might wonder what the press was doing while these events were taking place. The genuine sense of panic and anxiety that surrounded Reston is difficult to convey even after the passage of more than a decade. Yet while dozens of monkeys were being slaughtered for safety, most military scientists believed that they were dealing with the world's most dangerous virus, Ebola Zaire. What was their response, given that these infected animals had been in the US for almost eight weeks? Were nearby residents evacuated? No. Was a surveillance center opened to catch early cases of infection? No.

Instead, the military instituted a planned policy of disinformation, even though two men had already become ill, diagnosis unknown. One man was thought likely to have Ebola infection. He was taken to a local community hospital. By complete contrast with the Zaire government's policy of openhanded collaboration, the American response was to mislead. To stave off unwanted attention from the mass media, children were allowed to play freely around the Reston unit; press inquiries were complacently deflected; and local communities and hospitals were recklessly exposed to danger by medical authorities, who were portrayed as heroic when the story of the virus was finally released.

By a stroke of unbelievable and unexpected good fortune, the Reston strain of Ebola only affected monkeys. Four of the animal workers in the quarantine unit developed symptoms of viral infection, and three could have acquired the virus only through the air. If that virus had proven to be Ebola Zaire, the consequences for Reston—and Washington, D. C.—are unimaginable.

Richard Preston and Laurie Garrett both collected an impressive amount of evidence proving the global importance of newly emerging infections, of which Ebola and Marburg are, perhaps, the most dramatic instances. Preston adopts a narrative style of reportage which does not sacrifice scientific accuracy. His tale began as an article published in *The New Yorker* in 1992, and it benefits from expansion. By rooting the events of Reston in the lives of its central characters, Preston is able to convey the startling fears and uncertainties that these scientists felt as the crisis unfolded. He succeeds in translating the sober facts of research literature, which usually provide post hoc rationalizations and justifications for often hazardous decision-making, into a perceptive account of an emergency.

In describing the discovery of Marburg he has much to say about the lives (and deaths) of two victims who were infected by the virus in 1980 and 1987. Remarkably, a careful exploration of their histories suggested that both might have been infected in a single cave near Mount Elgon on the Uganda–Kenya border. Such odd events wrap further layers of mystery around the origin of these novel viruses. Garrett applies a more conventional, though no less persuasive, journalistic method to her subject, explaining step by step the discovery and evolution of particular viral and bacterial diseases, and considering the various possible ways of controlling them.

Still, in their praise of the physicians and scientists who work on these infections, Preston and Garrett ignore one striking truth: that the single occasion of a potentially species-threatening event in the US produced a disquieting response which exposed remarkable passivity and arrogance among the American research community. Little has happened since to suggest that this same mistake would not be repeated. The rule that secrecy equals safety still holds in the government's public health service.

The increasingly vociferous message about infectious disease is one of impending apocalypse. Here Garrett brilliantly develops her theme that rapidly increasing dangers are being ignored. Her investigations have taken over a decade to complete, and her findings are meticulously discussed and distilled. Her book is a manifesto for those who see our biological future from a somewhat pessimistic perspective. According to Garrett,

> While the human race battles itself, fighting over ever more crowded turf and scarcer resources, the advantage moves to the microbes' court. They are our predators and they will be victorious if we...do not learn how to live in a rational global village that affords the microbes few opportunities.

The recent outbreak of SARS in China only reinforced her argument. But what, one might ask, of cataclysmic epidemics of the past? If the ancient Athenians had understood the meaning of microbes, I suspect that they would have shared Garrett's gloomy view. In 430 BC, Thucydides wrote:

> Those with naturally strong constitutions were no better able

> than the weak to resist the disease, which carried away all alike, even those who were treated and dieted with the greatest care. The most terrible thing of all was the despair into which people fell when they realized that they had caught the plague; for they would immediately adopt an attitude of utter hopelessness, and, by giving in in this way, would lose their powers of resistance. Terrible, too, was the sight of people dying like sheep through having caught the disease as a result of nursing others. This indeed caused more deaths than anything else.[6]

The Plague of Athens originated in Ethiopia and spread rapidly to Greece. Victims were overtaken with violent fever and declined toward death within a week. By the end of the fourth year of plague, one quarter of the population had perished. The cause of the plague remains a matter of speculation, with smallpox, measles, and typhus the leading candidates. Its origin in central Africa—indeed, in the country neighboring Sudan—raises the additional possibility of a Marburg- or Ebola-like agent. The unusual velocity of physical disintegration, together with symptoms and mortality rates not dissimilar to those of Marburg, adds weight to this possibility.

Our most alarming notions of plague come from the two episodes of Black Death which cut through Europe from the Byzantine era onward. The Plague of Justinian arrived in Europe in 547 and continued to recur sporadically for the next two hundred years. As much as one quarter of the Roman Empire might have been wiped out during this epidemic. A second wave persisted for some four hundred years, beginning near the Caspian Sea in 1346.

Black Death, or bubonic plague, is caused by a bacterium—*Yersinia pestis* (named after Alexandre Yersin, a student of Louis Pasteur)—transmitted to human beings by fleas from the black rat, *Rattus rattus*. From eastern Mongolia plague spread to Constantinople and then to Europe across trade routes. Over half of those infected with bubonic plague died within ten days; if you contracted the pneumonic form of *Yersinia*—spread by airborne bacteria—the chance of survival was zero. The response of the Christian Church was to claim the plague was God's punishment and to accept death as unavoidable repentance. By contrast, the response of most people was summed up in Guy de Chauliac's suggestion to "flee quickly, go far, and come back slowly," advice that was heeded most eagerly of all by physicians.

The few doctors who remained conjured up some fanciful theories about the sources of the plague. When Philip VI of France ordered his chief physicians to investigate, the message came back that the conjunction of Saturn, Jupiter, and Mars at one PM on March 20, 1345, was the indubitable explanation. Endemic plague also led to some startling instances of improvisation. Perhaps the first recorded episode of biological warfare took place in 1346, when furious Mongolian soldiers hurled plague-ridden cadavers over the walls of a neighboring Italian trading post.

Despite the lack of any germ theory of disease (Galenic humors were still the fashion), Europeans understood the concept of plague's transmissibility only too well. The archbishop of Milan noted that "contagion can occur by contact or by breath." Primitive anti-contagion policies were widely introduced. Cities were quarantined (the word derives from the isolation of incoming vessels for forty days in port), the sick were separated from the healthy in pesthouses (lazarettos), trading was tightly regulated, and burials were carefully monitored.

Human losses remained calamitous. Italy had one of the most advanced public health systems in Europe—each city had a magistrate for health—and the effects of plague were recorded carefully. Between 1600 and 1650 the population of Italy actually fell from 13.1 million to 11.4 million. In Venice, an average of six hundred bodies were collected daily on barges. More than 50,000 Venetians died in the plague of 1630–1631, leaving a population smaller than at any time during the fifteenth century. The Baroque masterpiece that presides over the entrance to the Grand Canal, Santa Maria della Salute, was erected in 1630 and dedicated to health and salvation. On November 21 each year Venetians still cross a bridge of boats to celebrate mass and commemorate their deliverance from pestilence. It was Florence, however, that took the brunt of the epidemic. Giovanni Boccaccio wrote of the 1348 plague that

> many breathed their last in the open street, whilst other many, for all they died in their houses, made it known to the neighbors that they were dead rather by the stench of their rotting bodies than otherwise.... It is believed for certain that upward of a hundred thousand human beings perished within the walls of the city of Florence, which, peradventure, before the advent of that death-dealing calamity, had not been believed to hold so many.

During this entire period, the practice of medicine made little headway. Gastaldi—a Roman cardinal responsible for his local health board between 1656 and 1657—wryly commented that "the writings of doctors on the cure of plague produce much smoke and offer little light. Medical remedies against the plague have been proven by practice to be of no use and at times dangerous." Despite huge bribes, prosperous physicians refused to work in the lazarettos. When they did submit to the public authorities, they offered advice at a conveniently discreet distance: the surgeon would call out the patient's history from a window of the pesthouse, while the physician would shout back the treatment.

If epidemics are ancient phenomena, why the growing sense that there is an unprecedented threat now? Jonathan Mann, a former director of the World Health Organization's Global Program on AIDS who died, along with his wife, Mary Lou Clements-Mann (a noted AIDS vaccine researcher), in the 1998 Swissair Flight 111 crash, answered this question in his preface to Garrett's account:

> The world has rapidly become much more vulnerable to the eruption and, most critically, to the widespread and even global spread of both new and old infectious diseases. This new and heightened vulnerability is not mysterious. The dramatic increases in worldwide movement of people, goods, and ideas is the driving force behind the globalization of disease. For not only do people travel increasingly, but they travel much more rapidly, and go to many more places than ever before.

The threat from viruses has received the greatest attention, with HIV rightly demanding our deepest concern. But there are lesser dangers. Hantavirus arrived in the Four Corners area of the southwestern United States (where Colorado, Utah, Arizona, and New Mexico converge) in May 1993. As of June 2002, this rodent-borne virus has infected over three hundred people in the US, over a third of whom have died. There is no definitive treatment. Rabies, the most lethal virus affecting humans (death almost always follows soon after infection takes hold), has become widely prevalent among wild raccoons in the northeastern United States.[7] WHO records about 50,000 cases of human rabies annually, with 30,000 deaths; between 1990 and 2000, there have been only thirty-two human rabies cases in the US, although there are about seven thousand cases of rabies in animals reported each year. Infected insectivorous bats also pose a serious threat. The first rabid bat bite in the US was described in 1953. Since then, over five hundred cases of exposure to rabid bats are recorded annually.[8] Twenty-four of the thirty-two cases are thought to be due to bat-associated virus. The resurgence of rabies in a largely urban and suburban animal population raises new anxieties that most of the public (and many physicians) are unaware of. Many of those infected with rabies are misdiagnosed and their treatment is frequently delayed.

Ordinary bacteria also deserve scrutiny. The specter of tuberculosis continues to cast a somber shadow over global health. Not long ago many experts thought that TB would be controlled by antibiotics, but two million people die each year from TB and the global epidemic is growing. Between 2002 and 2020, WHO estimates that one billion people will be newly infected, and 36 million people will die from TB. Currently, about a third of the world's population is infected with the TB bacillus. WHO declared tuberculosis an international health emergency in 1993. The most dramatic increases in incidence have been in Africa, Southeast Asia, western Pacific areas, and the eastern Mediterranean. Ninety-five percent of cases occur in developing nations, where tuberculosis is now the major cause of disease. The economic effects on these low-income nations are devastating: 80 percent of cases are among working people between fifteen and fifty-nine years old. In these countries HIV is endemic and it continues to be largely responsible for the huge burden of tuberculous illness, since the breakdown of the immune system makes it vulnerable to TB. Such synergy between infectious agents is an especially worrisome feature of emerging modern infections.

More worrying still, particularly in developed countries, is the discovery of drug-resistant tuberculosis. With the incidence of HIV likely to double or even triple in nonindustrialized regions of the world, the global incidence of resistant strains of tuberculosis is rising substantially. Over two thirds of those with drug-resistant infection die. In addition to HIV and drug resistance, the third stimulus to recent tuberculosis outbreaks has been imported infection. For example, although rates of TB are falling in the US—there was a 7 percent decline in the number of cases between 1999 and 2000, to 16,377 new cases —the rates among people born overseas (almost half of all infections) is seven times greater than among US-born individuals.[9] The lack of adequate access to health care for these people raises the risk not only of widespread transmission but also of receiving inadequate treatment once diagnosed, a further factor in producing drug-resistant strains.[10] The problem of drug resistance also affects many other bacterial infections.[11]

The same story applies to fungi. A swelling diversity of infectious types of fungi, opportunistic infections in those with cancer or who undergo organ transplants, emerging resistance to the drugs usually prescribed to treat them, and lack of new antifungal agents—all these present dangers that parallel those for viruses and bacteria. The fungal threat is greatest in hospital settings. When CDC experts reviewed their figures from 1980 to 1990, they found that hospital-acquired fungal infections had doubled.[12]

Why have infectious diseases emerged again as such a major threat to the human species? Part of the explanation has come from Lee Reichman, the director of the National Tuberculosis Center at New Jersey Medical School, who, as Garrett points out, was one of the first to sound the alarm about a new epidemic of tuberculosis. He has described both medical and public complacency as a U-shaped curve of concern[13]: initial successes in improving public health usually give way rapidly to a rhetoric of false hope. The relaxation in surveillance of common diseases, such as tuberculosis, permitted their phenomenal resurgence. The decline between 1950 and 1980 in US tuberculosis rates eased the pressure on those responsible for funding tuberculosis elimination programs. The result was a dramatic rise in the incidence of TB in the US, which peaked in 1992.

The 1950s notion of a "health transition" to a new state of physical well-being was based on the almost continual success with which scientists developed new drugs and vaccines against common infectious agents. The eradication of microbial disease was widely foreseen;

hyperbole was piled on hyperbole by organizations that should have known better. For instance, WHO announced that a time was soon approaching when malaria would be "no longer of major importance." Such a statement would now seem laughable if it were not so tragically wrongheaded. Currently there are over 300 million new cases of malaria each year; many people suffer from strains of the malarial parasite Plasmodium that have developed resistance to antimalarial drugs. One and a half million people die from the disease annually, of whom two thirds are young children. Yet twenty years ago with the gradual eradication of smallpox, optimism did not seem so far-fetched. Only when HIV emerged into public consciousness in 1981 was the "health transition" finally proven to be an embarrassing myth. Today, malaria costs Africa $12 billion a year.

The history of HIV points to the second reason for a recrudescence of infection. Richard Preston claims that the paving of the Kinshasa Highway, which traverses sub-Saharan Africa, was one of the most significant events of the twentieth century. This transportation artery allowed HIV to be swept out of central Africa and to be distributed worldwide.[14] Our continued disruption and pollution of ancient ecosystems has led to the rapid displacement of unfamiliar organisms into more immediate human environments.

The huge population pressure that we face—we are likely to double our numbers between now and 2050—has produced our own global hot zone. The world's population currently stands at 6.1 billion but Ismail Serageldin, a former vice-president of the World Bank and now director of the Library of Alexandria, estimates that its population will stabilize somewhere between 8.5 and 12 billion during the next century. Ninety-five percent of these newcomers will live in the world's poorest countries. The convergence of these demographic trends, atmospheric warming, widespread chemical pollution, environmental destruction, the consequences of war (refugee populations exceeded

19 million by the end of 2002), and our own vastly increased mobility has created a boiling broth of infection.

Garrett quotes Rita Colwell from the University of Maryland, who estimates that we have identified only 1 percent of up to one million types of bacteria and only 4 percent of five thousand species of virus. A global redistribution of these organisms among biologically vulnerable animal populations, including *Homo sapiens*, with little herd immunity to new infectious agents will have profound effects. In truth, despite the recent awakening by many scientists to this threat, the coordinated effort that would be needed to control these organisms, together with the vast regulatory apparatus and enforcement strategies to quell persistent ecological imbalance, seem almost impossible to achieve. The threat is just too distant to be real, the world too fragmented to act as the "rational global village" Garrett hopes will come into being.

In any case, denial remains common. At a world gathering of over twenty thousand gastroenterologists in 1994, three plenary sessions were devoted to infectious diarrheal disease, which accounts for more than nine thousand deaths per day worldwide. Despite such prominence at an international gathering, fewer than thirty people attended each session, suggesting the lack of concern felt by these physicians and scientists about the most important public health issue facing their specialty.

Nonindustrialized countries are particularly ill-prepared to deal with these new (and old) infectious threats. Political instability, economic chaos, huge foreign debts, poorly developed health care systems, and the persistence of war have all led to what Garrett calls a "paradigm of perpetual poverty." Onto this background has been projected a process of relentless urbanization. A British scientist, John Cairns, has called cities "the graveyards of mankind," and with ample reason. Continuous rural depopulation had increased the number of city dwellers from 275 million in 1955 to three billion by 2001. The number of megacities with populations greater than ten million had risen to nineteen by 2001, including Tokyo (26.4 million), Mexico City (18.1 million), Mumbai (18.1 million), São Paulo (17.8 million), and Shanghai (17 million). This figure is projected to increase to twenty-three megacities by 2015. Urban growth is now often a sign of economic and social regress. Hand in hand with urbanization have come epidemics of diseases that heretofore were usually confined to rural areas, such as tapeworms, roundworms, schistosomiasis, trypanosomiasis, and dengue.

These social changes are also affecting industrialized countries. Poverty, unemployment, malnutrition, drug use, homelessness, and lack of access to health care have all led to a process of "third-worldization." The health effects are striking. In San Francisco, a 1991 study found that 11 percent of the homeless were HIV-positive. Immunization campaigns have stumbled and multidrug-resistant infections are common. For example, each year in the US, almost seventy thousand adults die from three illnesses that are largely preventable by vaccines: influenza, hepatitis B, and pneumococcal infection. Until the anthrax attacks of 2001 dramatically revealed the holes in American defenses against infection, the US public health system had been slowly and quietly falling apart. In 1988, a committee of the US Institute of Medicine concluded that "we have let down our public health guard as a nation and the health of the public is unnecessarily threatened as a result." Laurie Garrett examined this erosion of public health preparedness further in her 2000 book, *Betrayal of Trust*.[15]

What can be done? If the coming plagues are embedded in deep-rooted sociocultural trends and distorted economic development, the inevitable answer is, not much. This conclusion may sound defeatist, but it is implicit in the warning of Jonathan Mann quoted by Garrett:

> A worldwide "early-warning system" is needed to detect quickly the eruption of new diseases or the unusual spread of old diseases. Without such a system, operating at a truly global level, we are essentially defenseless, relying on good luck to protect us.

Luck? This sounds as if we are back in the court of Philip VI, and relying on celestial prophecy. Garrett devotes twenty-nine pages of her 622-page text to possible solutions. And rather thin they are too. The experience at Reston proved how unprepared the US was for a potentially lethal epidemic. In a laboratory scare on August 8, 1994, a scientist at the internationally recognized Yale Arbovirus Research Unit became infected with Sabia, a newly emerging insect-borne agent that had been discovered in Brazil only two years earlier. The scientist inhaled virus material from a leaking plastic centrifuge tube. An inquiry by the CDC charged the researcher with misconduct and the unit with poor emergency response protocols.[16] Shouldn't the public be informed about the dangers of this research before it is allowed to continue?

In India, the two epidemics of *Yersinia pestis* in the fall of 1994 (one in Maharashtra State and the other in Surat) both became more and more acute despite clear indications of their presence—widespread deaths among the local rat population—for many weeks.[17] Two hundred people died of plague before the disease was confirmed. Two hundred thousand people fled the area, some of whom were infected, spreading *Yersinia* to Delhi and Calcutta. Even though the large number of suspected cases has not been confirmed, poor surveillance combined with poor communication led to unwarranted panic. No single agency—CDC, WHO, the military, or a nongovernmental organization (such as Médecins Sans Frontières)—currently has the resources, staff, or equipment to act as a rapid-response strike force during a civilian health emergency. Any proposed early-warning system will require excellent surveillance in regions of highest risk (for example, in places where the ecosystem is severely disrupted, as by deforestation) and highly efficient communication. Surveillance will be hampered if there is poor indigenous primary health care or inadequate health education. Efforts to streamline communication systems have made some progress with the use of satellite technology. In January 1995, the CDC began an international on-line journal on emerging infectious diseases, receiving reports of new infections filed from the field. The collection and dissemination of information about new outbreaks of infectious disease will greatly help scientists to track, isolate, identify, and control these agents.

There is a continuing and urgent need for research and more research. Garrett argues for inquiries into ways to change social behavior (for example, how to empower women in the developing countries in their relations with men; how to introduce successful needle-exchange schemes) as well as into microbial ecology (patterns of disease that follow urbanization and "third-worldization"). Both kinds of inquiry cross traditional disciplines of sociology, biology, microbiology, and environmental science. This dual strategy has been forcefully endorsed in a 1995 report from the US Institute of Medicine:

> The lesson of history is that prevention of infectious diseases by prophylaxis or immunization will be only partially effective in the absence of changes in human behavior and ecology.[18]

It is also being recognized that past vaccine research has been misdirected.[19] In the rush to develop new vaccines, scientists have only belatedly understood that their technical ability to mass-produce vaccines has failed to match their knowledge about the cellular and molecular processes used by the body to protect itself from invading pathogens. The most appalling example of this failure was the abandonment of several clinical trials of candidate HIV vaccines in the US at a late stage in their development because of their poor efficacy.[20]

All these strategies—an anti-infective strike force, surveillance, education, improved health care systems, and research—depend on funding. And funding depends on politicians. Here is one of the worst fears associated with the prospect of a plague: any protection we might conceivably design depends on the foresight and commitment of politicians. As a recent report from the Brookings Institution accurately pointed out, politicians frequently have to make decisions under circumstances of deep uncertainty, and lack of information can produce disastrous consequences.[21] For instance, the swine flu vaccine program was authorized in 1976 after advice indicating that the US was soon to face a substantial epidemic. No such epidemic ensued, although fifty-eight people died from Guillain-Barré syndrome, an unforeseen complication of administering the vaccine. Effective reporting of the risks from infectious diseases is critical if politicians are to understand the seriousness of this threat. The Reston debacle provides a cautionary lesson here.

Finally, should we begin to confront the unthinkable? Are our efforts at prevention largely inadequate measures to deal with an increasingly destructive process over which we have little or no control? Why do we believe that we alone of all animals can alter the pace of change of this emerging threat? In a provocative analysis, Marc Lappé invites us to view the infectious epidemic in an evolutionary light. He writes:

> At the root of the resurgence of old infectious diseases is an evolutionary paradox: the more vigorously we have assailed the world of microorganisms, the more varied the repertoire of bacterial and viral strains thrown up against us.[22]

Lappé claims that our perception of man as the dominant and most successful animal species is mistaken. Rather than viewing organisms in relation to *Homo sapiens*, we could regard human beings as a part of *their* evolution. Our relentless reductionist scientific focus on the minute biochemical and genetic details of these organisms may prevent us from observing a larger truth: that our efforts to control the environment have produced challengers to our species that are more and more resistant to control. Human societies are responsible for the accelerated evolution of infectious diseases. It may be that only wholesale reversal of our social development, in a direction we can hardly imagine, would check this process. But such a reversal will never happen.

Yet we can also recall, however grimly, that bubonic plague once proved to have positive as well as negative consequences. The post-medieval public health tradition was strengthened, the impulse to care for the sick was initiated, a revolution in scholarship took place, and medical science was pursued with new energy. Ebola is still active; the latest outbreak came in 2003 in the Congo Republic. SARS took the world by surprise as well. Will it once again take a species-threatening epidemic to provide the opportunity for vigorous human renewal?

# 2

# THE PLAGUES ARE FLYING

NO OTHER DISEASE—indeed, no other force of nature—did more to shape the evolution of American life than yellow fever. HIV/AIDS may, in a century or so, come to be regarded as an equal influence. But it was yellow fever that set the modern rules of engagement—emotional, political, scientific, and medical—in confrontations between disease and humankind. As is often the way with pathologies suppressed and illnesses prevented, the threat that yellow fever posed to society is now largely and happily forgotten. The apparent victory over a temporarily prevalent mosquito is part of the gilt-edged human history of the New World. Such are the repressions of memory, the distractions of the present.

The inquisitive reader is therefore forced to rely on primary sources to recover the sense of terror brought about by yellow fever in nineteenth-century proto-urban America. One example: Elizabeth Drinker, a Philadelphia Quaker born in 1734. She wrote a diary until six days before she died on November 24, 1807.[1] Her chronicle of domestic living provides grisly insight into the drama of yellow fever in America's then most significant city.

The fever first struck Philadelphia in 1699. In September 1762, Drinker noted its comeback: "A Sickley time at Philada. many Persons are taken down, with Something very like the Yallow-Feaver." During the frequent epidemics of the 1790s, she called part of her diary the "Book of Mortality." In 1793, for instance, she described "an unusual number of funerals," the escape of families as the "fever prevails in the City," and the burning of tar in the streets to ward off disease. Five thousand people died during that single outbreak, 10 percent of Philadelphia's population. Drinker recounts stories of harrowing tragedy:

> G Hesser told a sad story, of Robt. Ross Broker that he died in the night of the Yallow fever, no Body with him but his wife who was taken in labour while he was dying, she opend the window and call'd for help, but obtain'd none, in the morning some one went in to see how they fair'd, found the man and his wife both dead, and a new born infant alive....

The number of dead exceeded all expectations. In September 1793, Drinker reported:

> It is said that many are bury'd after night, and taken in carts to their graves.... we have also heard to day that the dead are put in their Coffins just as they die without changing their cloths or laying out, are buried in an hour or two after their disease.... Coffins were keept ready made in piles.

The marks of these epidemics have been erased from the city's public exterior. When I was there recently the only visible memorial—pointed out to me by an elderly man sitting beneath the Bicentennial Bell—was a U-shaped depression in the ground beside Carpenters' Hall. An old sewer. And this for an epidemic about which, during fierce public petitioning for George Washington to declare war in support of the French Revolution, John Adams claimed that "nothing but the yellow fever...could have saved the United States from a total revolution of government."

* * *

Yellow fever is caused by a virus transmitted to human beings in villages and towns by a delicate-looking mosquito called *Aedes aegypti*, although the connection between mosquitoes and the fever wasn't established until 1900. When the yellow fever–infected mosquito enters a human settlement, outbreaks of disease tend to be explosive —and mortal. An epidemic in Ethiopia between 1960 and 1962 killed as many as 30,000 people. The disease itself is particularly horrible. Illness begins abruptly with fever, headache, and muscle pain. The victim is extremely ill with bleeding and violent episodes of vomiting. Within a few days, the pulse slows, blood pressure falls, and the kidneys fail. Blood oozes from every tissue surface. When the infection is severe, half of those affected die.

Margaret Humphreys, a respected historian of science, has shown how the human slaughter brought about by yellow fever almost by itself precipitated the creation of important US public health institutions, including the Public Health Service, which was set up, Humphreys argues, largely in response to yellow fever's effects on American commerce.[2] Each epidemic in the nineteenth century—and New Orleans took the brunt of the disease—"stopped trains and bottled up ports, keeping cotton from the mills and preventing the movement of basic merchandise from distribution points in cities to the countryside." Boards of health were set up to combat yellow fever's threat. Thus,

> Yellow fever was crucial to the expansion of federal public health involvement in the late nineteenth century, largely because, unlike any other disease that steadily afflicted the country, it was fundamentally a national problem.

In her powerful and original analysis, Humphreys tried to lay down universal criteria that any new health threat must meet in order to command serious political attention. Her conclusions remain relevant today. The theory surrounding the disease, she writes, should be agreed upon by scientists; proposed intervention measures should be affordable; the rights of citizens should be disrupted only minimally by those measures; the risk of disease should hang over a substantial proportion of the population; and the actions to be taken must be understandable and acceptable to the public. A public health movement arose in response to yellow fever. The Public Health and Marine-Hospital Service—marine hospitals were responsible for the seamen's well-being—was finally enacted into federal law in 1902. The disease was extinguished from North American shores by 1905.

Yellow fever also galvanized an unusually public debate about the epistemology of disease. The issue mattered because of a prevailing medical view that the yellow fever epidemic of 1793 had been imported from the West Indies. If correct, extensive quarantine measures at ports and in major cities would have been the only means of future protection. Such interventions would have seriously damaged expanding but fragile commercial networks. The dispute could not be left to sterile musings within the salons of academic medicine. Instead, Noah Webster, lawyer, journalist, lexicographer, and the first historian of epidemic diseases, took the debate out of doctors' hands and made it a public issue. He pieced together information from medical and philosophical societies to construct a new theory to explain yellow fever as depending "wholly on the constitution of our own atmosphere," and perhaps most of all on "the poisonous acids, extricated from every species of filth in hot weather."

As a layman with extraordinary forensic skills, Webster challenged physicians of the time—in particular, Dr. William Currie of Philadelphia, a man described by Dr. Benjamin Rush as "the oracle of our city upon the subject of yellow fever." Webster set out his contrary ideas in twenty-five letters published in the *New York Commercial Advertiser* in 1797.[3] It is one of the earliest and most important examples of investigative journalism provoking discussion about a subject of crucial civic and public health significance.

One freakish modern branch of this history concerns American enthusiasm for yellow fever as a biological weapon. In now declassified government documents, a glimpse can be had of the US biological warfare program between 1945 and 1960.[4] Yellow fever, together with its urban mosquito vector *Aedes aegypti*, was a great military hope. Work began on offensive mosquito strategies in 1953 at Camp Detrick. The advantages of a mosquito attack were plain—the virus is injected into the human body directly; as long as the mosquito is alive, the release area is dangerous; there is no known cure for yellow fever; the population of the USSR would be highly susceptible; and vaccination programs would be impossible to organize quickly enough. In 1956, field trials using uninfected mosquitos began in Georgia and Florida. These insects were good carriers: mosquitoes spread over several square miles. Fort Detrick could produce up to half a million mosquitos each month.

Part of this early work was completed by Dr. Lewis Gebhardt, a scientist at the University of Utah. Together with colleagues elsewhere, Gebhardt defined the requirements for a successful urban yellow fever attack. His team studied the advantages and drawbacks of several mosquito species, the complexities of Eurasian meteorological conditions (notably around Moscow, Stalingrad, and Vladivostok), and the defensive capacities of these regions, and they appraised plans for mosquito attack. Their analyses were followed by Project Bellwether and Operations Big Buzz and Magic Sword. Bellwether, conducted in 1959 and 1960, centered on studying the biting potential of starved female mosquitoes at various distances, wind speeds, temperatures, and humidities, together with experiments in several simulated urban settings. Big Buzz set out to assess the feasibility of mass production of mosquitoes and their use in munitions. (In these documents, China crops up as another US target.) Magic Sword took Bellwether a step further by detailing precise attack rates per thousand mosquitoes released. President Nixon eventually terminated US research into offensive biological warfare in 1969.

In *Mosquito*, Andrew Spielman, a distinguished Harvard investigator into mosquito-borne diseases and a professor of tropical public health, summarizes the history of yellow fever's discovery and the complex interplay of Cuban and American scientific rivalry that tied the infection to the *Aedes* species.[5] After twenty years of research and debate between scientists in Havana and Washington, D.C., it fell to Walter Reed in 1900 to announce yellow fever's true source of transmission. (The virus was eventually isolated in 1927.) A century later, as Spielman notes ruefully, "after a person is infected, there is little even today that physicians can do." Indeed, as the Ethiopia epidemic underlines, there was a fatal slackening of interest in yellow fever during the twentieth century, so much so that only in 1983 did the World Health Organization gather yellow fever experts together in Dakar, Senegal, to reach a consensus on how to deal with this emerging global menace.[6]

Since 1983, yellow fever has ignored the efforts of these scientists. In Africa, almost five hundred million people live at risk for the disease. The virus is endemic in nine South American nations, including much of Brazil, Venezuela, Colombia, Peru, and Bolivia. And the threat is spreading. Yellow fever epidemics are occurring more frequently and the numbers of mosquitoes are increasing. A yellow fever outbreak occurred in Kenya for the first time in 1992.[7] The worst outbreak in Brazil during the past twenty years took place in 1993. Yellow fever reemerged in Senegal in 1995. And the first instance of urban yellow fever in the Americas for half a century was described in 1999.[8] WHO reconvened its expert forces in 1998 to examine why the disease was reemerging.

The reasons are twofold. First, the relation between human settlements and the forests from which yellow fever emerges is changing fast. In the Kerio Valley, where the Kenyan epidemic began, a road had recently been cut through the bush. Opportunities for mosquitos to be transported out of the valley, or for humans to come into the region at risk, have widened significantly. With high birth rates in many of these regions, forests have been destroyed to make way for human habitation, thereby opening up new contact points between susceptible humans and virus-loaded mosquitoes.

Second, although there is an effective vaccine against yellow fever, coverage of the populations at risk is low. For successful prevention, vaccination rates need to exceed 80 percent. They never do. The outbreaks in Brazil and Senegal were largely owing to a lack of vaccination. Part of the difficulty is practical. The yellow fever vaccine contains a live but attenuated virus, and so has a short shelf life. It is easily damaged if removed from reliable refrigeration. But there is also the issue of political will. Vaccination campaigns are often poorly planned and usually do not form part of a coherent regional or national strategy against yellow fever. The motivation to deploy yellow fever vaccine is likely to be questioned still further with recent reports of serious (but rare) adverse reactions associated with the only vaccine currently available.[9] African and South American governments have repeatedly failed to appreciate the damaging effects of the disease on their own country's economic and social development. Meanwhile, WHO continued to report new outbreaks in Guinea, Brazil, and the Ivory Coast. The lessons of yellow fever in the southern United States remain to be learned elsewhere.

Search your house for the corpse of a common mosquito—*Culex pipiens*—and take a look at it under a microscope or a powerful hand lens. The image you will see is one of frightening beauty. The head is a compact black bullet from which emerge long thick spikes of hair, two segmented antennae, and clamplike mandibles. A thin rod of a neck joins the head to the thorax, which is hunched and anchors the wings firmly in place. These wings are variegated and flecked with pigment, taking on the radiant transparency of monochrome stained glass. The six legs are long, bristled, and jointed. The mosquito's back is arched into springlike readiness; the entire body is shaped for attack.

Whatever its human cost, Spielman clearly admires the mosquito. He is captivated by its power: "No animal on earth has touched so directly and profoundly the lives of so many human beings." He considers our position toward the mosquito nothing less than a "relationship." Indeed, "It may be difficult to love the mosquito but anyone who comes to know her well develops a deep appreciation." Spielman's adjectives are telling: the mosquito is, variously, iridescent, beautiful, exquisite, hardy, clever, relentless, elegant, fascinating, and bizarre. He eventually throws biological caution to the wind: this insect "*thinks* with her skin." Spielman is not naive in his admiration. He readily admits that the mosquito is brutally "self-serving." It lives to eat and copulate. Nothing more.

The mosquito is an evolutionary exercise in subtle biological engineering. Its anatomy boasts trumpets and siphons. *Culex pipiens* must beat its wings up to five hundred times a second to fly at a modest three miles per hour. Yet its life is visceral in the extreme. One New Zealand male mosquito loiters around developing adults in their pupae, awaiting the emergence of virgin females on which it pounces with only one thought in its insect mind—"essentially a rape," Spielman concludes. Sometimes a male *Culex* is so firmly engaged with its female partner that withdrawal can only be achieved by tearing off the male sex organ. Spielman also debunks common myths. While a female mosquito may like to feed on human blood, a more likely source of food is sugary plant nectar. Blood is only necessary to help drive egg production. (One myth that is true: only females bite.)

To such information one could add that there are well over two thousand species of mosquito (seventy-three of which live in Florida); salt-marsh mosquitos can migrate up to a hundred miles; a mosquito can smell a host up to thirty miles away; and there is a board game for children called "Know Mosquitoes."

But the theme of Spielman's book is far more than a natural history of the lives and loves of mosquitoes. He tells the story of how human beings have tried to control and eradicate mosquito-borne diseases, and how these campaigns have frequently failed. He does not revel in human defeat. Rather, he wishes to draw attention to the extraordinary adaptability of these insects. They live in a state of total war with predatory microbes, worms, ants, beetles, dragonflies, bats, and geckos. But human beings have become their chief enemy. And what we do commonly gives fresh life to mosquitoes and their accompanying diseases.

Spielman's best example is *Aedes albopictus*, the Asian tiger mosquito that transmits dengue and other viral encephalitides. The Asian tiger was discovered in the US in 1983. It had most likely traveled to its new home—Memphis, Tennessee—from abroad. By 1985, *Aedes albopictus* had taken root in Texas. The origin of this unusual mosquito species was the importation of billions of tires into the US from Asia. A disturbance in the ecological balance created the conditions for a new mosquito to bring new diseases before us. Spielman argues that the mosquito has a "remarkable ability to adapt and specialize," and that we humans are the main force behind this sometimes dangerous adaptation.[10] New species of mosquito are still discovered in the US every few years.

West Nile virus is a good example of how a new mosquito-borne infection can come from nowhere, or so it seems, to threaten an unsuspecting urban population. The virus leaped to New Yorkers' attention in August 1999. By September there had been sixty-two cases and seven deaths. The characteristic illness was an encephalitis, a meningitis, or both. Older people were especially vulnerable. Infections centered on northern Queens and the South Bronx, although the entire city was gripped with panic. Mayor Rudolph Giuliani promised "to wipe out the mosquito." Public health officials took thousands of specimens and isolated twenty-four species of mosquito. But Spielman believes that scientists should have done better: they "could have subjected the samples that were sent to more thorough testing." Indeed, these experts thought they were dealing with an entirely different virus. They were wrong.

The primary hosts for West Nile virus are birds. Human beings become infected incidentally when the infection spills over from badly stricken bird communities. In the Bronx Zoo, for example, a Chilean flamingo, a bald eagle, and assorted cormorants, herons, gulls, and mallards were all struck down. The message to the public during the outbreak of 1999 was to avoid bites. While New Yorkers were hastily rolling down their sleeves and covering up their ankles, the city's response was to begin ground and aerial insecticide spraying to reduce the density of adult mosquito populations. This chemical cull was readily embraced by politicians and the public alike. The criteria cited by Humphreys for mounting an acceptable response to these sudden mosquito attacks were all satisfied. By the end of the year, a survey of Queens residents suggested that as many as one in five people with evidence of West Nile virus contact had developed an abnormal fever in the previous months, a surprisingly high frequency. As a recent report points out, this outbreak of West Nile virus is the first ever to have been detected in the Western Hemisphere.[11] The virus was originally discovered in the West Nile district of Uganda in 1937. Genetic analysis of the New York strain indicated that it may have originated in the Middle East, brought over perhaps via an infected migratory or imported bird.[12]

By 2000, the New York public health department was ready for a return of the virus—and it came. But this time only twenty-one New Yorkers contracted the infection, although two people died. The epicenter of the outbreak shifted to Staten Island, and the virus spread out to New Jersey (six cases) and Connecticut (one case). The smaller number of infections may have reflected successful efforts to control mosquito populations. Insecticide spraying schedules began early to cut down the numbers of adult mosquitoes. To allay additional public anxiety about an atmosphere full of toxic insecticide, advance warnings of spraying were given on local radio stations. Whatever the reason for the smaller outbreak—and it could have been natural variability in infection rates—nobody took any chances in 2001. New York State set aside $20 million for West Nile virus research and control programs, and the Centers for Disease Control and Prevention added a further $4 million.[13] A new research group was established near Albany.

Since birds are the natural hosts for West Nile virus, a dead bird is an ominous warning—an indicator that the virus might be prevalent once again. When a dead bird is stumbled across and tests positive for West Nile virus, the area around the site becomes a center for intensive mosquito-control strategies. In 2000, dead birds were discovered in late June, and virus-carrying mosquitoes were subsequently found in July.

On May 8, 2001, I attended a lecture given by Roger Nasci, a research entomologist at the Centers for Disease Control and Prevention. He was speaking at the annual Washington, D.C., conference of the American Mosquito Control Association. To the audible gasps of an obviously agitated audience, he announced that the first two dead West Nile virus–positive crows had recently been found in New Jersey —one in Bergen County on April 30, and one in Middlesex County on May 2. The West Nile virus season had started early. Pennsylvania expected West Nile virus to spread across its state borders too, and in 2000 spent over $11 million on West Nile virus detection and eradication schemes.[14] Eastern seaboard newspapers carry regular articles on how to keep the virus at bay.[15] In the summer of 2002, 169 cases were reported from thirteen states—with nine deaths. The hardest-hit area was Louisiana, where seven people died out of eighty-five who contracted the infection. America's most severe recent episode of mosquito attack was in 2002.

Is it time to award victory to mosquitoes? Not quite yet, perhaps, although the outlook for human beings is far from encouraging. Take malaria. Ronald Ross pinned the blame for malaria transmission on the *Anopheles* mosquito in 1897, and he received the Nobel Prize for his efforts in 1902. By the 1930s, leading malaria experts were focusing on the mosquito as the target for disease control. According to Spielman, they "had come to see the mosquito as a formidable but vulnerable enemy that should be subjected to an all-out war."[16]

But public health policies of zero tolerance toward mosquitoes—the principal instrument being the insecticide DDT—failed. Spielman's experience working for the Tennessee Valley Authority in the 1950s taught him that "economic development, especially improvements in rural communities, had been the keys to a positive cycle of wealth and health." The mosquito was too simple a target:

> In reality, mosquitos are a pest and a threat that require people to mount a consistent, sophisticated, and even strategic defense. The impulse to smash the enemy must be measured against the knowledge that, in the case of a weapon like DDT, it is possible to go too far.

The 1990s have seen a return of optimism to malaria control programs. Facing an annual death toll of one million people, together with three hundred million new acute infections each year, the director-general of WHO, Gro Harlem Brundtland, launched a Roll Back Malaria campaign in 1998. Her target is more modest than the earlier goal of total eradication—to halve the world's malaria burden by 2010. This will be immensely difficult. Ninety percent of deaths take place in

Africa, and so commitment from African nations is an absolute prerequisite for success. The 2000 Abuja Declaration was signed by forty-four African governments. It advocated new efforts to strengthen health systems, thereby assisting anti-malaria initiatives, such as drug treatment, provision of insecticide-impregnated mosquito nets, and other preventive measures.

April 25, 2001, was designated Africa Malaria Day to reinforce the promises of a year earlier. The signs are hopeful for this renewed global effort.[17] But hubris is always close at hand. Writing almost a decade ago about anti-malaria programs, Spielman cautioned that grandiose "global solutions tend to be the most dangerous."[18]

One variable is outside even WHO's control—namely, climate change. Despite President Bush's wobbling on the subject, glaciers are shrinking, permafrost is thawing, Arctic ice is thinning, the land surface is warming, and ocean temperatures are rising.[19] Climate clearly influences malaria, together with many other mosquito-borne infections. Higher temperatures support the malaria life cycle. The amount, intensity, and timing of rainfall affect breeding sites. Humidity shapes mosquito behavior. Strong wind stops mosquitoes from biting. It is not surprising that some scientists have predicted a heightened threat from "vector-borne" diseases such as malaria with the acceleration of global warming. But is there any substance to these claims?

Paul Reiter, a respected American entomologist, calls forecasts of this sort "indefensible."[20] A federally mandated review of climate change and health concluded that "the levels of uncertainty preclude any definitive statement on the direction of potential future change.... Most of the US population is protected against adverse health outcomes associated with weather."[21] But in a recent study of how malaria will be affected by a warmer planet, the zoologists David J. Rogers and Sarah E. Randolph find changes, although small, in expected malaria distribution.[22] By 2050 malaria may have spread northward into the southern United States, southward in Brazil, westward in China, and across into Central Asia. Malaria transmission may also be enhanced by the El Niño Southern Oscillation, a periodic variation in Pacific Ocean temperature and atmospheric pressure that occurs every two to seven years.[23] The UK government issued a warning in 2001 that malaria could return to the English landscape by 2020. And dengue, another mosquito-borne disease, which currently places 1.5 billion people at risk of infection, is projected to put 4.1 billion people at risk by 2055.[24]

What new measures might be taken to block the mosquito's incursions on human health? Inevitably, much fashionable emphasis is being placed on genomics. In March 2001, an international group of scientists met in Paris to agree on principles for sequencing the genome of *Anopheles gambiae*, the most important carrier of malaria in sub-Saharan Africa. The hope is that the mosquito's DNA sequence, which stretches the length of about one large human chromosome, will open up new possibilities for neutralizing the increasingly drug- and insecticide-resistant malaria parasite. A first draft of the genome was reported in 2002. A similar research project is planned for the genome of *Aedes aegypti*.

Spielman is not especially impressed by these initiatives. As an old entomological hand who learned his craft in swampy salt pools and on exotic islands rather than in the laboratory, he writes:

> For nearly twenty years, those who set the agenda for science funding have taken an optimistic view of the myriad obstacles to the genetic approach to disease-bearing mosquitos. They felt that the power of modern science is limitless. The practice of molecular biology is wonderfully exciting, involving ingenious experiments based on technology that can, at times, seem almost magical. But laboratory work is reductionist.

So while he supports realistic programs like Roll Back Malaria, Spielman wants to plan for a "permanent fix" beyond 2010. The answers will lie in reversing poverty and encouraging intelligent development—education, primary health care, housing, and roads. In the end, it comes down to our "relationship" with the mosquito, and the key to this relationship "is getting to know it better." Research is important, but it should aim "to create fundamental changes in the relationship between human and mosquito populations." In a paper written in 1994, Spielman said: "Efforts to suppress or contain a vector-borne infection should select research directions on the basis of health relevance rather than technological opportunity."[25] In his recent book he argues that simple measures work well, such as quickly detecting and diagnosing new outbreaks of mosquito-borne infection. They must form the basis for any successful public health strategy.

Ronald Ross would probably have agreed with Spielman. A hundred years ago, Ross wrote:

> It is, of course, very desirable to make as many theoretical investigations as possible on the mosquito theory, but we must not forget that while we are considering academical details valuable lives are constantly being lost and that we are already in possession of facts solid enough to form a basis for practical action.... The duty...is distinctly one which belongs to the Governments of our malarious dependencies.[26]

With the launch in 2002 of a global fund to fight AIDS, tuberculosis, and malaria, this lesson is a timely reminder of the urgent challenge ahead.

# 3

# WAITING FOR THE BIOWAR

A POWDER PUFF seems an unlikely weapon. Yet records released by the British government in 2002 revealed that powder puffs had indeed been used forty years earlier in biological warfare experiments as a possible means of distributing infectious agents. The puffs were dipped in talcum powder loaded with spores of the harmless *Bacillus globigii* and then thrown from a train on the London Underground's Northern Line onto the station platforms. At least two tests were conducted, one in July 1962 and the other in May 1964. All the stations on the line were contaminated, but scientists at Porton Down, the UK's biological warfare center, concluded that the experiment was a failure. The powder puffs didn't disperse the spores very well at all.[1]

But recently we have seen that there are other, more effective ways of dispersing biological weapons. Robert Stevens, a physically fit photo editor working for a tabloid newspaper in Boca Raton, Florida, was admitted to a hospital on October 2, 2001, with a fever, nausea, and muscle aches. As his condition deteriorated, confusion and vomiting ensued. Doctors made an initial diagnosis of bacterial meningitis. A lumbar puncture suggested otherwise. Anthrax was considered, and he was treated aggressively with intravenous antibiotics. Anthrax was subsequently grown from his spinal fluid. He suffered a seizure, then respiratory failure and collapsing blood pressure. His kidneys stopped working. Stevens finally died of cardiac arrest several days later.[2]

The fear surrounding anthrax, if indeed that is what it was—no terrorist-associated case had ever been described in the US before—persuaded doctors caring for Stevens to defer a press announcement until local public health authorities had confirmed the diagnosis. There would be, in the words of the doctors, "serious ramifications"—panic was inevitable, they seemed to believe—once such a disclosure was made. There were. When the first report of this successful bioterrorist attack was released on October 4, alarm spread throughout the US, and beyond. Anthrax had been discovered in the building in which Stevens worked. Regional and local postal centers were scoured for traces of the organism and several of them also tested positive. Anthrax spores were then found in letters in a number of federal buildings, and parts of the US government were forced to shut down while offices were searched and decontaminated.

Investigation of the facility handling government mail revealed that *Bacillus anthracis* had been dispersed through the postal system in an aerosolized form. Four additional cases of inhalational anthrax—two of them fatal—occurred in people who had handled letters that were mailed on October 9 and arrived in Senate offices on October 15.[3] Despite public knowledge about the Florida case, anthrax was not high on the list of possible diagnoses for doctors seeing these four patients. The two who died remained untreated for anthrax for seven and five days, respectively. In all, there were five deaths from anthrax, and eighteen nonfatal cases of the rare disease. This bioterrorist act had been highly effective: fear had spread across much of the country and normal government business was disrupted.

The first lesson for doctors from this series of events was that the transfer of information through complex public health networks—from detection anywhere within a community to action somewhere perhaps quite distant from this point—has to be fast, faster than the system seemed capable of achieving. Early diagnosis and treatment are likely to save lives. A second lesson concerned the capacity of the public health system. If the bioterrorist threat is to be resisted, diagnostic facilities must be in place for proper appraisal of these unusual but lethal infections. Finally, the entire medical community needs to educate itself about infections that could be used for bioterrorist acts. For the first time in the history of the Western world, such infections need to be considered seriously in any patient with an unusual or atypical illness. Rather chillingly, as Thom Mayer pointed out, the scientific reality is that in the case of anthrax, "only further experience with this devastating disease can clarify its precise natural history and optimal treatment."

Reviewing this "new challenge for American medicine," H. Clifford Lane and Anthony S. Fauci, two leading infectious disease scientists (Fauci is director of the US National Institute of Allergy and Infectious Diseases), wrote of a "new era" in their country's history of public health.[4] Fear had led well over 30,000 people to be treated preemptively with antibiotics because of concern about possible exposure to anthrax. Lane and Fauci emphasized the critical importance of distributing information through reputable Internet sites, not only for physicians but also for the public. For an immediate and important health impact of these bioterrorist attacks was on psychological well-being. A measure of the likely effect was described in a national survey of stress reactions after the September 11 attacks on New York City and Washington, D.C.[5] Two out of five adults surveyed described one or more symptoms of stress, such as feeling very upset on being reminded of the September 11 events; disturbed memories, thoughts, or dreams; difficulty concentrating; sleep disturbance; or irritable outbursts. These indicators of stress also affected children. The degree of anxiety, a symptom that was pervasive, seemed to be linked to watching television coverage of the terrorist incidents. And bioweapons are justifiably to be most feared. Nuclear material is hard to get hold of and chemical weapons require large quantities of whatever agent is being deployed. By contrast, bioweapons can be easily constructed and grown in a garage.

These events had an instant effect on government research policies —and funding. After an initial $5.1 billion was committed to bioterrorism defense and research in 2001, a further $11 billion was promised in 2002. This money was spent on stockpiling vaccines and antibiotics, building new laboratories, funding basic research, and designing drug and vaccine discovery programs, although vocal dissent about how a new Department of Homeland Security would manage this broad mandate has come from many scientists with substantial knowledge of civil defense.[6]

The freeing of funds was as sudden as it was unexpected. D. A. Henderson, the man who led the smallpox eradication campaign, was summoned to meet Tommy Thompson, the US secretary for health and human services, at 7 PM on September 16, 2001. After a five-hour conversation, he was given $3 billion only a few months later—although he was told to spend it carefully.

The European Union has also raised civil protection from biological attacks higher on its list of funding priorities, with special attention being given to detection and diagnosis, surveillance, vaccines, and pooling of knowledge among member states. Michel Tibayrenc, a longtime advocate of greater European collaboration over emerging infectious threats, has argued for the creation of a European Center for Infectious Diseases.[7] Such a body would coordinate surveillance of biological threats and study their effects and treatment. He described the existing European efforts at controlling infection as "a distressing cacophony, like an orchestra with no conductor." Within the space of a few months, protecting the public from bioterrorism had assumed a position of unprecedented political importance, where previously few people had taken the threat seriously.

* * *

With the move to create a Department of Homeland Security, the US government officially designated the country as vulnerable. Security experts had long ago pointed out the lack of American preparedness for terrorism. Joseph S. Nye, dean of Harvard's Kennedy School of Government, wrote in *The New York Times* of the astonishing complacency that greeted a study he conducted with James Woolsey, a former director of the Central Intelligence Agency, into the US capability to respond to terrorist threats.[8] While he was reassuring in his belief that biological weapons were difficult to make and thus an unlikely terrorist tool, he emphasized the need for civilian cooperation between agencies and across national governments. Nye warned that a purely military strategy against terrorism would be a serious mistake. The CIA, FBI, immigration authorities, custom services, and Defense Department all had parts to play.

The political failure to devise systems to protect the public from terrorist, and especially bioterrorist, attack is widespread. A survey of 456 US cities with populations of more than 100,000 revealed that a third did not have a terrorism response or prevention plan in place.[9] Half of all cities had no antiterrorism training. Most remarkably of all—and this survey was conducted after the September 11 attacks—48 percent of cities had no intention of conducting an overall reassessment of their preparedness.

The lack of an effective antiterrorist plan produced an unsystematic and disorganized domestic response when terrorists did strike. For example, fear of biological and chemical attacks led the Federal Aviation Administration to cause a temporary agricultural crisis by grounding crop-dusting planes once it learned that at least one of the September 11 hijackers had downloaded information from the Internet about the aerial distribution of pesticides. And yet experts on weapons of mass destruction argued that these aircraft were far more likely to be used as flying bombs, carrying explosives rather than biological or chemical agents.

One domestic strategy was a financial war on terrorism. An effort to freeze terrorist assets included key figures in al-Qaeda and groups that channeled money to the Taliban regime in Afghanistan. The effect of this response was highly symbolic—in the words of one US government official, "It sends a powerful signal to al-Qaeda that we know who they are, who their friends are, and who supports them financially."[10] Perhaps more importantly, given the initial faltering government response, this statement sent a signal to the American public that despite the attacks on major cities and the fears of bioterrorism, the Bush administration thought it knew exactly who its enemy was. This counterterrorist measure was designed as much to calm public nerves as it was to stop terrorism.

An emphasis on securing and parading reliable information about individual terrorists was clearly intended to compensate for what was seen as the US's greatest failure of intellligence since Pearl Harbor. Since one of the goals of any terrorist operation is to induce a state of pervasive fear and anxiety among those who are its target, countering that mental state must be a major antiterrorist strategy. This approach therefore becomes an important aspect of the public health response to terrorism: reducing mass public anxiety by offering reassurance, often false, that the government has all the necessary intelligence to protect its people. Thought of in this way, the CIA and FBI have features of a public health agency as much as they do those of an intelligence service, and thus their responsibilites include providing both the government and the public with as much information as possible during crises like the anthrax attack.

But there is another interpretation of these events, one that has important implications for public health responses to bioterrorist threats—namely, that the failure to react quickly and effectively when an attack occurred was due not to a lack of information but rather to ignored information. An aversion to evidence creates the climate for inaction, and to see this one only has to look at recent US press and government responses to escalating terrorist threats. On August 7, 1998, two US embassies in East Africa were bombed, killing over two hundred people and injuring thousands. In retaliation, President Clinton authorized the bombing of a pharmaceutical plant in Khartoum on August 20, 1998. The basis for the US attack was evidence of chemical weapons collected from a soil sample at the site of the plant. Yet this response was largely seen as unjustified and as one of Clinton's most serious foreign policy errors, in large part since it occurred at a time of intense public scrutiny of the ongoing investigation into his personal sexual affairs.[11]

Al-Qaeda admitted responsibility for the bombings in Nairobi and Dar-es-Salaam. Evidence later secured from a witness in the trial of those responsible for these attacks confirmed that al-Qaeda had tried to acquire components of chemical and nuclear weapons in Sudan, thus lending support to Clinton's order to bomb the plant. The intelligence services had gathered sufficient information to alert them to the threat from al-Qaeda. Given the evidence that Osama bin Laden's network was attempting to build such weapons, dismissals of a bioterrorist threat by US Health and Human Services Secretary Tommy Thompson and his predecessors as an exaggerated overreaction were, with hindsight, complacent. For the greatest danger to intelligence and public health agencies trying to protect citizens from biological attack is a climate of skepticism—even apathy—about the prevailing risks, and the resulting failure to prepare for possible attacks.

But the most important political and perhaps even public health consequence of the September 11 attacks and anthrax deaths has been a reassessment of America's place in world affairs. In order to build a coalition against terrorism, the US has had to embark on its biggest global diplomatic effort since the Gulf War. In doing so, it has forged alliances with countries that had previously been anathema to its foreign policy interests, notably Pakistan. America needed the world on its side. A Republican administration at least temporarily discarded its own unilateralist policies to achieve new aims. It will have to maintain an enlarged commitment to global cooperation for years to come if its war on terrorism is to succeed. In the long term this shift in policy might have a profound impact on US attitudes toward issues that go beyond bioterrorism in their relevance to public health (for example, climate change, environmental policy, and issues of international human rights and criminal law). President Bush's veto in July 2001 of a draft protocol adding enforcement and verification mechanisms to the 1972 Biological and Toxin Weapons Convention, which had prohibited the development, testing, production, and stockpiling of biological weapons, was an example of how US isolationism harmed not only global efforts to reduce terrorist threats but also homeland security. Will national sovereignty now come second to global security and public health? The early indications are that although the US government recognizes that there are global issues to be resolved, its own national interests will not be diluted by larger strategic or humanitarian concerns. Quite the contrary.

The war in Iraq, which opened with bombings in Baghdad in March 2003, after a diplomatic failure that left the UN struggling to regain credibility and Europe more divided than at any time since World War II, has reopened fresh concerns about US unilateralism. Weapons of mass destruction, and bioweapons in particular, have been the core motivation behind America's new doctrine of preemption. In the 1980s, US laboratories—specifically the American Type Culture Collection of Manassas, Virginia—supplied anthrax, botulinum toxin, and other agents of biowar to Iraq. Documents show that the US and France together sent seventeen types of organism to Iraq. A spokeswoman for the American laboratory that shipped these materials to Iraq told *The New York Times* in 2003 that any bioagents were for research purposes and must have been authorized by the US Department of Commerce.

Iraq admitted to UN weapons inspectors in January 2003 that it once possessed 8,500 liters of anthrax. But it claimed to have destroyed all its supplies in 1991, although the government provided no evidence to verify this assertion. Hans Blix, the chief UN weapons inspector, also noted that the Iraqi government had failed to declare 650 kilograms of bacterial growth medium and had deliberately altered documents to conceal its existence. This amount of culture material would enable the production of 5,000 liters of anthrax. Amid fierce and unresolved debates among experts about the shelf life of anthrax, a war was launched. Many military and intelligence observers seemed to agree that Saddam Hussein posed no immediate threat to anybody. But the fear of bioweapons after the anthrax assault on Washington, and in the context of September 11, had transformed US foreign and security policy. The risk of disease was shaping the exercise of geopolitical power like never before.

The threat of biowar is not new.[12] Some of the first fears of bioweapons in a Western country began after a July 1934 report by the former editor of *The Times*, Henry Wickham Steed, that German spies had tested biological agents in the London Underground. This matter was viewed mainly as a problem for public health and referred not to the Ministry of Defence but to the UK Medical Research Council. In contrast with modern perspectives on bioterrorism, respectable opinion at that time was that any biological threat lay in public health service disruptions caused by conventional warfare. A breakdown in sanitary services could leave many people vulnerable to crippling epidemics of infectious disease—such as from bacteria, especially tetanus, that cause wound infections, as well as anthrax and typhoid. The political response was to strengthen existing public health services. Direct attacks with bacteria or viruses were judged improbable. But the threat of epidemic diseases as a consequence of air attacks on the civil population was real. After a great deal of protracted committee debate, it was agreed that the time had come for an Emergency Public Health

Laboratory Service (PHLS). Sparked by the threat of biological warfare seen through this broad public health perspective, the PHLS, established in 1947, today "protects the population from infection by detecting, diagnosing, and monitoring communicable diseases."

With the advent of World War II, an explicit research effort into biological warfare was launched. By 1943, a prototype anthrax bomb had been built. In 1947 UK biological weapons research achieved equal priority with nuclear research. But this offensive effort soon switched to more defensive goals when the British military establishment canceled its order for a biological bomb. Although research has continued, it has never reached the level it had in the immediate postwar period.

After the Gulf War, politicians and scientists shared renewed interest in biological weapons. In 1999, the UK Royal Society, together with the US National Academy of Sciences and the French Académie des Sciences, met to consider the control of biological agents.[13] The Royal Society's report urged "a scientifically sound and realistic assessment" of the effects of potential biological agents. It also recommended that medical staff be trained to recognize diseases caused by biological weapons and that limited national vaccine banks and stockpiles of antibiotics be created. Most importantly,

> To manage the consequences of a BW attack on civilians, an overall structure is needed within which attacks by specific agents can be handled. Collaborative plans should be set up between the police, public health authorities, the clinical and hospital services, the intelligence agencies and the military. The authorities who would co-ordinate the local and national responses should be made clear. These plans should be tested in simulated attacks.

None of these measures was ever implemented. Thus, when the UK Parliament's Defence Committee met in November 2001 to consider the threat from terrorism, there was little evidence to draw on for substantive public inquiry. Still, a crucial shift in policy emerged during this gathering of evidence:

> In the past the level of resources put into the defence of the UK has been set principally to reflect the perceived level of threat rather than through an assessment of the weak points in our society. Provisionally we have concluded that in the UK we will have to do more to focus our capabilities on defending our weak points.[14]

The conclusion of the Defence Committee was that the threat of nonstate terrorism was increasing, especially from terrorists using weapons of mass destruction. Bioterrorism is the greatest danger of all, although its effects are uncertain. Biological weapons may be used in small quantities, are low in cost, and have high strategic impact. They have the weakest international controls of any weapon. What limited evidence exists suggests that terrorist organizations are trying to secure biological materials. Presently, the UK could not respond to a large-scale bioterrorist attack. An urgent military review will be required, including an appraisal of homeland security and the place of the military in civilian protection.

When the British Parliament's Home Affairs Committee[15] took evidence to underpin the Anti-Terrorism, Crime and Security Act 2001,[16] there was a specific interest in protecting the public health from bioterrorist threats. Politicians were most concerned with the need for a proportionate response and with the careful construction of rules of detention without trial of suspected terrorists. The balance between protecting the public (health) and protecting individual rights was not easily achieved. Eventually, it was reluctantly agreed that detention when there was no prospect of extradition, deportation, or prosecution was allowable in rare circumstances. Provisions covering data sharing, racial and religious offenses, hoaxers, powers of identification (such as fingerprinting), aviation security, police authority, and freezing financial assets were all covered in the act.

But it was the bioterrorism-inspired PHLS that provided the immediate anchor for efforts to construct a practicable and responsive public health strategy. By October 31, 2001, less than a month after the first anthrax-laced letter was opened in the US, the PHLS had issued interim guidelines for health professionals dealing with packages suspected of containing anthrax. The advice began with the comment that the threat of bioterrorism in the UK remained low. It acknowledged the genuine public anxiety about biological weapons and argued that the PHLS guidance was a proportionate response to this anxiety. Yet the advice, together with its implications, was stringent. It recommended that every business review its procedures for handling mail. It also suggested that any suspicious envelope or package should trigger a call to the police, evacuation, and isolation of the person who opened the mail.

In January 2002, the UK's chief medical officer, Liam Donaldson, published a national strategy document for dealing with the threat of infectious disease.[17] This investigation had long been promised, but now took account of the risk posed by biological weapons. The report was withering in its criticism of current anti-infection arrangements in the UK. There was no integrated approach to the problem of infectious disease, no clear lines of responsibility, no reliable infrastructure, no standardized diagnostic criteria for infections, and poor laboratory security procedures. To counter these profound weaknesses, Donaldson recommended the creation of a National Infection Control and Health Protection Agency. The threat from bioterrorism, he argued, had been judged low because of the technical difficulty of launching a biological attack. In the light of the terrorist attacks in the US,

> the possibility of a much more extensive terrorist operation, the absence of a specific warning, the deployment of terrorists who have no fear for their personal safety or survival, and the use of

> multiple simultaneous points of attack must now form part of the planning for countermeasures to protect the health of the population against deliberate release.

His analysis ended with a recommendation that dealt directly with one of the central criticisms of intelligence services in the US after September 11—namely, a failure of imagination. He advised "forward thinking and innovation in identifying and protecting against vulnerability." The UK's Health Protection Agency opened for business on April 1, 2003.

The anatomy of the public health response to the reality of bioterrorism is part medical and part political. The necessary public health measures to tackle biological weapons had been discussed before the October 2001 incidents in the US, but government authorities, while paying lip service to this advice, did little to engage with these measures seriously. Since that October, this advice has been reiterated and enlarged—and now money is at last moving to shore up public health defenses ($1 billion for states to improve bioterrorism defenses, and $3 billion for the Department of Health and Human Services to begin preparedness planning—ten times the department's budget in 2001). But bioterrorism also substantially widens the scope of public health. By the very nature of the threat, protecting the public's health involves intelligence-gathering, strengthening criminal justice, and reassessing defense and foreign policy initiatives. There are few contemporary issues that require such a broad conception of public health, yet public health has much to offer in each area.

The response of the medical and scientific communities to the events of September 11 and the subsequent anthrax attacks showed that doctors and scientists believe they have an important part to play in limiting the risks of bioterrorism. Writing in *Science*, Christopher F. Chyba, director of Stanford University's Center for International Security and

Cooperation, described public health as "a kind of homeland defense that is applicable to both unintentional and intentional disease outbreaks."[18] He noted that health care workers were likely to be the first to respond to a biological attack and so disease surveillance, together with domestic and international networks for notification, were crucial defensive counterterrorist measures. Senior scientists and administrators at the PHLS drew attention to guidance on covert pathogen releases and wrote that the UK's "excellent public health systems and infrastructure give us a good start" in laying down a preventive system to combat bioterrorist threats.[19]

The view that further biological weapons use is inevitable is now commonplace. Yet the equally common view is that countries are ill-prepared for a biological attack.[20] The fact that a biological incident would begin silently—no explosions, no warnings—makes effective preparation almost impossible. D. A. Henderson, now director of the Center for Civilian Biodefense at Johns Hopkins University, has argued that there is "no comprehensive national plan nor any agreed strategy for dealing with the problems of biological weapons." Antibiotics and vaccine stocks are simply inadequate to deal with such an attack. This impression was borne out by a study of disaster preparedness in New York City on Y2K.[21] Fewer than two thirds of directors of emergency receiving hospitals had protocols for dealing with biological attacks and only a third felt very or moderately confident about managing victims of a biological incident. Early mistakes by senior American politicians —for example, in failing to rely on health officials to act as key information sources for the public—seemed to bear out this uncertainty.[22]

Yet the escalating threat of biological weapons had been predicted by the public health community. A US working group on civilian biodefense, supported by the Department of Health and Human Services Office of Emergency Preparedness, had been publishing regular consensus statements on potential biological agents, such as anthrax,[23] smallpox,[24] plague,[25] botulinum toxin,[26] and tularemia.[27] This careful process of defining the threat and drawing up guidance on diagnosis, vaccination, treatment, prophylaxis, and decontamination stemmed from the failure of the Biological and Toxin Weapons Convention to contain the threat successfully. The US Centers for Disease Control and Prevention played a critical part in strengthening public health defenses,[28] although a lack of ability to respond to surges in demand remained a serious weakness.[29]

Moreover, once the first anthrax case was reported in October 2001, health officials quickly secured supplies of the antibiotic ciprofloxacin at reduced cost, after the US government put pressure on Bayer, the drug's manufacturer, to cut its price. Scientists at the Centers for Disease Control and Prevention acted immediately to determine how the first patient contracted the disease and which genetic strains of *B. anthracis* had been used. Thus, while it might be true that, as *The New York Times* claimed, "the nation has short-sightedly allowed its public health agencies and facilities to weaken in recent years,"[30] it is also true to say that those same agencies acted remarkably quickly and effectively to deal with the threat once it became real.

Some critics might even argue that the US government is reacting too quickly. Was it appropriate, for example, for the government to accelerate safety trials of a new smallpox vaccine? Vaccine manufacturers were asked to rush through clinical trials to have a vaccine available by the end of 2002.[31] Can safety reasonably be marginalized in the interests of national security? And, in any case, at what cost to other social programs? The increases in US bioterrorism budgets have forced a rebalancing of welfare priorities—services for the elderly and uninsured are likely to be cut and CDC's non-bioterrorism spending to fall, with likely adverse effects on public health generally.

What can those concerned with public health achieve globally? In 1997, Joshua Lederberg argued that "the medical community does indeed have a primary role in institutionalising the prohibition of biological weapons as a global commandment, as well as in mitigating the harm from infractions."[32] This international imperative could be achieved through a new global coalition against terror. But

> For many nations that were born out of what was once labelled terrorism, efforts to eradicate totally a method of protest that was part of their own historic political struggle are likely to be resisted.... Diplomacy will be confronted by histories that cannot be separated from politics.[33]

Public health—through ideas such as harm reduction, human rights, population approaches to health, and social medicine—has a central role in disarming the terrorist: "Attacking hunger, disease, poverty, and social exclusion might do more good than air marshals, asylum restrictions, and identity cards."[34] Transnational communities of doctors, scientists, and other professionals can do much to foster tolerance between countries.[35] Medicine acts as a bridge between societies since it sets out shared concerns for prevention, care, and healing.[36] The World Medical Association has called for the creation of an international consortium of medical and public health leaders to monitor the threat of biological weapons, to identify actions to stop bioweapons proliferation, and to develop a plan for surveying the worldwide emergence of infectious diseases. All that is now lacking is leadership to convert these ideas into reality. Public health approaches to counterterrorism also cannot ignore the development debate. Unstable states afflicted by poverty, disease, inequality, debt, poor infrastructure, lack of effective administrative capacity, weak governance, and state violence can become a breeding ground for terrorism. Public health therefore has a political, economic, and social, as well as a medical, agenda to follow. Constructing or rebuilding health services in poor nations—for example, Afghanistan—is one practical goal.

The most radical opportunity for the public health community to develop this role came with the report published in 2001 by the Commission on Macroeconomics and Health.[37] The commission was established by WHO's director-general, Gro Harlem Brundtland, in 2000. Its aim was to place the health of the poor at the center of the development agenda. The argument underpinning this effort was that disease is inherently destabilizing for economies and entire political systems. The stability of the global economy depends, therefore, on an effective program to reduce disease burdens and improve the health of the poorest people. The commission concluded that by focusing on only a few diseases—for example, TB, malaria, and HIV/AIDS—eight million lives per year could be saved by 2010. At a total annual cost of $66 billion ($34 per person per year in low-to-middle-income countries) the economic benefit could be $360 billion per year by 2020. Present donor contributions are about $6 billion per year. That figure must increase to $27 billion per year by 2007 if these benefits are to be realized. If one accepts the twin assumptions that investing in health will encourage political stability and economic development, and that state instability fosters terrorism, investment in health may be an important counterterrorist measure. But whether the causes of terrorism—and the remedies—are so simple remains to be seen.

Is the threat of bioterrorism illusory? Simon Wesseley, a respected British psychiatrist who specializes in the psychological consequences of war, has claimed that the main purpose of biological weapons "is to wreak destruction via psychological means—by inducing fear, confusion, and uncertainty in everyday life."[38] He argues that the long-term psychological and social consequences of the threat are likely to be more serious than the physical risk itself. This argument is not new. However, the experience with anthrax is too brief and inconclusive to make such confident claims. D. A. Henderson would certainly disagree with him. The fact is that biological weapons have been made, are being designed, and are likely to be used again. The accidental outbreak of anthrax in Sverdlovsk, in the Soviet Union, on April 2, 1979, which caused at least sixty-six deaths, showed that this agent was being prepared within a military facility in a country that had signed an international agreement not to do so.[39] The risk of bioterrorism is credible.

Indeed, once smallpox was eradicated, Russia saw a military opportunity within a medical victory and began stockpiling the virus. Even today, according to Henderson, Russia maintains a major smallpox production laboratory in Sergiyev Posad. The US government sees the greatest threats coming from smallpox and anthrax, especially in aerosol sprays disseminated via ventilation and mail systems, as well as crop dusters. For an increasingly urbanized global population, the risks of aerosol attacks are great. Henderson is "not optimistic" that international exchange of biological agents can be limited.

From a public health perspective, therefore, a key issue is good surveillance. One approach that might amplify the ability to report, confirm, or prevent outbreaks is the use of the Internet as a means of civil defense. The American scientist and Internet enthusiast Ronald Laporte believes that the "existing international public health system is not sufficiently agile to compete with bioterrorists." He advocates devolving surveillance to citizens who would become "the first and most important line of defence."[40] The capacity of the public health system would expand enormously, fear might be averted by sharing responsibility among a larger community, and the necessary communications network would also double as an effective mechanism for distributing information. This argument has been implicitly accepted by US government agencies. The FBI sent half a million letters to New Jersey and Pennsylvania residents inviting their help in identifying the anthrax assailant. "Look at your neighbor and see if he fits this profile," one postal inspector said. But would such an initiative simply turn us all into a nation of busybodies and informers?

Indeed, the failure to pass on accurate information to the public about the anthrax incident showed how weak and unreliable public health systems of communication really are. When news of the first anthrax case was initially reported, Health and Human Services Secretary Tommy Thompson described the case as one of natural origin with no evidence of underlying terrorism, instead of acknowledging the possibility of bioterrorism, admitting uncertainty, and reassuring the public that the incident was being urgently investigated. The agency in the nation most able to give authoritative advice on bioterrorism—the CDC—was blocked from commenting, on the grounds that an anthrax attack fell under criminal, not public health, jurisdiction. As a result no consistent message was being given by a respected and reliable public health source.[41]

There are signs that the US government is now taking the domestic threat of biowar seriously. In January 2003, the Bush administration announced that the CDC will lead a new surveillance system in eight cities to identify infectious disease outbreaks. This alerting service will be highly sensitive. Information will be collected from physicians, pharmacists, and emergency rooms. A shift away from military to civilian leadership is a good sign—homeland defense is an issue for every citizen.

But when does information become propaganda? Is the threat of biowar being talked up or talked down? The immediate government response in 2001 was to talk down the threat. The result was that when a case of anthrax was confirmed, there was widespread and unnecessary fear and panic. Either the government did not have a grip on the situation or it was being complacent. It is perilous to speculate on the motive behind the initial Thompson denial. Certainly, he would have wished that what he said was true. But maybe also, since there was nothing the government could do about an anthrax attack (a reality that the public still seems not to have appreciated), his immediate denial bought the government time, and masked national uncertainty about the extent of the attack and how to respond. That uncertainty will always remain, no matter how good the government's surveillance systems are.

# EPILOGUE TO CHAPTERS 1, 2, AND 3

CAN LIFE BE created in a test tube from its constituent chemicals alone? The incredible complexity of even the most unsophisticated bacterium would be hard to reproduce from a few simple molecules. The structure of anything that resembles a cell is just too refined—almost civilized—for such crude assembly.[1] Not so a virus, which is little more than a protective protein coat surrounding a more delicate piece of genetic material. And in 2002, an important line in the biological sand was crossed, creating a storm of angry dispute. A team of scientists from the State University of New York at Stony Brook reported the creation of the world's first synthetic virus. They had gathered the building blocks of a poliovirus together in a test tube and, to cut a longish story short, stirred. The result? A particle that behaved in all ways like a natural poliovirus. When the synthetic virus was injected into mice, they fell ill with a disease indistinguishable from polio. The implications of these findings were not lost on the New York scientists:

> The global population is better protected against poliomyelitis than ever before. Any threat from bioterrorism will arise only if mass vaccination stops and herd immunity is lost. There is no doubt that technical advances will permit the rapid synthesis of the poliovirus genome. . . .[2]

Polio will soon be eradicated, perhaps in the next three years or so. Could an enterprising terrorist cause mass paralysis of the population by introducing synthetic poliovirus into a community? Critics of the Stony Brook team described their efforts as little more than a cheap stunt. One slammed the journal *Science* for giving this work its stamp of authority.[3] Poliovirus is not especially contagious, so it will never be a practical biological weapon. The editor of *Science*, Donald Kennedy, agreed that any "national security concerns are not worth serious consideration." But he also commented that "sticking one's head in the sand and hoping that unpleasant realities will go away has never been a fruitful approach to science or to public policy." Although polio may not be an immediate bioterrorist threat, an important principle had been proved. Viruses that cause human disease can be created in the laboratory—from scratch. Polio today—smallpox, when?

This work conjures up the prospect of imminent human self-annihilation from technologically adept terrorists. But the threats are far more real than these playful experiments in the laboratory. The World Health Organization estimates that 56 million people died in 2000. Over 14 million died of infection. The major killers were chest infections (3.9 million deaths), HIV/AIDS (2.9 million deaths), diarrheal disease (2.1 million deaths), tuberculosis (1.7 million deaths), malaria (1.1 million deaths), and measles (800,000 deaths). To put these figures in context, 6.9 million people died of cancer and coronary heart disease each, and 5.1 million people died from stroke.[4] In other words, infection today continues to pose the greatest threat to human survival.

The diseases that get all the attention—in the media and from multilateral institutions, such as WHO—are HIV/AIDS, TB, and malaria. So it might come as a surprise that a condition as mundane as a chest infection kills so many people. Certainly pneumonia does not attract the interest of presidents and prime ministers. And yet pneumonia is one of the leading causes of death among children under five years old, and 40 percent of these deaths take place in Africa. A further complicating truth is that these diseases are not independent of one another. Chest infections and pneumonia coexist with measles, malaria, and HIV, all among people who may also suffer from severe malnutrition and anemia. Separating out these conditions for the neat and tidy purposes of research does little to convey the mix of forces that shape the conditions for creating illness. To isolate one disease from another is to miss their essential interdependence in their constant pressure on human life.

Listening to doctors debate how they can tackle these diseases, one can be left feeling that the outstanding issues are largely technical. If this were true, the burden of human disease would be straightforward to combat. It is not. What scientists have been less keen to investigate is the messier questions about the social, even behavioral, aspects of disease. These cannot be studied in a sterile laboratory or in a carefully controlled clinical trial. And because they are messy, such questions are frequently ignored.

Take HIV/AIDS. Many detailed studies in Africa, Asia, and Latin America have shown that most people are only too familiar with this disease—more than nine out of ten men and women in most settings.[5] The more cases there are, the more people know about it. And the better educated people are, the more they know too. But despite this high level of awareness, perceptions of risk are surprisingly misguided. In most countries, 80 percent of men believe that they are at little risk of acquiring AIDS. Two thirds of women think the same. And while most men say that they have changed their behavior to avoid AIDS, in many countries less than half of all women have either started using condoms or confined sex to one partner. Condom use is a particular problem. Less than one in ten women in countries where AIDS is taking its greatest toll use condoms.

These findings reveal huge and dangerous gaps in the global response to HIV/AIDS. Most people in Africa—over 80 percent—live in rural areas, where knowledge of AIDS is lowest. And even when knowledge is high, far too few people have changed their behavior to stop the spread of infection. For countries such as Botswana, Zimbabwe, Swaziland, Lesotho, Namibia, South Africa, Zambia, Kenya, Malawi, Djibouti, Mozambique, Burundi, the Central African Republic, Ivory Coast, Ethiopia, and Rwanda—all of which have over 10 percent of their population infected with HIV—no matter how many drugs are delivered, doctors and nurses trained, or hospitals and clinics built, unless people change the way they live, HIV/AIDS will destroy what remains of their national social fabric.

Malaria is a good example of how Western demands for continuous technical progress entirely miss the far greater problem facing developing countries—namely, how to implement the knowledge we already have. Scientists constantly seek better and better evidence, but they are usually far less interested in translating what has already been discovered into practice. And while many scientists avoid such practical concerns, malaria's effects accelerate. About 300 million people are infected annually, out of 2.5 billion people at risk. Deaths from malaria are projected to double over the next twenty years. And the slow warming of our climate is extending that risk still further.

In 2002, Las Vegas was the scene of an announcement that was hailed as a "milestone" for malaria research—a preliminary draft genome of the parasite was at long last reported. The project had taken six years to complete and involved the identification of 30 million base pairs on fourteen chromosomes. One scientist who took part in this sequencing project said that this latest discovery would "accelerate [the] timetable of developing . . . these new therapies and new vaccines."[6]

The advent of genetically modified mosquitoes, an even more imaginative technological feat, was also hailed as a milestone. Mosquitoes expressing genes that block malaria development have been successfully bred in the laboratory.[7] These mosquitoes are less susceptible to malarial infection. Those that are infected carry a smaller amount of parasite, and are far less able to pass malaria on to—well, mice, in this instance. But nowhere is it explained how those new genes could be safely introduced into mosquitoes in the environment where they usually live. And there is no reason to believe that mosquitoes resistant to the effects of this gene will not evolve quickly by natural selection. Is it true, therefore, that the birth of the transgenic mosquito "represents a new era of malaria-related research"?[8] Not quite yet.

What we do need, undisputably, is a vaccine against malaria, or rather vaccines. One type of vaccine is necessary to protect infants and pregnant women. A different vaccine is needed to stop transmission of malaria from mosquitoes to human beings. Finally, travelers to malaria-endemic areas will need their own vaccine. Because of the complexity of malaria's life cycle, these three vaccines will most likely have to target different stages of the parasite's life cycle. There are several encouraging examples of vaccines in development.[9]

Yet this technological vision of modern medicine is desperately short-term. None of these vaccines will be completely effective. And it is here that malaria is likely to get the better of man. In a remarkable series of calculations performed by Sylvain Gandon and his colleagues at the University of Edinburgh, the catastrophic dangers of imperfect vaccines have become all too clear.[10] Gandon and his team applied the rules of evolution to their studies of how malaria would spread and its virulence—its capacity to kill—would change if an imperfect vaccine were introduced. They found that vaccines designed to diminish the growth of malaria led to long-term increases in virulence and more severe infections in those who did not receive the vaccine, such as nonimmune travelers and unvaccinated children. Any short-term benefits were outweighed by these adverse long-term effects, which together would be likely to increase, not decrease, deaths from malaria. The time scale for these damaging consequences is well beyond the usual period studied in vaccine clinical trials. Gandon's team estimated that a mutant malaria parasite twice as virulent as any that exists today would emerge thirty-eight years after the introduction of a vaccine. Nobody presently thinks this far ahead.

How can we sum up the present state of progress in malaria vaccine research? The Drugs for Neglected Diseases group, a part of Médecins Sans Frontières's campaign for Access to Essential Medicines, has concluded:

> Vaccine research over the past three decades has been characterised by lack of funding, a serious underestimation of the complexity of the parasite, faith in technology above scientific understanding, lack of appropriate models, and above all a lack of adequate knowledge about the immune mechanisms underlying protection.[11]

Indeed, although the global malaria crisis seems insurmountable—one billion people in the world carry malaria parasites—the drugs are available right now to treat sick people. Flailing around in the swamps of disillusion means that we delay saving the lives of millions of people in sub-Saharan Africa, Asia, and South America. The reason why we delay is sadly obvious. Drug manufacturers that could provide effective treatments—notably Novartis, who makes the only artemisinin-based combination (Coartem) for treating the now well-established acute multidrug-resistant malaria—for free to the most vulnerable populations at risk do not do so.

In 2002, Coartem was added to WHO's list of essential medicines and the company promised to provide tablets at cost: $2.40 per dose for an adult (four doses are usually needed). But what seems like a generous offer—the cost is $40 per dose in developed countries—has a terrible catch. Most of those at risk of malaria are already living on less than $1 a day; $2.40 is still simply too expensive for those at most risk.

And now, thanks to anthrax, infections are viewed as part of the threat to global security. Globalization has fostered the conditions that will permit acts of biowar to flourish. There is no simple cause-and-effect relation between terror and increasingly obvious economic and social inequality. Yet these inequalities and the anger they foster pose an acute threat to global security. Twenty-four-hour news media, for example, provide an ideal stage for terrorists to act out their grievances. The goal of the terrorist, after all, is to create maximum and pervasive fear. Inadvertently, CNN has become the world's leading terrorist propaganda machine.

A new generation of influential and less democratic global institutions, which beat to the rhythm of US foreign policy (most prominently the World Trade Organization), is replacing older and weaker, but internationally more legitimate, bodies within the UN system. Decades of criticism by governments and activists alike have eroded the authority of the UN, allowing a creeping marginalization to take place with barely any effective protest. At best, the UN functions after the fact, cleaning up after organized state (Indonesian terrorism in East Timor) or nonstate (in the former Yugoslavia) violence has taken its toll.

Infectious disease, regardless of the threat of bioterrorism, adds a further substantial global security threat. Andrew Price-Smith, a respected American analyst of international affairs, has done the most to make the case for treating infection as an issue of defense policy. In his important book *The Health of Nations*,[12] Price-Smith argues that infectious disease will

> simultaneously increase poverty and misery throughout these societies, erode and/or prevent the consolidation of endogenous human capital, and (through the erosion of state capacity)

> increase the probability of social unrest, governance problems, and political violence within states.

This view received strong political endorsement in January 2000, when the UN Security Council met to discuss HIV/AIDS. US Vice President Al Gore then defined HIV/AIDS as a security crisis, as well as a humanitarian crisis. What of solutions to the problem of an escalating risk of infectious disease, whether from conventional means or biowar? There are at least three avenues of direct action.

First, the inequalities between and among peoples, which help to foment social unrest and draw a veil of popular protection around terrorists, must be confronted. The usual approach is to tackle disease. The far more difficult challenge, so far mostly ignored by the developed world, is to deal with the risk factors of disease—those structural issues in society that frame all aspects of human living. When such risk factors were quantified in 2002, the three most important global predicaments were underweight, unsafe sex, and high blood pressure. Not surprisingly, variations in risk factors across the world are huge. In sub-Saharan Africa, malnutrition dwarfed all other risks. This understanding of what causes disease must provide a springboard for new concerted action.

Second, global information flows will help to inform national and, more important, transnational communities of emerging threats. For countries in the developing world, the challenges of sending and receiving information are immense. How to build information capacity as a means to strengthen communities across continents and civilizations should be a priority for those concerned about global public health and security. The solution will be far more complex than simply installing computers and connecting them to the Internet. There may be no sustainable research infrastructure within a country, making its intellectual capital merely a well of talent to be exploited by developed nations.

Finally, the institution that has a global coordinating role in public health efforts to diminish risks of infection is WHO. The main instrument at WHO's disposal is a document called the International Health Regulations. These regulations are binding on all 192 member states of WHO and authorize the agency to "ensure the maximum security against the international spread of diseases with a minimum of interference with world traffic." The diseases that most concern WHO are cholera, plague, and yellow fever. But the widespread view is that these regulations have failed—they are too narrow and do little to build a global coalition to prevent the spread of infection.

New regulations are planned. WHO has promised to send out a first draft of these new regulations in 2003, with a final version planned for late 2003, and approval by the World Health Assembly, its governing body, in May 2004. The world needs better surveillance for emerging infectious diseases, a means to provide rapid alerts to governments, more coordinated exchange of information between countries, and expanded public health capacity within countries. The global politics of disease are now firmly on world leaders' agendas.

But what if nothing is done? There are other ways of protecting ourselves from infection. We can establish immunity among those at risk by means of vaccination—where vaccines exist, that is. A security threat begins to impinge on the freedoms we presently take for granted when governments extend their powers to isolate individuals or communities, thereby restricting the movement of potentially infected individuals. The confinement of newly arrived refugees in hostels or camps is current government policy in the UK—aside from being discriminatory and stigmatizing, it is also a policy born of fear of infection. An even more extreme solution is for a government to eliminate those who pose a threat to noninfected individuals, thereby creating a cordon sanitaire around the healthy population. Elimination could simply mean evacuation or deportation—or it could, through passive neglect, and in not unthinkable circumstances given the history of the past century, mean a new form of genocide.

Whatever approach to the continuing threat of infection is taken, dealing with these diseases in isolation will surely fail. Confronting infection means confronting the conditions that enable infectious diseases to flourish. These conditions can be reduced to one word—poverty. With 1.2 billion people living on less than $1 a day, the burden of poverty is of a scale almost too vast for the human mind to conceive. Disease goes hand in hand with failures in human development. The next two chapters look at these health and development challenges in more detail: in one instance, a region recovering from a post-Communist war and, in another, a country that represents many of the difficulties facing the part of the world most oppressed by poverty and infection—sub-Saharan Africa.

# 4

# SURVIVING CONFLICT

*Zaklela se zemlja raju da se tajne sve saznaju*
(The earth swore to heaven that all its secrets would be revealed)

AS THE FORMER Yugoslavia emerges from yet another war, people's health and the region's health care, scientific research, and medical education have been seriously damaged and disrupted. There are lessons to be learned from the recent Balkan wars, lessons that might help doctors, international relief organizations, and governments do better than they have done elsewhere during the long reconstruction period that will follow this savage conflict. An analysis of the medical legacies of the war may also raise issues for doctors worldwide to consider as part of their responsibilities in a larger public health community. For a week in May 1999, I traveled to Croatia and the Croat-Muslim Federation of Bosnia-Herzegovina to meet doctors working in peace but next to war. In the first part of this essay, I briefly survey some of the medical consequences of the Croatian and Bosnian conflicts. In the second part, I consider plans for and obstacles to reconstruction, and try to identify possible opportunities for prevention of the adverse health effects of war in a newly enlarged Europe.

The dispute in the Balkans had a long and troubled gestation—dating back more than one thousand years—and the twentieth century witnessed its extraordinarily bloody climax. Tensions among the people of Croatia rose in August 1990, with a clash between Serbs and Croats in the southern city of Knin. An appalling nadir was reached a year later in Vukovar on the border between Croatia and Serbia, a dividing line marked by the gentle twists of the Danube. Vukovar was besieged and bombed for three months, falling to Serb forces on November 18, 1991. Almost every house and public building was demolished, including the city's school, and the hospital was badly damaged.

Before the war, the Vukovar hospital was a center for primary and secondary care: 120 doctors had four hundred beds to serve a population of more than 80,000. During the bombing, up to 12,000 shells hit the city daily (eight hundred hit the hospital complex alone), killing thousands and driving away all but 12,000 of Vukovar's people. While the shelling continued, the hospital admitted eighty patients a day, and the staff, a mix of Serbs and Croats, treated the two communities without exception. Damage to the upper floors of the hospital forced doctors to shift care into service corridors underground. The intensive care unit was moved to an antinuclear bomb shelter. One pediatrician, who later visited Serbia and asked why the hospital was bombed, was told, "Because you held wounded Croatian soldiers there."

When the Serb army took over the hospital, the Croatian staff, including the hospital's director, Dr. Vesna Bosanac, were forced to leave for Zagreb. One night during the occupation, a Serb soldier toured the hospital with a surgeon, also Serbian. According to at least two witnesses, the surgeon identified about 260 wounded patients as Croat soldiers. The next day these wounded men were taken away, driven at night to the small town of Ovcara nearby, and shot and buried in a rye field. One man escaped, and he was subsequently able to identify a mass grave that contained two hundred bodies. That place is now a simple and fittingly bleak memorial on the desolate landscape of eastern Slavonia. The hospital's Croatian staff were not able to return until November 1997, and many now live in hastily reconstructed hostels or hotels.

Only in recent years has the full story of medicine during the Croatian war been revealed in personal testimonies and published academic papers. The entire health system became geared to the needs of the conflict. For example, mobile surgical teams were created to support special forces of the Croatian police during battle. These units aimed to train surgeons in generalist skills so that they could save lives and salvage limbs directly on the front lines.[1] The broad range of injuries inflicted during the campaigns has been documented,[2] and the experience of hospitals has also been carefully recorded. At the Osijek University Hospital from May 1991 to November 1992, more than 4,500 war victims were admitted and had surgery.[3] A third were civilians, with a mean age of thirty-three. Postoperative mortality was 3 percent. Seven hundred and eighty corpses were taken directly to the pathology department. A similar pattern was found at the Slavonski Brod General Hospital, which admitted more than seven thousand wounded between September 1991 and December 1992.[4] For medical centers, digital wireless communication systems—a personal computer, a digital signal repeater, and a radio station—were vital for exchanging "information on casualties, forcibly displaced, detained or missing persons, gross breaches of Geneva conventions and war crimes committed by enemy soldiers, on-site epidemiological and toxicological reports, and the changing needs for medical supplies and drugs in endangered and besieged cities and villages."[5] One hundred and ten thousand confidential files were transmitted in this way.

Although the war in Bosnia-Herzegovina started in 1992 and was over by 1995, the structural damage to its major cities is still apparent today. In Sarajevo, the nearby Mount Trebevic provided a base from which Serb forces targeted government buildings, civilian homes, and public institutions (such as the university and newspaper offices). A huge program of reconstruction is now visibly under way, partly assisted by grants from the European Union. But damage remains severe. Mostar was the site of an especially violent conflict, first between Serbs and an alliance of Muslims and Croats and then, for another two years, between Muslims and Croats. The newer of Mostar's two hospitals, exposed at the pinnacle of one of its hills, was hit by shells six times and, as in Vukovar, patients had to be moved underground. Despite the intensity of the fighting between different ethnic groups, all wounded combatants were admitted to the hospital.

Two main factors determined patterns of health care needs during the conflict.[6] First, the physical trauma of war itself. In Bosnia, for instance, more than 150,000 people were killed and 20,000 were physically disabled permanently, including five thousand who had amputations. Few data have been published on these and other casualties. However, forensic reports on 874 bodies taken to Split University Hospital indicated that more than 70 percent died as a result of severe battlefield injuries, most from the effects of shell fragments and gunshot wounds.[7] Numbers of civilian deaths were not small, and women, children, and older people were all deliberate targets of sniper fire (in the Split report, the youngest victim was a five-year-old boy).

The second main factor influencing health care during the war was the risk of communicable disease. In Bosnia, rates of tuberculosis increased by half, and outbreaks of hepatitis A were reported. In view of these dangers, particular attention was given to public health efforts to preserve essential sanitation services. In one setting—Lika-Senj County in the center of Croatia[8]—doctors scoured territory that had been won back from Serb occupation to ensure that water supplies and food depots were clean, animal carcasses safely disposed of, and public buildings (hospitals, schools, shops) free of infestation by disease-carrying animals. Mines, which had been laid around the main water pump in the area, had to be cleared before a secure water supply could be assured.

The mix of populations within Bosnia and Herzegovina and the conflict among them produced a severe refugee crisis. By 1994 about 300,000 Bosnians had left for Croatia. The network of health care available to them was fragile. Although Croatia was able to supply basic services, specialist care could not be given, except in emergencies. For Bosnian patients with cardiovascular disease who traveled to Zagreb, the supply of pacemakers and valve replacements was severely rationed, with serious consequences.[9] In one group of refugees, for example, the overall prevalence of heart disease was twice that of the local Croat population. Rates of hypertension, ischemic heart disease, and cerebrovascular disease were also substantially higher among refugees. The burden of chronic illness in these displaced populations may be high and perhaps overlooked while the immediate concerns of more acute conditions take precedence.[10]

The experience of war can lead to important improvements in trauma care. Descriptions of these advances range from detailed case reports[11] to substantial case series.[12] Although it is difficult to conduct rigorously controlled studies in a war zone, short-term and long-term follow-up investigations provide useful clinical data. Zvonimir Lovric and his colleagues, for example, assessed the results of reconstructions of major limb arteries after war injuries. Debate has continued about the use of grafts in vessel injury management. Although joining vessels end-to-end is the preferred technique of repair, grafts are usually necessary because of the extensive vessel damage associated with battlefield injuries. Some surgeons believe that synthetic grafts are inferior to vein grafts. In their early results, Lovric and his colleagues reported successful placement of both vein grafts and synthetic prostheses in highly contaminated wounds.[13] Longer-term follow-up showed that the forty-month cumulative limb salvage rate for vein grafts and synthetic grafts was 92 percent versus 87 percent, a difference that was not significant. The investigators concluded that "we consider our data a good step forward in changing the opinions of synthetic prosthesis use."[14] Such opportunities to advance learning are one of the perverse advantages of war. They are few.

The drive from Zagreb to Split takes five hours, weaving through broadly cut valleys to Karlovac, skimming the border of the Croat-Muslim Federation of Bosnia-Herzegovina, passing through Knin, and finally circling around mountain roads into the 1,700-year-old former Roman port. The way is marked by clusters of abandoned houses, many burned out, which have been left by Croats and Serbs alike—families driven from their homes during army occupation. Four to five million people live in Croatia; 600,000 of them were "displaced" as refugees, and about the same number eventually entered the country as refugees from Bosnia.

On May 4, 1999, one of Zagreb's largest hospitals opened a National Center for Psychotrauma. Hundreds of thousands of Croatians are living with some form of post-traumatic stress disorder (PTSD). It is difficult to find someone who has not been affected. A common mistake is to think of PTSD as a condition with a consistent set of symptoms. But Croatian psychiatrists have discovered that cases of PTSD among tortured prisoners of war—guilt, psychic numbing, headaches, and lethargy—differ strikingly from those among soldiers with combat-related illness (mainly panic attacks and aggressive behaviors).[15] Definitions of PTSD have mostly come from studies of men. But many of the cases of PTSD in Croatia have been reported in women and children. Here, again, the clinical picture is different—fewer symptoms of panic and aggression and more of avoidance and silence.

Treatment of PTSD usually involves a multidisciplinary team of doctors, psychologists, and special educators, together with a brief stay in a day hospital and a mix of group, work, and relaxation therapies. I watched therapeutic work with ten women who had been raped, bereaved, or displaced. The team of psychiatrists at the Zagreb clinic—Dragica Kozaric-Kovacic, Dubravka Kocijan-Hercigonja, and

Vera Folnegovic-Smalc—believe that it will take two to three generations before the psychological effects of the war pass.

The stories from children are the most wrenching. One boy, displaced at the age of seven in 1991, was moved with his family to a camp in Zagreb when his father, a soldier, went missing in Vukovar. The father, a prisoner of war, was eventually exchanged for a Serb and returned to his family—a hero in their eyes. But he was by now an alcoholic, withdrawn and depressed. The war was transferred to his family. At ten years of age, this young boy took an overdose of whichever pills he could find. He survived, only to say that his family was no longer his family, his father a father no more.

As Vesna Bosanac, the reinstalled director of the Vukovar hospital, told me, "The hardest thing is to face the loss." Psychotrauma is a serious problem for the former inhabitants of this burned-out city—in Osijek too, where outpatient psychiatric attendance has risen from 15,000 per year before the war to 26,000 per year today (PTSD was 5–6 percent of this number before the war; it now accounts for 27 percent of visits). Professor N. Mandic, who runs the psychiatric service in Osijek, argues that he needs another ten psychiatrists to meet clinical demand (he already has a team of fifteen specialists). Unemployment rates as high as 25 percent and a ruined primary care system do not help his work.

Research is difficult to do when the service needs are so great. But in Split, Slavica Jeroncic is studying the organization of medical and psychological care for children and their families. She is trying to find a way to unlock bereavement in settings in which someone remains missing. Her aim is to compare reactions among an experimental group of parents whose sons disappeared in the war and remain missing today with a control group consisting of parents who know the fate of their children through postmortem identification. In another Split–Zagreb collaboration, the emotional responses of displaced individuals have been described and linked with positive or negative clinical outcomes.[16] The traits most likely to ensure future mental health were found to be self-control, self-disclosure, and altruism. Many exposures to war were intense: among 199 children, 85 percent experienced shooting, 67 percent shelling, and 24 percent bombing. And the reactions to these traumatic events were highly age-dependent. How they combined to produce the different patterns of stress disorder remains unexplored.

Analysts of modern war, such as Chris Gray, agree that rape "is hardly a new war strategy but it seems to be increasing."[17] Evidence to support this view was amply available in the Croatian and Bosnian conflicts, during which as many as 25,000 women may have been raped. For example, one report from Zagreb described eighteen women (thirteen Muslim, five Croatian) who were under psychiatric care in 1993 for the consequences of rape.[18] All had PTSD, ten were depressed, four had attempted suicide, and eleven became pregnant. Seven had undergone repeated sexual torture. The practical difficulty for care is to separate the effects of bereavement, violence, and displacement from those of rape.[19] In one study of fifty-five rapes that took place in Bosnia-Herzegovina, most (thirty-two) had occurred while the victims were held in captivity.[20] Others were perpetrated randomly when homes were attacked, broken into, and looted. "Rape camps" have been described in which women were gang-raped by soldiers and subsequently expected to wash clothes and prepare food. Libby Arcel and those who worked for the International Rehabilitation Council for Torture Victims concluded that the main aim of systematic rape is political—namely, to hasten the expulsion of national groups by spreading terror, fear, humiliation, and stigmatization.

Two hundred and forty-eight children were killed during the Croatian war, almost half through injuries caused by explosions.[21] Nine hundred and one were injured, including eighty-six who were permanently disabled. Few of these children received immediate or adequate medical assistance. Well over four thousand children in Croatia lost at least one parent, and fifty-four lost both. By 1994, 72,000 children had become refugees, and 6,725 had been evacuated abroad. The psychological effects this trauma will have in the decades after the war is barely being addressed, although there is, at last, an effort to document the different ways in which children have been harmed.[22]

Some of the traumas experienced by children are almost inconceivable. I heard of one girl who was six years old and living in Vukovar in 1991. Her father had been killed, and she and her mother were in a prisoner-of-war camp along with her seventeen-year-old sister and her one-month-old brother. In this camp, Serb soldiers raped her sister daily, leaving the six-year-old to watch while holding her brother in her arms. The troops continually threatened her and eventually she was raped too. It took another five years for the effects of that incident to surface. At school, she became detached and absent. Only after several further months of drawing and playing with psychologists was she able to tell her full story.

Older people were often a forgotten group during this war. Yet they were badly affected and frequently less able to cope with their experiences than their younger counterparts. Older people had the homes they had worked for all their lives destroyed, their families torn apart, and their routines disrupted. These events often took place on a background of undiagnosed or worsening chronic disease.[23] There were isolated examples in which older people were in especially vulnerable settings. One such instance occurred in four UN Protected Areas within Croatia during 1995. These regions were occupied by Serb forces and were later won back by the Croatian army. After reoccupation it was clear that elderly people made up a large proportion of the remaining population. More than 75 percent of ten thousand people in 524 villages were over sixty. Their ethnic mix was diverse: Serbs (70 percent), Croats (27 percent), and Muslims (1 percent). Half were living without electricity, a third had no income, and 6 percent needed emergency care. A team of doctors conducted a "humanitarian census," interviewing every one of the ten thousand abandoned people, and provided immediate medical and social care, irrespective of ethnic status. Slobodan Lang and his colleagues agreed that "this operation was based on a premise that the present warfare was targeted against the civilian population, which resulted in a total social collapse requiring a planned and coordinated effort to regain control."[24] The elderly continue to be one of the most understudied groups affected by war.

On November 21, 1995, after signing the Dayton Accord with representatives of Serbia and Croatia, the Muslim leader Alija Izetbegovic said, "And to my people I say, this may not be a just peace, but it is more just than a continuation of war." The search for a way to end a war comes inevitably, no matter how bold the initial calls to arms and despite every convincing justification for fighting. The attrition of fatigue and death eventually silences even the most ardent of warring voices. When one surveys the legacy of the Croatian and Bosnian wars across their populations, among their most vulnerable peoples, and in the health care teams that were deployed to look after them, the patriotic enthusiasm for battle can seem hollow. Croatians would disagree. They won the right to a long-sought-after self-determination. Those living in Bosnia-Herzegovina may take a different view from their Croatian neighbors as the cantonized Federation struggles haphazardly on.

Modern wars, some politicians say, are fought on grounds of humanitarian need, liberal philosophy, and progressive politics. Some writers, such as C. H. Gray, go so far as to claim that the conduct of war also differs today from in the past, and point to new, more precise technologies of warfare, changes in the role of the media, and the increase in conflicts between different cultures rather than competing nations. These interpretations are revealing, but they obscure the truth of war's brutal legacy. The subject of land mines easily erases fashionable and convenient rationalizations. In Croatia, there are at least two million live mines yet to be found, preventing the safe return of thousands of refugees. In one study of fifty-seven land mine victims, the mean age of those injured was twenty-eight. The injuries were carefully recorded: foot or lower-leg amputation (19); splenectomy (2); hip fractures (4); internal organ damage (16); abdominal, pelvic, and thoracic damage (33); nerve lesions (9); and head and face wounds (11).[25] The lowlands of eastern Slavonia, where those mines were laid, saw a violent front line between Serbs and Croats. Here, there was no debate about the meaning of a "just war." The aim was simply to kill, disable, or maim.

Emile Zola's novel *The Debacle* describes the hopeless course of the 1870 Franco-Prussian War and begins with one of its main characters, Maurice, a well-educated intellectual, asking whether "the very condition of nature [is not] a continuous struggle, the survival of the fittest, strength maintained and renewed through action, life rising ever young out of death." Maurice recalled the "great fever of excitement" in Paris at the start of the war. Even today we still see war as a matter of victory or defeat, and we are often encouraged to do so by those who lead us into it. But a view across the health of a country that has recently been through—and claims to have won—a war reveals a different, more entangled story.

* * *

> Europeans are coming to resemble one another more and more . . . an essentially supernational and nomadic type of man is slowly emerging, one that is distinguished, physiologically speaking, by having a maximum of adaptive skills and powers.
>
> —Friedrich Nietzsche, *Beyond Good and Evil*

In the thick of the Bosnian war, Ivan Bagaric, a doctor, a former member of the Bosnian parliament, and in 1993 chief commander of the health section of the Croatian Defense Force of Bosnia-Herzegovina, wrote a memorandum to the Spanish battalion of the United Nations Protection Force (UNPROFOR). It read:

> Republic of Bosnia-Herzegovina
> Croatian Community of Hercog-Bosnia
> HVO [Croatian Council of Defense]
> Department of Defense
> Health division
> No: 02-5/1-570/93
> Mostar. 16.09.1993
>
> Request
> Hereby we are kindly asking you to be the interface in our offer to the Muslim side for the accommodation and medical treatment of civilians—especially women and children—in the war hospital of Mostar as well as the other HVO hospitals. To the ill and wounded persons of Muslim nationality we guarantee the same treatment and healing as for our civilians and wounded persons. We propose that our work is controlled by the International Committee of the Red Cross, European Community, and UN observers. We are doing this for only one reason, which is a humanitarian reason, so we kindly ask you not to read anything political into this request.
> With respects,
> Assistant to the Chief of Defense,
> Department of Medicine and Health Care,
> Dr. Ivan Bagaric[26]

UNPROFOR did not reply.

Bagaric's difficulty was that Bosnia had only three large hospitals —in Sarajevo, Tuzla, and Banja Luka. The first two were in Muslim-held territory and the third was under Serb control. The one remaining medium-sized hospital for Croatians was in Mostar. From almost nothing, therefore, Bagaric and his team had to create a new health system for Bosnian Croats. They established a network of thirteen military hospitals in whatever space they could lay their hands on. They converted a Franciscan church in Nova Bila, a Catholic chapel in Orasje, a school in Zepca, a tobacco factory in Grude, a hotel in Neum, and a computer company in Rama. Bagaric recruited staff from Croatia, Italy, the UK, and international relief organizations. He employed two Serb surgeons in Mostar. Forty thousand wounded people went through these makeshift hospitals—Croats mostly, but also Muslims and Serbs.

Bagaric had good reason not to seek reconciliation on the battlefield. On April 12, 1992, his brother—married and the father of two children—was killed during an attack by Serb tanks on the town of Suica. Bagaric blames the war, not the Serbs, for his brother's death. His work propelled him, at the age of thirty-seven, into the role of special adviser to Bozo Ljubic, the Croat-Muslim Federation's minister of health.

Minister Ljubic is a slight figure and, on the day I met him, he was in an oppressively somber mood. A former professor of orthopedic surgery in Sarajevo and once director of Mostar's largest hospital, his task then was to steer health care in the Federation through the administrative checks and balances of the Dayton Accord. Ljubic was open about the Federation's prospects. He admitted that Dayton "is not a stable political settlement" and that the country's policies are "very often imposed by international factors." He believed that the new Croat-Muslim Federation did not work. "Is it ungovernable?" I asked. "Yes," he replied, "a lot of laws are unimplementable."

The most important tasks Ljubic identified were health financing and rebuilding the country's broken health care system. His main difficulty was with regard to the division of the Federation into semi-autonomous cantons, each of which has its own parliament and minister of health.[27] Coordination across the region is almost impossible. Doctors and the hospitals at which they work are not divided equally between regions (rural areas have especially poor services). The future is uncertain because the Dayton Accord handed over responsibility for the Federation's economy to the World Bank. In return for monetary loans, the Bank is demanding cuts in subsidies for welfare and health. If the Federation's government refuses to comply, the Bank is authorized to stop credit and end aid. That's blackmail, I suggested. "Yes," Ljubic replied. He believes that in the short to medium term, his country's standards of medical care and the health of its 2.5 million people will inevitably worsen.

Ljubic sees the Federation's prospects as being utterly dependent on the rest of Europe. Bosnia's richer neighbors could help, he argued, by providing health supplies and greater assistance with hospital-building programs. But Europe seems resistant to doing more. At the end of our conversation I asked him what he thought the solution was. "I don't know," he replied. "To escape the country!" He smiled, but thinly. The minister's twenty-three-year-old daughter recently completed a philosophy degree in Zagreb. He encouraged her to seek a job there rather than return to the Federation.

Ljubic's analysis is supported by the experiences of many medical practitioners. Ante Ivankovic and Zoran Rebac, in their study of dental care services for the Federation, conclude that

> available regular funds for health care are not sufficient to bring us to international standards.... Without foreign financial support the improvements will be slower than needs [demand].... However, there is less and less help since we are expected to

> develop as economic subjects and be potential [contributors].... The process of health care restructuring will thus directly depend on solving the political crisis in the country.[28]

Mostar, seen by some observers "as a barometer for a return to normalcy in other areas of Bosnia and Herzegovina," is an example of this political paralysis. Three competing interests—Bosnian Muslims, Croats, and the European Union—have often engaged in "hostile obstructionism," blocking health reforms aimed at securing an overall health plan for the region's people.[29]

Despite these difficulties, Ljubic has set three priorities for Federation health policy.[30] First, he wants to control communicable diseases through mass vaccination programs. By 1997, vaccination coverage had increased to prewar levels (it fell by at least 50 percent during the war).[31] Second, Ljubic is focusing on maternal and child health, notably through education. And third, he is seeking renewal of certain health sectors, especially rehabilitation of war victims, both psychological and physical; essential hospital services (eight more cantonal hospitals); and basic community health services—that is, primary care and public health. For Ljubic, "strengthening of primary health care represents the cornerstone of health reform." A fourth priority, not listed by Ljubic but carefully calculated by Bagaric and others, will be to train adequate numbers of physicians.[32] During the war, nearly half of all health workers left the country. By 1997, the number of doctors in the Federation (adjusted for total population) was less than half that in Croatia.

Croatia faces many of the same health issues as the Federation but under more favorable circumstances, since the country is politically stable and was less assaulted by war. The relative sparing of the Croatian health system has meant that, according to public health planners, "the highest priority and needs are now related to coping with unhealthy behaviour of the population, such as smoking, accidents, physical inactivity, and nutritional problems...."[33]

Vukovar is the one exception. When Vesna Bosanac returned to the Vukovar hospital in 1997, there were no surgical instruments, no operating room facilities, no X-ray equipment, and no provisions for dialysis (thirty-eight patients were traveling three times a week to Serbia). She faced an epidemic of tuberculosis and a backlog of patients with suspected (and subsequently confirmed) cancer. Maternal mortality had risen to 12 per 1,000 (elsewhere in Croatia the number was 0.1–0.5 per 1,000) and infant mortality rates were 23 per 1,000 live-births (12 per 1,000 in other regions and 5.7 per 1,000 in England and Wales). Those who remained in the city and those displaced who were now returning also had high rates of PTSD. A practical difficulty was that staff who were returning, mostly Croats, found themselves working alongside Serb colleagues who had stayed ("It's different from before the war; there is nothing personal going on," one pediatrician told me).

Bosanac found neglect everywhere. On one ward she discovered three patients in their beds and seven nurses sitting drinking coffee, indifferent to their needs. One man with a fractured hip was starved, dirty, and unshaven. She called her entire staff together and told them that "from this day on, nobody should die in this hospital." Bosanac invited her colleagues "to leave their problems at home and act strictly professionally." Nobody was asking Croat and Serb staff to be friends, but they had no alternative but to work together. She embarked on an ambitious program of retraining Vukovar doctors and nurses in Osijek; she insisted on detailed and accurate medical record keeping; and she refused to pay salaries unless these rules were followed. Within three months, her plan was starting to work. Staff now followed hospital codes of practice, and they had begun to rediscover a sense of professional pride. The hospital is still recovering—newly arrived boxes of X-ray equipment were waiting to be unpacked on the day I was there—although beds are often empty, reflecting the emptiness of the city itself.

Zagreb, by contrast, is a bustling, cosmopolitan Central European capital with twenty-five hospitals serving one to two million people. Construction began on a large university hospital on the south side of the city in 1985, but the project was put on hold during the war. Although hospital services today are stretched, existing facilities are reasonably good, and they are in great demand. Calls have been made to restart construction on the university hospital, its existence being seen as "indispensable for both the city of Zagreb and the Republic of Croatia."[34] But money is short—Croatia lost over $1.5 billion in tourist revenue annually because of the war in Kosovo.

Over the entire country, causes of death and hospital morbidity are little different from those in other Western European nations. One major strain was the influx of one million refugees from Bosnia and its surrounding areas during the 1991–1992 war. By 1997, there were still 300,000 refugees living in Croatia. Vaccination coverage must be improved, and psychosocial care for patients with PTSD is an important priority. The key requirement for long-term gains in health care is a stable income. In a region that endures the politics of unpredictability, that goal is likely to remain elusive for some time to come.

This interpretation of future health needs is vigorously contested. Derek Summerfield, for instance, has tried to expose the weaknesses of arguments that claim "war as a sort of mental health emergency." He believes that PTSD is "the flagship of this medicalised trauma discourse"; it "has become important for many in civil society who are competing for victim status." Summerfield criticizes psychological trauma programs because they depend on Western models of illness and often fail to take account of the unique local conditions under which "stress" takes place. Diagnoses of PTSD, for example, are made from what he calls "a naive application of unvalidated checklists." Even the subject of rape, "given a voyeuristic slant by the international media," is open to misrepresentation. Summerfield concludes:

> There is little in the medical literature to justify the conviction that rape per se is a discrete cause of psychological vulnerability in conditions of war, and that there is a therapy specific and effective enough to justify actively seeking out women who would not normally come forward.

Summerfield rejects the individual medical approach to the consequences of war and prefers instead sociological and political approaches. His view leads to a radically different strategy for post-war restoration: "Perhaps the primary task of interventions is to identify patterns of social strength and weakness, and reinforce local capacities."[35]

This focus on the social history of war and the social world of those affected is an important and valuable counterweight to the bulk of existing opinion that emphasizes personal psychological trauma. But that is all it is—a counterweight, not a disproof. For individual lives were harmed during the Croatian and Bosnian wars, and some of these individuals are more vulnerable to psychological sequelae than others. Lack of data to support the efficacy of trauma programs is a fair criticism but doctors who face a vast demand for limited health services and have little research experience are only now beginning to collate their findings into a coherent and publishable form. And just as Summerfield asks for proof that diagnostic criteria are valid and that counseling services are effective, so he must demonstrate that a social model is a more powerful explanatory and therapeutic approach than one based on the individual. The truth almost certainly includes both perspectives.

Croatia has four medical schools, in Zagreb (240 students admitted annually), Rijeka (120), Split (50), and Osijek (50). These schools were largely spared serious wartime damage. At Osijek, a new faculty of medicine was opened in March 1999, with modern facilities for teaching anatomy, physiology, and pathology. Computer-based learning is standard. An on-line Croatian academic network has been established among the four teaching centers. And a medical video conference was recently held—a first for Croatia.

The conditions in the Croat-Muslim Federation of Bosnia-Herzegovina could not be more different. Again, there are four medical schools, in Sarajevo (240 students admitted per year), Tuzla (200), Banja Luka (100), and Mostar (50). During the 1992–1995 war, medical school attendance fell by at least 50 percent, and there is now an acute shortage of physicians. In early 1997, I. Sarac and his colleagues proposed that the creation of a new medical school was central to the long-term interests of health care in the Federation. They proposed Mostar as the ideal location. In the autumn of 1997, the first fifty students were admitted to the Mostar medical school. They were taught in a newly built, one-story building next to the hospital. A second building was constructed for the 1998 class. The medical school is so far a success, but only because of the enormous efforts of scientists and doctors in Zagreb and Split, who visit Mostar to teach and offer mentorship. Nearby European countries have provided additional assistance—for example, Germany has given microscopes for histology classes. Still, one has the feeling that Europe could do more.

In view of the tremendous pressures on health care delivery, one might imagine that research is a low priority in Croatia and Bosnia. Not so, although there are predictable difficulties. For example, a new basic sciences research building on the Zagreb University campus was completed in December 1998. Currently, only four research groups occupy its thirty-four laboratories. Nevertheless, since 1980, Matko Marusic, an immunologist and co-editor of the *Croatian Medical Journal*, has sent seventy students to complete postdoctoral training in the US and Germany[36]—he calls it the "strategy of scientific leap," designed "to help my best students develop into scientists who would enable Croatian science to make the 'leap' from the mediocre to a respectable level." Thirty-four trainees did not return to Croatia, many preferring to stay in the US, and Marusic judged that he had eleven "failures." But fourteen of his students were "successes," and several of these are now leading research departments in Croatian medical schools. For example, Zeljko Dujic is a professor of physiology in Split. He has developed a small but effective research department,[37] which also has a substantial teaching commitment. And Dragan Primorac is laboratory head in the Department of Pathology and Forensic Genetics at the Clinical Hospital in Split. His work concerns DNA typing to identify the remains of war victims.[38]

During the rebirth of Croatian medicine after 1992, one journal became synonymous with a new national medical consciousness—the English-language *Croatian Medical Journal*.[39] Although born out of war, it now acts as a forum for collaboration. In 1999, the journal published its first paper from Serb scientists.[40] Croatian journals—there are over forty in print—have a long heritage. *Lijecnicki vjesnik*, for instance, was founded in 1877, and played a part in creating the first medical school in Croatia in 1917. Croatian-language journals have an important role in the continuing education of doctors.[41] Bosnia, too, has its own national periodicals—for example, *Medicinski Arhiv*—although these are more precariously supported and appear only erratically. Partnerships with more financially secure Western journals might be a way to assist scientific communication in Bosnia.

At Ovcara, there are two dedication stones on the square of land that commemorates the lives of two hundred wounded soldiers and civilians who were taken from the Vukovar hospital and murdered. One is an official memorial that sits toward the center of the ground. The other is smaller and lies at the edge of the square, with flowers arranged beside it in the form of a Croatian flag. The second stone reads:

> In the midst of the International Committee of the Red Cross's attention and in the presence of the European Community Observer Mission, in this place on November 20, 1991, the Yugoslav Federal Army and its helpers perfidiously killed 200 patients, medical staff, and civilians from the Vukovar hospital. With faith that the righteous never die, this memorial stone is erected by the Association of Croatian Homeland War Volunteers and the APEL center.

Concern about the passivity of international organizations during the Balkan wars has come from many quarters. Slobodan Lang, a professor of public health and a former adviser on humanitarian issues to the president of Croatia, is one of their most persistent critics. In a series of papers published during the 1990s, he produced a devastating analysis of the mercurial attitudes and atrocious weaknesses of existing agencies.[42] Lang points out the absence of the International Red Cross at crucial moments of the conflict—in Kosovo (1988), in Croatia (1990 through 1993), and in Bosnia (1992). Of Vukovar, Lang writes:

> The inefficiency of the International Red Cross and other humanitarian organisations in the protection of hospitals, medical staff, patients, wounded, civilians, and prisoners-of-war resulted in killing of Vukovar patients, civilians, and prisoners-of-war in the marshes of Slavonia and Baranya and torture in Serbian prisons.

Lang's conclusion is that doctors have a duty to assemble knowledge from these experiences. We must learn these lessons because, as he notes in one of his favorite phrases, "morality without knowledge is inquisition." An international "hate watch" should be initiated since it is inciting people to hate that creates the conditions for war.

We should identify access to a home as a fundamental human right. And hospitals ought to be regarded as centers of peace, caring for all sides in a conflict, and protected by the UN in the way envisioned by Ivan Bagaric.

Humanitarian intervention is easy to demand, but less easy to achieve. Kofi Annan, secretary-general of the UN, argues that a coherent strategy for deciding when and how to intervene is now urgently required since civilians are, more than ever before, targets in war. An effective UN Security Council is essential because "only the Council has the authority to decide that the internal situation in any state is so grave as to justify forceful intervention." To achieve that effectiveness, representation in the Security Council should be extended, decision-making must be streamlined, and the creation of a UN rapid reaction force could help stem emerging conflicts. Annan also argues that past UN resolutions allow, even encourage, intervention—despite there being no specific Security Council mandate—to support "the overriding right of people in desperate situations to receive help, and the right of international bodies to provide it." Responsibility, therefore, is shared beyond the UN and "All of us should recall how we responded, and ask: what did I do?"

Annan pointed to Kosovo as a key test for the UN's future. "All our professions of regret," he said in June 1998, "all our expressions of determination to never permit another Bosnia, all our hopes for a peaceful future for the Balkans will be cruelly mocked if we allow Kosovo to become another killing field."[43] Some critics have claimed that "the [recent] NATO bombing of Yugoslavia also signals the end of any serious role for the UN and Security Council; it is NATO, under US guidance, that effectively pulls the strings."[44] The political commentator Noam Chomsky has written that "there is no serious doubt that the NATO bombings [in Serbia and Kosovo] further undermine what remains of the fragile structure of international law."[45]

Many observers already had misgivings about the UN's effectiveness.

In 1995, Lang noted that the "UN did not make a single report on the functioning of the medical institutions during the conflict [in Croatia] or on the health conditions of the people in the occupied areas." The UN failed, WHO has been and remains largely invisible during these wars (a strange irony given that Andrija Stampar, a Croatian, was one of WHO's founders and its first president), and there is confusion about which international agency should do what.[46] By default, humanitarian leadership is left to national party politicians, whose principal responsibility is their own national interest. Worse still, existing humanitarian institutions have often been poorly supported by some of the very countries that have been engaged in war with Serbia—for example, the US, "the world's leading deadbeat in its debt to international organizations," according to Myron E. Wegman.[47] Many of these same criticisms about lack of will to intervene on humanitarian grounds have been aimed at governments that, despite warnings, failed to make adequate preparations for refugee relief in Kosovo and neighboring nations before beginning an air war on March 24, 1999. Nongovernmental organizations worked hard to catch up, but they still lacked adequate food, water, and shelter for 1.4 million people.

What can doctors do to prevent future conflict in the Balkans and elsewhere? The six former Yugoslav republics—Slovenia, Croatia, Bosnia and Herzegovina, Serbia, Montenegro, and Macedonia—together with the two previously autonomous regions of Kosovo and Vojvodina make up part of the southeastern border of Europe. These territories share common intellectual cultures with their European neighbors. Their future integrity and safety depend not only on the protection or realization of their independence but also on the understanding that security will only come through an interdependence with the rest of Europe. As Kosovo fades from international news agendas, the financial generosity of European nations must increase to fill the inevitable void in our attention.

Health care and medical research are powerful catalysts for promoting collaborations to foster such interdependence. The work of individuals such as Ivan Bagaric, Vesna Bosanac, and Slobodan Lang shows that medicine can encourage tolerance, cooperation, and peace among peoples at war. Those who work in the arena of health can even assist democratic reform by creating an infrastructure of care, thereby weaving the social fabric necessary for political stability.

In Croatia and Bosnia after their wars, doctors have taken up important positions of civil leadership. Apart from Ljubic, Bagaric, and Lang, for example, Ivica Kostovic, a neuroscientist and former dean of the Zagreb University School of Medicine, became head of the Croatian president's office. Why have doctors assumed these roles so successfully? Kostovic told me that he had a unique political independence because of his academic medical background, which gave him credibility in an often incredible political process.[48] Certainly, such independence seemed to explain why Ljubic could feel so free to criticize existing political arrangements in Bosnia. This special position for doctors also makes them vulnerable; reports of Albanian physicians being killed as a strategic objective of Serb forces in Kosovo were an unwelcome reminder of that vulnerability.[49]

The war in the Balkans is over—for now at least, although land mine injuries continue to cause death and disability to adults and children alike. Many Western leaders have proclaimed a military triumph despite a desperate humanitarian catastrophe. British prime minister Tony Blair emphasized "that we did have the resolve to see it through." But this brief survey of the physical, psychological, and social imprints of war on children, women, the elderly, and those who took a more active part in the conflict shows, I hope, that "to see it through" means making a commitment to more than simply short-term military success, Serb troop withdrawal from Kosovo, the introduction of a peace implementation force, or the return of refugees to their homes. The problems facing Kosovars and Serbs will affect several generations to come. And these difficulties—medical and political—may be even more intense than they have been in Bosnia since Kosovo lacks the civil institutions of government to implement a regional policy of reconstruction. The same potential for Bosnian-style paralysis also exists, this time between the competing interests of Serbs, Albanians, the European Union, the United Nations, and Russia. And how will Western countries show ordinary Serbs and Kosovars that they are welcome partners in a peaceful and prosperous Europe, irrespective of their political leadership?

Over a century ago, Nietzsche saw Europe moving naturally toward unification, a result that has been slower—world wars being unforeseen in 1886—to emerge than he predicted. However, the potential for conflict in Europe was perhaps anticipated by Nietzsche. He argued that the process of nurturing the "evolving European" may produce an environment for "men of the most dangerous and attractive qualities" to exploit. He wrote that "the democratization of Europe is at the same time an involuntary contrivance for the breeding of tyrants." And tyrants we have certainly seen. But it need not be so, and doctors have an important part to play in laying those first preventive foundation stones.[50]

# 5

# THE AFRICAN CHALLENGE

IN WARD D3 of Komfo Anokye Teaching Hospital in Kumasi, Ghana, Professor T. C. Ankrah, professor of medicine and recently elected Fellow of the Royal College of Physicians of London, leads his team to a sixteen-year-old male patient who has massive swelling on the left side of his face. The boy can barely speak. He whispers that the swelling has been present for only three weeks. He lives in a village thirty-six miles from the city and has been out of school for four months. On examination there is a disfiguring mass on his left upper jaw, together with several clearly visible abdominal masses. A fine needle aspiration of one of these superficial abdominal swellings had revealed a mixture of large and small lymphocytes.

The treatment of Burkitt's lymphoma, from which he suffers, should be straightforward. The drug cyclophosphamide commonly causes rapid tumor dissolution. Professor Ankrah has started a steroid, dexamethasone, to reduce the surrounding swelling. There is a difficulty, however. The hospital pharmacy has no cyclophosphamide. Instead, the parents of this boy will have to find and pay for the drug at one of several hundred private pharmacies in the city. Standard treatment for Burkitt's lymphoma is 1,000 milligrams of cyclophosphamide per square meter of his body every two to three weeks, and then continued beyond complete remission for another two courses.

That would work out at roughly 1,500 milligrams per course for this young man; at least five courses will be needed.

We go to meet the hospital's chief pharmacist to find out whether cyclophosphamide is expected to arrive anytime soon. If the drug were in stock, it would cost 24,000 cedi per gram (5,000 cedi is about seventy-five cents). The pharmacist tells us that none is expected. He is reluctant to stock cyclophosphamide because demand for it is irregular. Komfo Anokye's accountant stands at his side. I am told that as many as two in five patients abscond from the hospital without paying. Clinicians and pharmacists have been urged to collect their fees before offering care or giving treatment. A new patient must give 100,000 cedi to the hospital on admission. Each dressing, syringe, needle, and set of disposable gloves is recorded by a nurse on the patient's chart. Accommodation, sanitation, food, and diagnostic investigations all have to be paid for. This is the pernicious world of user fees—or "cash and carry," as Ghanaians call the system.

Professor Ankrah next leads us out of the hospital to two private pharmacies nearby. One does not have cyclophosphamide. The other does—1 gram of the drug costs 35,000 cedi, which would cost the parents of the sick boy a minimum of over 250,000 cedi. For a village farming family that grows crops and tends livestock for a subsistence living, and which has already spent 100,000 cedi for the privilege of occupying a bed at Komfo Anokye, this further sum may well be far out of their reach. Will the boy get the treatment he needs? The medical team agrees that his prospects are not good.

A cursory review of Ghana's history shows a path leading to hard-won success. Formerly called the Gold Coast when it was under British rule, Ghana became independent on March 6, 1957. Kwame Nkrumah led this independence movement to victory and today is seen as a Pan-Africanist hero. He was voted the greatest African of the second millennium in 1999 by African listeners to the BBC, ahead of Nelson Mandela. In December 2000, for the first time in Ghana's history, an opposition party won office through democratic elections rather than armed force. Analyses of Ghana's development by international institutions seem to bear out this history of liberal progress. The *Human Development Report 2002*[1] ranks Ghana in its medium development category—129 out of 162 countries, above Kenya, Congo, Nigeria, Sudan, Uganda, and Ethiopia. This position has been calculated by combining measures of life expectancy at birth, adult literacy rate, school enrollment, and GDP per capita. Ghana is held up as a model of World Bank policy.

But the legacy of Ghana's history is more ambiguous than raw dates and numbers suggest. The Portuguese staked their interest in the region in 1472, followed by Dutch, Danish, French, and British naval adventurers. An enormous traffic in gold and slaves ensued, producing a prosperous colony. Exploitation had no respect for traditional cultural boundaries. According to the historian Thomas Pakenham, the Gold Coast was "a colony knocked together, like most of the colonies of the Scramble [for Africa], from an incongruous ragbag of territories."[2]

In the twentieth century, the success of Nkrumah as politician and revolutionary led to a hideously repressive counterreaction. Ghana steadily collapsed after he came to power. Debts grew, Soviet-style purges were common, detention without trial was introduced, and corruption was endemic. Ghana became a centralized one-party state. In 1966, while Nkrumah was abroad, a coup ended his increasingly paranoid rule. He died in Romania in 1972. Nkrumah's biographer, Peter Omari, argued that this African dictator was an "evil genius" who "sacrificed Ghana on the altar of Pan-Africanism."[3]

Six governments followed between 1966 and 1981, reflecting a painful cycle of military interventions and thwarted democratic elections. Stability of a sort finally came when Flight Lieutenant Jerry Rawlings ushered in an era of socialism marked by violence. But an economic crisis in 1983 forced Rawlings to embrace structural adjustment. Although Ghana's economy grew, the poor became even poorer under the influence of World Bank strictures. Rawlings found that the only way to retain power was by submitting himself to a popular vote. Rawlings the dictator became Rawlings the democrat. He won presidential elections in 1992 and 1996. In 2000, John Kufuor beat Rawlings's anointed successor in new elections. Seven people died in political killings during the election campaign. Rawlings has since questioned the army's confidence in Kufuor.

Pakenham's view of Ghana as a "ragbag of territories" is unkind. But it is true that it encompasses the Akan people (including the Ashanti, based around Kumasi), the Mole-Dagbani in the north, the Ewe in the east, and the Ga in Accra. The country divides naturally into a southern coastal plain around Accra, a central (much denuded) rain forest region, and a northern "wilderness" (Pakenham again) of savannah grassland. The long fingerlike extensions of Lake Volta, thickened by the Akosombo Dam, reach across the country, making it the world's largest artificial lake.

These divisions have tended to concentrate wealth and attention on Accra and Kumasi. The north has been persistently neglected. Yet the Northern Region is 70,000 square kilometers—by far the largest of the ten regions that make up Ghana, comprising almost a third of the country's land surface—and its population is 1.9 million. By contrast, the Ashanti region around Kumasi is only 24,000 square kilometers, supporting a population of three million. The capital of the Northern Region is Tamale. Most people live in rural settlements averaging about five hundred in number, and these are more thinly dispersed the farther one moves from Tamale.

The most striking feature about Ghana's public health system is the vast inequality between its north and south. According to 1993 figures, 59 percent of water in the Northern Region is drawn from unsafe open surface collections, compared with only 10 percent in greater Accra. There are toilet facilities for 10 percent of the northern population compared with 76 percent for those living in the Accra region. The infant mortality rate in 1998 for the Northern Region was seventy per one thousand live births; in Accra, the figure was forty-one. In the entire Northern Region there are seventeen Ghanaian doctors in practice (greater Accra serves a population of four million people and has around five hundred doctors). There is a regional hospital in Tamale, but five northern districts are without local hospital services. Yet the need is huge. In mid-1999, a government scheme started exempting certain groups—children, the elderly, pregnant and postnatal women, and victims of snake and dog bites—from paying for district-level health facilities. Outpatient attendance for children under five years old more than doubled (from 51,000 in the first six months to 136,000 in the second half of the year). For those over age sixty, figures for the same periods were 9,000 and 17,500. This is further evidence that the imposition of user fees severely inhibited families from seeking hospital care. Where there are no hospitals, or where the distances to travel are too great, villagers simply have nowhere to go.

If you drive ten kilometers north of Tamale to the town of Savelugu, turn off the main road and into the bush, then follow a track through dry grassland for several more kilometers, you reach the village of Tibale, which contains about twenty-five mud-and-thatch houses—small compounds of four or five separate buildings for living and working—with a population of about 640 people. The village has nine hand-dug wells and two primary schools. There is no electricity and there are no toilets. The main religion is Islam. A clinic is one kilometer away by foot, and the nearest district health center is in Savelugu. There are neither doctors nor nurses readily available.

Dr. Sylvester Anemana, the regional director of health, recognizes the difficulties of delivering health care in such a setting. But he also has ingenious solutions—the villagers themselves and motorcycles. Since 1989, district health centers have begun to implement outreach programs. The initiative only started to pay dividends when about two hundred motorcycles were donated to the area in 1996. Now a nurse and a medical assistant can visit each village once a month via the rough bush paths. Motorcycle outreach has helped vaccination coverage to rise from 40 percent to 75 percent. But the greatest difference to village health has been made by Tibale's own people. Instead of waiting on a perpetual promise of new resources, Dr. Anemana's team identified village volunteers who could do the work of trained health staff. Volunteers live in the village and are respected within their communities. At first, villagers were allowed to nominate a person to represent them. All the early nominees were men, an outcome that was not well received by international aid donors, who may well be out of touch with local cultural attitudes. But instead of insisting on equal proportions of men and women, Dr. Anemana decided to appoint two community surveillance workers, a man and a woman, for each village.

In Tibale, I met Sumani Issifu, a village health worker since 1989. He could neither read nor write, yet his first task was to record figures for births and deaths in his village. He did this by using a picture-based community register for vital events. The monthly register has drawings depicting meningitis, polio, guinea worm infection, measles, and neonatal tetanus. Sumani Issifu shades in open circles for each case he sees. He uses a similar system to document male and female births and deaths in infancy, pregnancy, or at other times. For example, in 2001, he had recorded sixteen births in Tibale, two infant deaths, and twelve further deaths from, variously, "old age," "chest pain," anemia, and snake bites. The register provides a means to measure the success of prevention programs. When filters were introduced to protect water supplies from guinea worm infection, the number of cases fell from thirty-nine during the peak incidence months of January and

February 1999 to three cases in 2000 and zero cases in 2001. The volunteers act not only to monitor outbreaks of infection but also to educate villagers about disease prevention. Posters reminding villagers of the risks of HIV/AIDS were pinned on walls of homes.

I asked Sumani Issifu what changes he had seen in the village since he had become a volunteer in 1989. He said that guinea worm eradication had reduced the time lost through illness for farming the land and that villagers were now more willing to go to the hospital. The major challenge for the village remained access to water. When the hand-dug wells dried up, women in the village had to walk four kilometers to the nearest supply.

The volunteers' work is complemented by trained traditional birth attendants. Half of all births in Ghana are assisted by untrained birth attendants. But a fifth of these attendants are now skilled in aseptic technique and safe obstetric practice. I met Madame Damata, one of Tibale's trained attendants, along with many of the children she has delivered. She looks after prenatal care as well as the delivery itself. In a white wooden box, battered from much use, she carries soap, spirits, a plastic sheet to cover the ground, a cloth, cotton wool, and ligatures. Madame Damata has seen only one birth-related death in Tibale since 1999.

Nanton-Kurugu is a larger village of almost two thousand people lying deeper in the Savelugu bush than Tibale. Susana Kumah, the community nurse, visits monthly to supervise a child health clinic. In addition to diphtheria, pertussis, tetanus, polio, BCG, and measles vaccinations, yellow fever vaccine is now routinely given to children three years of age or older. Weights of children are measured monthly for the first year. Unfortunately, the health district had run out of new growth charts. It would be harder to track progress of these children without them.

But the biggest obstacle faced by the village chief was more practical, and revealed just how great the impact of these outreach schemes had been: How could he ensure that sick villagers were safely transferred to the Savelugu health center or Tamale for care when needed? The expectations of villagers are now high, and only partly satisfied.

District and regional hospital services in northern Ghana are desperately short of trained medical and nursing staff. Walewale Hospital, a busy district-level center northeast of Tamale, is run single-handedly by Dr. Kofi Issah. He completed his undergraduate medical studies in Moscow. (Many Ghanaian doctors owe their skills to the education they received in the former Soviet Union and Eastern Bloc countries.) Dr. Issah continued his postgraduate training in England. He is now the district director of health services and head of Walewale Hospital.

Dr. Issah's day had begun at six that morning in the operating room. He has an experienced nursing sister who assists him and the morning is filled with a dozen patients admitted with hydrocoeles and hernias. According to the hospital's operating register, common procedures also include evacuation of the uterus for partial abortion and cesarean section. Dr. Issah obtains consent for surgery by taking thumbprints from the patient, a relative, and a witness. There is no anesthetist. Pethidine provides pain relief and xylocaine is the local anesthetic.

Wards are clean but packed with patients—local demand for hospital care is beyond what Walewale can provide. From the operating table, Dr. Issah proceeds to complete ward rounds and clinics. He spends evenings leading mother-and-baby groups or prevention programs for sexually transmitted diseases. He rarely sees his young family, who live some distance from the hospital.

Walewale's hospital laboratory is small—a single cramped room and a back office—but well organized. Ernest Dakurah, head of the laboratory service, needs new equipment urgently. He pipettes by mouth, a practice that, given the uncertain prevalence of HIV/AIDS, he would stop if only the hospital were provided with a proper mechanical pipetting device. The lamp for the hospital's one functioning microscope is broken. A lightbulb is propped up facing the microscope's mirror. Sometimes the bright sunlight is a better source of illumination.

There is no in-service training for staff at Walewale. Dr. Issah is struggling to raise the standards of his hospital team. On a wall in Ernest Dakurah's laboratory is a recent reminder to staff about their appearance at work: "Having supplied material for at least one uniform per staff, it is sad to notice that some of you come to work in casual/other wear."

Tamale regional hospital must have been an impressive building with modern medical facilities when it opened in 1974. There were thirty-eight doctors employed there. X-ray machines and elevators worked. Morale was high. Now, the hospital has "really deteriorated," according to one of the few remaining Ghanaian doctors. Staff have moved away, abroad to Germany and the UK, and elsewhere within Ghana itself, especially to Accra and Kumasi. Services have been bolstered by visiting doctors—a German specialist in tropical medicine, Egyptian and German pediatricians, and Cuban surgeons and pathologists. A surgeon and a senior surgical theater sister were in Tamale to give in-service training. The living conditions for medical staff are poor—facilities for nurses even more so. Often there is no clean water. Since 1974, there has been no major maintenance work on the hospital and equipment has not been repaired or replaced. There are no resident doctors in training. When the hospital opened, ten house staff from Accra rotated through Tamale, but no more. The hospital is no longer recognized for training. "Everything has collapsed," says Dr. Anemana. Ghana's government has promised a program of renovation, but that promise has been made each year for the past six years. Staff at Tamale are waiting for this promise to be fulfilled. Overseas aid donors are more interested in paying for new buildings than restoring an old and failing hospital.

Given that the hospital is the main referral point for the entire

Northern Region, clinical services are disconcertingly unpredictable. Drug supplies are haphazard, there are too few beds, and simple diagnostic measures (such as blood glucose, serum potassium, and blood cultures) are often unavailable. The admissions area is well equipped and wards are spacious but dilapidated, with no clean bedclothes. Peak admissions take place from July to February, with up to 550 new patients per month. Pediatric admissions run between seven hundred and nine hundred each month.

North of Tamale, Bolgatanga is the capital city of the Upper-East Region of Ghana. The regional hospital's medical director is a Hungarian-trained surgeon, Dr. Aduko Amiah. The main causes of morbidity and mortality in Bolgatanga are malaria, anemia, and pneumonia. Although malaria is the greatest burden on clinical services, meningitis has the highest death rate (31 percent). There is no pathology service. The hospital library, such as it is, remains unused and wrapped in cobwebs. Four Cuban doctors have been sent to strengthen the surgical service in Bolgatanga. They come as part of an arrangement organized by the previous government. But their presence causes resentment rather than relief, for these Cuban visitors are exempt from on-call work, do no outpatient clinics, provide no pre- or postoperative care, speak little English (the common language among many health workers), and are paid more than locally trained doctors. Perversely, the presence of the Cuban team only acts as a further incentive for Ghanaian doctors to leave the region or, worse still, the country.

Professor Ankrah trained in Accra, graduating in 1969. He was one of Ghana's first group of thirty-four medical graduates, and their success was greeted with the "congratulations of the whole country."[4] When these new doctors stepped out of medical school, they found themselves without either accommodation or food in the hospital—in "no-man's land," according to the *Ghana Medical Journal*. The journal's editorialist acidly noted that the government had "to face urgently and squarely" the lack of postgraduate training and declining standards in Accra's Korle Bu Hospital. Professor C. O. Easmon, then dean of Ghana's first medical school, challenged his colleagues to have "imagination, dedication, sacrifice and effective leadership ... [to provide] total health to the total population."[5]

Returning to Komfo Anokye Teaching Hospital in Kumasi, Professor Ankrah specialized in respiratory medicine and traveled to the UK in 1975 for further training to pass the examination for membership in the Royal College of Physicians. But, as an award citation in the *Ghana Medical Journal* noted, "you then did what the majority did not do at that time, in that you demonstrated patriotism and an undetachable bond to the land and place of your birth by returning to Kumasi."[6] He now presides over an effective medical school, producing about sixty new medical graduates each year.

The School of Medical Sciences is presently expanding, with a large new lecture theater and a new department of physiology under construction. The two-room library is well stocked with general and specialty medical journals, together with several copies each of textbooks in key subjects. Students publish their own magazine, *Mediscope*, which includes a student personality of the week ("Any final lines for the fellow citizens of cadaver land?"), editorials about student issues ("Members will however not tolerate any act of insolence, corruption, and dictatorship on the part of the executives"), news (donations to the child and maternal health clinic), opinions ("Freedom of speech and access to information are fundamental human rights which should not be repressed"), and commentaries ("How far should we stretch gender issues?").

The school has its difficulties. The department of community medicine is struggling to recruit staff, facing impossible competition from nongovernmental organizations that, with larger salaries and better resources, attract some of the best Ghanaian academics.

Reports of this continuous drain on Ghana's physician and scientist community are repeated many times. Donors and aid organizations too often target Ghana with their own Western-style agendas. They mean well: development, human rights, and equity seem obviously worthwhile causes to invest in. But when these groups take time and talent away from local staff to work on often unsustainable projects, the aid community does great harm. Certainly, this is the case for medicine and public health in Ghana.

This picture of mostly progress and vigor is once again starkly contrasted with the perilously positioned medical school in Tamale. The School of Medicine and Health Sciences at the University of Development Studies was founded in 1996. The size of the annual preclinical entering class in the next five years (students go to Accra and Kumasi for clinical training) was eleven, twenty, thirty-five, nine, and four. Since the founding dean died in office and his successor retired, the past two years have seen a collapse in organization, staff morale, infrastructure, and funding. The school was on a direct course to closure. A final chance has been handed to Dr. Jehu Iputo, the new dean, who has a one-year contract with the university arranged through WHO. Dr. Iputo trained at Makerere University in Uganda and was most recently at the University of Transkei in South Africa. He was attracted to Tamale because he had "a feeling for what they are trying to do" and because "there is a need for a medical school" in the region. He wants to redesign the curriculum to emphasize the community basis of care in the north. But he is aware of the "101 problems" he faces, and he wants to popularize the issue of medical education to motivate his colleagues (who were on strike when I met him). Dr. Iputo's chief problem is lack of money. In meeting with his senior associates from the university, one could sense the great hopes they had in both his presence and WHO's renewed interest in Tamale.

Research might seem to be an indulgence, given not only the endemic poverty of resources for health care within Ghana but also the immense inequalities across the country. Yet many overseas researchers do come to Ghana to do laboratory, field, and clinical work. Investigators in Ghana have focused on malaria, maternal and child health, HIV/AIDS, filariasis, and diabetes. Part of the research conducted on the benefits of vitamin A supplementation in children was based in Ghana,[7] and the northern reaches of the country have been important areas for malaria and meningitis studies.[8] The staff of the medical schools have strong overseas collaborations. For example, in Kumasi two research groups from London are coordinating a clinical trial to determine the safety and efficacy of a new treatment for patients with Buruli ulcer. The trial is small with a short follow-up, but the desire to find evidence of a low-cost, simple-to-apply treatment is strong. A pity, therefore, for the patients giving their consent and for the Ghanaian doctors giving their time that the protocol insists that "no publication in any form will be issued without the prior authorisation of ——— Pharmaceuticals Ltd." African patients are being used as guinea pigs for untested Western medicines, a scientific exploitation that one rarely hears about.

Noncommunicable disease is a much-debated yet important new priority for research in sub-Saharan Africa.[9] A team from St. George's Hospital, London, and Komfo Anokye has designed a study to investigate whether intensive nutritional education could diminish blood pressures in a random sample of adults.[10] The research practicalities present formidable challenges. The project lasts for three years and involves six rural and six semiurban communities. The first step was to construct a complete age-sex register of these villages—almost 17,000 people. The study began in June 2001. Heights, weights, blood pressures, blood samples, and twenty-four-hour urine collections will be repeated at three-month intervals. The lessons of this particular collaboration have been enormously positive[11] and are likely to encourage others to look beyond their own immediate clinical and research environments.[12]

Ghana's research culture has developed rapidly during the past forty years. The *Ghana Medical Journal*, for example, was launched in 1962. In his opening message, President Nkrumah said, "Your observations, analysis, management and discoveries in the problems of Health in Africa, and in Ghana in particular, will be making important contributions to man's quest for good health."[13] (His son, Dr. Francis Nkrumah, is a senior Ghanaian academic pediatrician.) But the problems facing the research community today are common to many countries in the South—lack of funding, poor facilities, little training, weak peer networks, donor-aid projects that absorb available time and resources, and erratic communication with the world outside Ghana. One impediment remains lack of access to information. When I asked a group of Kumasi doctors to describe their information difficulties, the answers were sadly familiar. The high cost of journals and books was a universal complaint. Doctors want personal rather than library copies of the latest editions of textbooks and access to specialist and subspecialist titles. Journals arrive irregularly and are commonly delayed. Access to the Internet is limited, and even when PubMed is available, how was a physician to obtain a hard copy of the article being sought? The solution these doctors wanted centered on a better information technology infrastructure, improved library facilities, and subscription prices that reflected the economic realities of Africa.

There are many schemes designed to get health information to doctors in the developing world. Few are as targeted and technically well-developed as the US National Library of Medicine's (NLM's) journals project for the Multilateral Initiative on Malaria, led by NLM's chief of international programs, Julia Royall. African scientists began by selecting their twelve most needed journals. The publishers of these journals are now working to provide their content via a satellite (Intelsat801) and a VSAT (very small aperture terminal) antenna to give permanent Web access to seven hundred researchers in Ghana, Uganda, Kenya, Tanzania, and Malawi.

Despite the plea for improved access to information from beyond their own country, researchers I spoke with said that publication in the *Ghana Medical Journal* is still an important goal for any aspiring investigator. The journal is published quarterly and receives about one hundred submissions annually, 90 percent of which come from Ghana. Two thirds of all submitted articles originate in Accra. Papers are selected for review by an editorial board and are usually sent to two Ghanaian reviewers. The journal accepts about three quarters of submitted papers. The editor in chief, Dr. David Ofori-Adjei, wants to create a thriving research culture by teaching Ghana's doctors how to write scientific articles.

There is something almost neocolonial about an editor from a medical journal with offices in London and New York visiting Ghana and attempting to give a personal analysis of the country's health system. What of the views of Ghana's doctors themselves?

Dr. Anemana lists four constraints to his program for rejuvenating health in the Northern Region. First, he faces an exodus of doctors, nurses, and technicians to the south of the country. Second, he has few training facilities to offer the staff who choose to remain, although his initiative with the UK's Tropical Health and Education Trust to develop in-service training could well help to retain them. Third, he has no material incentives to draw doctors back to the most deprived areas of Ghana. Finally, he has no medical infrastructure in the north to support doctors even if they could be persuaded to return. The government, he believes, has to decentralize resources to the regions, establishing a permanent career structure, if inequalities are to be tackled. Dr. Anemana has lobbied parliament through the northern caucus of regional representatives. But they argue that the administrative capacity to manage large health budgets is just not present in the region.

Professor Agyeman Badu Akosa, the current president of the Ghana

Medical Association, is more optimistic. He returned to Ghana from the UK in 1995, and believes that "for most of our colleagues, they wish to be here." The Ghanaian diaspora is large—900 doctors and 200 residents-in-training in the US, 200 doctors each in the UK and South Africa, and 150 in Canada. The medical association plans to use its new Web site (www.ghanamedassn.org) to attract colleagues back home. The Web site reports news and events, and posts abstracts from the *Ghana Medical Journal*. Most interestingly, the association is offering residential plots of land for sale in Accra at $1,500 apiece for members, not only those living in Ghana but also those living abroad. But Professor Akosa is not blind to the challenge. Ghana is training marketable doctors to a very high standard, who are welcomed elsewhere. Perhaps only half-jokingly, he suggests that Ghana needs to produce less accomplished physicians. The only substantive strategy that is likely to retain his colleagues is a strong program of postgraduate education.

The incentives needed to keep doctors in Ghana are also seen as being more material. Doctors in Tamale told me that they should not have to pay rent for housing, that after three years they should be given a car, and that all utility bills should be paid by the government. At the medical school in Kumasi, doctors expressed a larger view, reflecting perhaps their own relatively well-funded state. The future health of Ghana's people depends on comprehensive primary care, better hospital services, cheaper drugs, and, last of all, material incentives for staff.

Health was not a central issue in Ghana's December 2000 election. But the newly elected president, John Kufuor, did promise "positive change," together with "development and prosperity." Kufuor campaigned on the idea that poverty was Ghana's greatest enemy. Eighty percent of Ghana's population live in rural settings. In 1998, according to national surveys, 40 percent of children under five years old were growth-retarded, 13 percent suffered from wasting, and 38 percent were underweight. Hospitals are unable to provide much more than symptomatic relief for patients with HIV/AIDS, renal failure, and cancer. Efforts to create exemption programs for the poorest Ghanaians are either bureaucratically complex or underfunded by government. Ghana's difficulties have been compounded by corrupt and ineffective administration, poor responsiveness to popular demands for health reforms, and a lack of commitment to devolving budget responsibility to regions and districts.[14]

The latest government report on the health of the nation reviews the country's "Vision 2020" strategy—namely, its plan to develop maternal and child health services, rural health care, and programs to control risk factors for communicable diseases. A list of priority interventions—from vaccinations to trauma services—was drawn up in 1996 and implementation began in 1997 as part of a five-year program. The government's own report is brutally honest in its appraisal of Ghana's progress: "Gains have been slow and unequal." North–south inequalities in poverty, disease, and services are emphasized; the financial barriers to health care are underlined; and the staffing problems starkly laid out:

> There is a major problem of staff recruitment, distribution, and retention generally within the health service and particularly in deprived areas.... Korle Bu Teaching Hospital [in Accra] had 285 doctors (25.6 percent) and Komfo Anokye Teaching Hospital had 184 doctors (16.5 percent) compared to 6.8 percent of medical doctors available in the three Northern Regions.... Despite policies to increase staff numbers, there is a large outflow of staff that is accelerating.[15]

The government sees the next five years as a time for "bridging the inequalities gap." The means to do so will be a mix of public-private partnerships, prepayment systems, safety nets, professional development programs, community-based services, and the resources that will flow back to the country from taking part in the Highly Indebted Poor Countries initiative (the government spends more on servicing its debt than it does on education and health).

Aid donors contribute about 40 percent of the total health budget for Ghana. In his Accra office, Rod Pullen, the British high commissioner, explained to me that the health program for Ghana is a model being replicated by the UK across Africa. Instead of supporting individual donor projects, the UK's new policy is to agree on a long-term strategy with Ghana's government and then to fund that plan. The strategy is agreed upon by all development partners and aid money is transferred directly into the government's budget. The UK Department for International Development (DFID) has committed £32 million for the next five years. Pullen's view is that this sector-wide approach is a better way to influence policy than simply working in parallel, almost in competition, with the national government. However, there is no evidence that this new attitude is delivering better health care to Ghana's poorest people.

Staff at the high commission are sensitive to any claim that the UK is stealing Ghana's doctors to work in its own health service. Pullen has written to Ghana's minister of health asking for specific examples of locally trained doctors leaving their country to work in Great Britain. None has so far been forthcoming. When I ask about primary health care, postgraduate training, and access to medicines for treatable conditions, such as Burkitt's lymphoma, the high commissioner and his principal health adviser, Liz Gaere, repeat the official Ghanaian government line, but with a hint of uncertainty, even skepticism. Primary care is indeed a priority (although "something has to give" in the budget); a postgraduate medical college has been promised (although no date for construction has yet been set); and a prepayment system should help to fund access to drugs (although the government has "definitely not got it right at the moment").

UK collaboration with Ghana is not wholly without controversy. DFID has commissioned a team at the University of York and within Ghana's Ministry of Health to study geographical resource allocation in Ghana's health sector.[16] They examined how resources might be targeted to regions of greatest need. Devising a formula for resource allocation must take account of population size, health status, the proportion of people living below the poverty line, and cost of care. A pilot method has been produced—the Northern Region would gain most, while the main "losers" would be Volta and greater Accra. Resources cannot be redistributed immediately, of course. The authors of the report estimate it will take at least five years, if their plan is implemented, to enable appropriate adjustments to take place.

The debate about human development remains radically and damagingly unresolved. Those skeptical of the forces of globalization argue that development is conceived by Western governments only as the creation of wealth through free trade—the "hegemony of capitalism," as political development theorist Paul Cammack puts it.[17] The World Bank, by contrast, believes that poverty will be reduced by building effective markets and strong institutions to support those markets.[18]

Yet the fact is that poverty, expressed as the needless deaths of thousands of people from treatable diseases, requires actions well beyond what markets and existing World Bank policies alone can achieve. Prevention, access to care, diagnosis, treatment, training, information, and food security are not amenable to market solutions. However, it is also true that the creation of sustainable local systems over time to support the health of a population depends on economic growth. Those who try to fit development practice into a single political ideology by adopting the vocabulary of either Marx or the market do not serve the poor well.

There is no simple blueprint of success for a country like Ghana. Instead, there is a framework of ideas, an orthodoxy of definitions about development and health, which governs debates and policymaking. These definitions must be strictly tested by empirical evidence if countries are to transcend the representations imposed on them by others. For example, development is presently standardized by the Human Development Index, a composite measure of life expectancy, literacy, schooling, and standard of living. This index is grossly misleading. Illiteracy is, as Sumani Issifu showed, no barrier to improving village health; education is no help to a country if qualified doctors leave rather than stay; average measures of GDP per capita are meaningless if they hide important geographical inequalities; and life expectancy estimates explain little if they fail to reveal the slowly shifting burden of disease from communicable to noncommunicable causes. Today's calculus of human development is badly distorting. Perhaps the entire concept of development as a means to imitate Western nation-states is wrong. Is Oswaldo de Rivero, the former Peruvian ambassador to the UN, correct when he claims that the future for the world's poorest countries is better thought of in terms of survival than development?[19]

Health is also an idea in need of revision. Alicia Fentiman and her colleagues have studied the relation between health and education among children in eastern Ghana.[20] Two thirds of six-year-olds were not enrolled in primary school. These nonenrolled children were substantially shorter than those attending school. Adolescent nonenrolled boys were also more heavily infected with *Schistosoma haematobium*. Parents decide about schooling according to a complex mix of factors, one of which is height, itself determined by the health of the child. The use of height as a trigger for school enrollment produces a wide age range of children attending primary school (about a third are adolescents). Through schooling, therefore, health is an important influence on long-term educational ability. Health cannot be isolated in any analysis of Ghana's present or future development. Health is woven into many aspects of the country's culture and beliefs.

Those who designed Ghana's first medical school had the highest aspirations for their nation. In the words of the minister of health at the time, Ghana's future doctors "will be the pride of the people and the Government of Ghana... [providing] limitless scope for unobtrusive service to the community... their worthy example will blaze a trail to be followed by other Ghanaian youth...."[21]

Ghanaians are working hard to improve the lives of fellow Ghanaians. Although resources are thinly stretched, the primary care network presently being laid down is probably the best example of what can be done to make a measurable difference to the health of rural people. The contrast with the country's cities is stark. Driving through Accra, there are obvious signs of Ghana's new market economy: hotels under construction, garage forecourts packed with secondhand European cars for sale, and advertising boards promoting Nestlé, Pepsi, Coca-Cola, Guinness, and British American Tobacco. The test is now whether Ghana's government will continue to turn to global trade for solutions to its people's health problems or whether it is ready to address directly the immediate future of its poorest people. It is a choice that many African nations face.[22]

# EPILOGUE TO CHAPTERS 4 AND 5

WHAT DOES GLOBALIZATION—and with it our increased awareness of war and poverty—mean for medicine? For individuals, its impact is likely to be gradual—for example, the application of evidence from globally organized research programs to local practices. But for the institutions that influence medicine and the people doctors serve, the changes brought about by globalization are more pressing. The inertia of large organizations, such as the World Health Organization, is being challenged by nongovernmental bodies whose advocacy has genuinely changed the way in which issues such as access to medicines in resource-poor settings have been confronted. Outward-looking nation-states with fairly elected political leaders (for example, Ghana) are flourishing and making health a priority, while violent tyrannies (for example, Zimbabwe) are doing exactly the opposite. Vast migrations of people—the Office of the UN High Commissioner for Refugees currently puts the number of displaced people at 20 million—are straining the capacities of national health systems. Inequities in health information between the rich and poor worlds have become starkly apparent. Yet the notion of health as a product to be bought and sold is now giving way to the notion of health as a universal human right.

Amid a debate about globalization that has too often dwelt on its threats, three important areas of broad consensus have emerged.

First, the eight Millennium Development Goals, together with their eighteen targets and forty-eight indicators of success, mark an agreed-upon strategy supported by the world's governments, as expressed through the United Nations at the 2000 Millennium Summit (see Table A, page 191). Health is by far the most important theme binding this strategy together—four goals, seven targets, and eighteen indicators are health-related. Second, the political framework for achieving these goals is unquestionably one of strengthened democracies.[1] And third, the economic case for the critical part that health plays in development has been argued and, for the most part, accepted.[2]

The difficulty faced by those who see this tripartite consensus as the means to pull 1.2 billion people out of the grinding poverty that less than $1 a day affords is that there is no institution to implement it.[3] Globalization lacks governance. Without some sort of global development organization (GDO) there is no prospect that UN development goals will be met. Indeed, things may get worse rather than better. For example, a decade of governmental paralysis and institutional fragmentation has seen the number of people living in poverty in sub-Saharan Africa rise from 242 million to 300 million.

Current institutions have failed to make progress on human development. It is true that Secretary-General Kofi Annan has provided strong leadership of the UN system since he took office in 1997. He has placed Africa's predicament at the heart of the UN's work, repeatedly underlining its special needs. But even he admits that the world continues to do far too little to help the continent. The widely acknowledged leading candidate to run WHO from 2003 onward was Pascoal Mocumbi, the prime minister of Mozambique. Yet the thirty-two members of WHO's executive board were clearly not ready for an African to lead the UN *and* WHO, despite Mocumbi's qualifications (he has been a respected physician, public health worker, minister of health, and minister of foreign affairs). This failure of commitment is all the more abject given the respect in which Annan and Mocumbi are held. If so little can be achieved with an effectively led UN, it is time to ask how much the world can expect from an organization designed for an era long past.[4]

WHO has done more than any other UN body to make health the cornerstone of development policy. But the regional structure and politics of WHO prevent it from being effective in the field. All it can do is fight important, but limited, skirmishes, such as its healthy environments for children initiative launched at the 2002 World Summit on Sustainable Development. The UN Development Program faces the same problems. Mark Malloch Brown, UNDP's administrator, has few powers to act. He can, for example, do no more than emphasize that the annual, independent, and impressively researched *Human Development Report* is "not a formal statement of UNDP or UN policy." His hands are tied when it comes to fresh thinking, policy development, and advocacy.

The failures of the World Bank and the International Monetary Fund in development policy have been well documented, most acutely by Joseph Stiglitz, the World Bank's former chief economist. He paints a picture of the IMF as an organization driven by an unbending free-market ideology, unable to take account of evidence pointing to policy failure, mired in a culture of arrogance and obsessive secrecy, dismissive of external criticism, blindly applying the same economic medicine to countries with very different histories and problems, biased in favor of its rich donors, and staffed by economists who have little specialized knowledge of the countries whose financial fate they are deciding. The IMF micromanages, denies countries opportunities to make their own choices for economic and social development, and fails to assess the impact of its policies on the most vulnerable people affected by them.[6]

The 2002 *Human Development Report* also points to "a crisis of legitimacy and effectiveness" in these organizations. Its authors argue that a severe "democratic deficit" exists at both the IMF and the

World Bank, where almost half the voting power on the executive board is exercised by just seven countries—the US, Japan, France, the UK, Saudi Arabia, China, and the Russian Federation. These important and influential financial institutions are not set up to meet the development needs of the world's poorest nations.

Meanwhile, the G8 leaders have failed to match their much-publicized rhetoric—led by British Prime Minister Tony Blair's claim that Africa is a "scar on the conscience of the world"—with the funds needed to finance development. And only in June 2002 did the European Union launch a health and development policy initiative, including a call for debate about how Europe could better target its aid for poverty reduction. Programs have fared little better than institutions. The report of the UN secretary-general about progress in the run-up to the World Summit on Sustainable Development concluded that "there is undoubtedly a gap in implementation."

The UN and Bretton Woods financial institutions still have important parts to play in world affairs. But none has the mandate, legitimacy, or means to make the advances in human development demanded by the Millennium Development Goals. Indeed, the world already lives in a post-UN and post–Bretton Woods era. The recent birth of two new global organizations shows that we need to think beyond existing political structures. Since 1995 the role of the World Trade Organization has been to deal with trade rules between nations by ensuring "that trade flows as smoothly, predictably, and freely as possible." The WTO is quick to deny that it ignores development issues, but its main function is to guarantee its members' trade rights, not to alleviate poverty. The Global Fund to Fight AIDS, Tuberculosis, and Malaria was launched in 2002. Its purpose is very much development-oriented; the fund aims to contribute "to poverty reduction as part of the Millennium Development Goals."[7]

Both organizations have their weaknesses. The Global Fund's decision-making is opaque and its focus is narrow, while the WTO frequently excludes developing country members from its negotiations. The *2002 Human Development Report* calls on the WTO to make its decision-making more participatory, to be demonstrably impartial, and to welcome open debate about the impact of trade liberalization.

The case for creating a new institution, one that conceives development as more than an economic process, is strong. Like Georges Canguilhem's view of health, development is about building adaptability. A country and its people need to have the capacity to withstand prevailing economic, environmental, and epidemiological threats. A key element of adaptability is information, the ability both to create it and to have access to it. A GDO must be an organization that gathers and disseminates knowledge.

Joseph Stiglitz has done much to work out this information-driven approach to development. In a series of lectures given while he was at the World Bank,[8] Stiglitz advocated a more scientific perspective on theories of development. This scientific attitude—one of constant questioning, sifting of data, measuring uncertainty, drawing tentative inferences, and repeating the process again and again—aims to discard the previous neoliberal consensus of minimal government, trade liberalization, privatization, and fiscal austerity. In its place, he sees development as nothing less than a complete transformation of society. Strong governments must create effective institutions (for example, a civil service), a legal and regulatory infrastructure, and health and education systems. Transformation must take place in the private and public sectors, in communities and families, and among individuals. Stiglitz wants to put control of development processes within countries, not have them imposed by the IMF or World Bank. Change must be society-wide, not directed at small elites. Governments can be the catalysts of change, building consensus through maximum participation.

This analysis is not shared by all economists. One of the most cogent critiques that has stood the test of time—judging by its three printings in 1983, 1997, and 2002—is Deepak Lal's *The Poverty of Development Economics.*[9] Lal, an economist with wide experience in development policy-making across India, international institutions (such as the World Bank), and academia, argues against the view that imperfections in the market are inevitable limitations to economic development. In more graphic language, he writes:

> It is easy to suppose that these half-starved, wretched and ignorant masses could not possibly conform, either as producers or consumers, to the behavioural assumption of orthodox neoclassical economics . . . [and] that some ethereal and verbally sanitised entity (such as "government," "planners," or "policy-makers") which is both knowledgeable and compassionate can overcome the defects of these stupid or ignorant producers and consumers. . . .

Easy, maybe, but wrong. Lal argues that imperfect markets are superior to imperfect planning. Even more trenchant language was used by Charles Calomiris, a professor of finance and economics at Columbia University. He criticized the "self-interested and self-righteous anti-globalists" who launch "farcical demonstrations" at international summits.[10] Calomiris believes that "the poor residents of developing economies . . . understand better than anyone that the entry of foreign firms into their economies and the opening of export markets translate into more food on their tables and a chance for a better life for them and their children."

Development remains a territory stained by the blood spilled in decades of ideological warfare. Differing theoretical perspectives—"alternative discourses" is the common term used to dignify the confusion[11]—abound: postcolonialist, feminist, social, neoliberal, sustainable, and participatory. Extreme positions are preferred to those that actually try to incorporate the messy complexities and compromises of real life. Strong views are seen as bold and necessary to resist the trampling momentum of the twin Western orthodoxies, democracy and modernization. Empiricism as a method of testing any one of these approaches is rarely discussed. Yet the diversity of opinion about development seems to prove the importance of systematically collecting evidence about the impact of development theory and practice.

A GDO could oversee this collaborative effort to acquire evidence, foster implementation, and measure results. It would function as an institution that sets standards for best practice, helps to avoid duplication of work across existing agencies, and coordinates the activities of all national government departments for international development. The purposes and possible functions of a GDO are shown in Table B (page 196). In particular, it would aim to reverse the fragmentation, strategic incoherence, and continuing resource overconsumption that have slowed down the global development process. The notion of a GDO as a scientific and technical agency could protect it from the political turf wars that do so much damage to existing UN and Bretton Woods institutions. A GDO would aim to improve the quality and range of information available to partner agencies, such as the World Bank and the IMF, and hold those institutions accountable for the impact of their work on development.

The rapidity of globalization has outstripped the capacity of existing organizations to provide effective strategies for human development. A greatly expanded global effort is now required. An organization to strengthen and coordinate the expertise, resources, and networks that are presently distributed across many different multilateral institutions—and to counter the exclusively trade-oriented mandate of the WTO—would fill an unmet need.

It would also help to confirm one high-minded assertion in the constitution of WHO, namely, "The health of all peoples is fundamental to the attainment of peace and security and is dependent upon the fullest co-operation of individuals and states." Can health really be an instrument of foreign policy, either to bring about an end to war or to prevent armed conflict from taking place at all? The argument for linking health and peace practically as well as conceptually is not new.[12] And the logic is straightforward. War kills and wounds combatants and civilians alike. Conflict is therefore a major medical and public health issue. But the trickier question is whether health workers can contribute uniquely to peace-building. I think the answer is that they can, and efforts to do so have been partly successful in Bosnia. Since 9/11, the threat of terrorism and our apparent inability to deter terrorists through conventional political and military means have made violence even more important in this public health agenda. In WHO's constitution, health is famously described as "a state of complete physical, mental, and social well-being and not merely the absence of disease or infirmity." One could similarly define peace as a state of complete political, economic, and social amity between peoples, together with their mutual cooperation to achieve physical, mental, and social well-being, and not merely the absence of war or conflict.

This linkage is not only made by liberal sentimentalists (if that is what you think I am). President George W. Bush's *National Security Strategy of the United States of America*, signed on September 17, 2002, says:

> The events of September 11, 2001, taught us that weak states, like Afghanistan, can pose as great a danger to our national interests as strong states. Poverty does not make poor people into terrorists and murderers. Yet poverty, weak institutions, and corruption can make weak states vulnerable to terrorist networks.... The United States will deliver greater development assistance... [and] we will also continue to lead the world in efforts to reduce the terrible toll of HIV/AIDS and other infectious diseases.

America's security strategy also encompasses nutrition, safe water, and sanitation systems. A key part of building an "infrastructure of democracy" is to secure public health. The US government's security strategy offers a strong and welcome commitment to reinforcing effective health systems:

> The scale of the public health crisis in poor countries is enormous. In countries afflicted by epidemics and pandemics like HIV/AIDS, malaria, and tuberculosis, growth and development will be threatened until these scourges can be contained. Resources from the developed world are necessary but will be effective only with honest governance, which supports prevention programs and provides effective local infrastructure. The United States has strongly backed the new global fund for HIV/AIDS organized by UN Secretary General Kofi Annan and its focus on combining prevention with a broad strategy for treatment and care. The United States already contributes more than twice as much money to such efforts as the next largest donor. If the global fund demonstrates its promise, we will be ready to give even more.

These themes were more clearly developed in President Bush's State of the Union address in 2003. Iraq was certainly a preoccupation, and the lessons of the Croatian and Bosnian wars may well have been on his mind when he said that "we will bring to the Iraqi people food, and medicines, and supplies, and freedom." Here was a strategy not merely of reconstruction but of nation-building, and establishing health systems is a central element of that work.

Two issues received particular attention in Bush's address—terrorism, especially bioterrorism, and global health. He backed up his aggressive policy toward Iraq by pointing to evidence that 25,000 liters of anthrax and 38,000 liters of botulinum toxin were unaccounted for in Saddam Hussein's dealings with UN weapons inspectors—as was the location of several mobile biological weapons laboratories. Given these uncertainties, Bush announced a $6 billion program to produce vaccines and drugs against anthrax, botulism, ebola, and plague. He called this "major research and production effort to guard our people against bioterrorism" Project Bioshield. And in a section of his speech called "Combating AIDS," he announced $10 billion in new investment over five years "to turn the tide against AIDS in the most afflicted nations of Africa." He did not, as he had done in his national security strategy, make security the justification for pursuing global health through US foreign policy. Instead, he seemed to be making a moral argument, and a moral argument only:

> Today, on the continent of Africa, nearly 30 million people have the AIDS virus including three million children under the age of 15. There are whole countries in Africa where more than one third of the adult population carries the infection.... A doctor in rural South Africa describes his frustration. He says, "We have no medicines. Many hospitals tell people, 'You've got AIDS. We can't help you. Go home and die!'" In an age of miraculous medicines, no person should have to hear those words. AIDS can be prevented. Anti-retroviral drugs can extend life for many years.... Seldom has history offered a greater opportunity to do so much for so many.... And to meet a severe and urgent crisis abroad, tonight I propose the *Emergency Plan for AIDS Relief*—a work of mercy beyond all current international efforts to help the people of Africa.

WHO welcomed Bush's initiative, underlining the fact that $10 billion *annually* will be needed if the AIDS pandemic is to be slowed—and most of that money should be targeted to the Global Fund to Fight AIDS, Tuberculosis, and Malaria, the multilateral body charged exclusively with tackling these diseases, rather than an entirely new organization. Am I being too optimistic in thinking that a fundamental schism from a past view of Africa as an impossible continent, full of corruption and conflict, is taking place? Quite possibly. After Bush's announcement, his AIDS program became stalled in Congress amid a partisan fight over whether money should be barred from clinics that also perform abortions. And there is also argument over how much of his $10 billion should go to the Global Fund—Bush wanted to channel only $200 million to the fund, while Democrats sought $1 billion.

There are many examples of how cooperation between resource-rich and resource-poor worlds can create the necessary institutions to form a national public health fabric, whether they be specifically disease-oriented or more concerned with building technical capacity.[13] The construction of a new medical school in Malawi is a good example of what can be achieved. When Malawi became a nation in 1963, its prospective doctors were trained overseas, where, sadly, many of them remained. There were few incentives for them to return home where they were most needed. By 1986, the German, British, and Malawian governments agreed to build a new college of medicine to retain the doctors so desperately needed to build a health care system for the country. Twenty-five students began their training in the UK, and they eventually returned to Malawi to complete their final year of clinical work, which emphasized, quite properly and by contrast with Western curricula, community medicine. The first group of students qualified in July 1992. By 2002, 168 doctors had graduated, 112 of whom were still working in Malawi, with the rest in postgraduate training abroad and expected to return. Only nine doctors had left the country for good. This program has been a small but stunning success.

Development aid, then, can raise the amount of money a government spends on health, which in turn, and with good stewardship, can produce better health care, improve health, lead to greater individual wealth, and so lessen the burden of poverty. The political, economic, and security case for investing in health is overwhelming. Politicians seem to understand this argument but none has so far stepped forward to truly make it happen.

## Table A

## THE MILLENNIUM DEVELOPMENT GOALS, TARGETS, AND INDICATORS

| GOAL | TARGETS | INDICATORS |
| --- | --- | --- |
| 1. Eradicate extreme poverty and hunger | 1. Halve, between 1990 and 2015, the proportion of people whose income is less than $1 per day | 1. Proportion of population below $1 per day<br>2. Poverty gap ratio [incidence × depth of poverty]<br>3. Share of poorest quintile in national consumption |
| | 2. Halve, between 1990 and 2015, the proportion of people who suffer from hunger | 4. Prevalence of underweight children under five years of age<br>5. Proportion of population below minimum level of dietary energy consumption |
| 2. Achieve universal primary education | 3. Ensure that, by 2015, children everywhere, boys and girls alike, will be able to complete a full course of primary schooling | 6. Net enrollment in primary education<br>7. Proportion of pupils starting grade one who reach grade five<br>8. Literacy rate of fifteen- to twenty-four-year-olds |
| 3. Promote gender equality and empower women | 4. Eliminate gender disparity in primary and secondary education preferably by 2005, and to all levels of education no later than 2015 | 9. Ratios of girls to boys in primary, secondary, and tertiary education<br>10. Ratio of literate females to males fifteen to twenty-four years old<br>11. Share of women in wage employment in the nonagricultural sector<br>12. Proportion of seats held by women in national parliament |

| GOAL | TARGETS | INDICATORS |
|---|---|---|
| 4. Reduce child mortality | 5. Reduce by two thirds, between 1990 and 2015, the under-five mortality rate | 13. Under-five mortality rate<br>14. Infant mortality rate<br>15. Proportion of one-year-old children immunized against measles |
| 5. Improve maternal health | 6. Reduce by three quarters, between 1990 and 2015, the maternal mortality ratio | 16. Maternal mortality ratio<br>17. Proportion of births attended by skilled health personnel |
| 6. Combat HIV/AIDS, malaria, and other diseases | 7. Have halted by 2015 and begun to reverse the spread of HIV/AIDS | 18. HIV prevalence among fifteen- to twenty-four-year-old pregnant women<br>19. Condom use rate, as a proxy for the contraceptive prevalence rate<br>20. Number of children orphaned by HIV/AIDS |
| | 8. Have halted by 2015 and begun to reverse the incidence of malaria and other major diseases | 21. Prevalence and death rates associated with malaria<br>22. Proportion of population in malaria risk areas using effective malaria prevention and treatment measures<br>23. Prevalence and death rates associated with tuberculosis<br>24. Proportion of tuberculosis cases detected and cured under Directly Observed Treatment Short Course |

| GOAL | TARGETS | INDICATORS |
| --- | --- | --- |
| 7. Ensure environmental sustainability | 9. Integrate the principles of sustainable development into country policies and programs and reverse the loss of environmental resources | 25. Proportion of land area covered by forest<br>26. Ratio of area protected to maintain biological diversity to surface area<br>27. Energy use (metric ton oil equivalent) per $1 GDP<br>28. Carbon dioxide emissions (per capita) and consumption of ozone-depleting CFCs<br>29. Proportion of population using solid fuels |
| | 10. Halve by 2015 the proportion of people without sustainable access to safe drinking water | 30. Proportion of population with sustainable access to an improved water source, urban and rural |
| | 11. By 2020, to have achieved a significant improvement in the lives of at least 100 million slum dwellers | 31. Proportion of urban population with access to improved sanitation<br>32. Proportion of households with access to secure tenure (owned or rented) |
| 8. Develop a Global Partnership for Development | 12. Develop further an open, rule-based, predictable, nondiscriminatory trading and financial system [includes a commitment to good governance, development, and poverty reduction—both nationally and internationally] | |

| GOAL | TARGETS | INDICATORS |
| --- | --- | --- |
| 8. Develop a Global Partnership for Development, *cont'd.* | 13. Address the special needs of the least developed countries [includes tariff and quota-free access for LDC exports; enhanced program of debt relief for HIPC and cancellation of official bilateral debt; and more generous ODA for countries committed to poverty reduction] | 33. Net ODA, total and to LDC's, as percentage of OECD/DAC donors' GNI<br>34. Proportion of total bilateral, sector-allocable ODA of OECD/DAC donors to basic social services (basic education, primary health care, nutrition, safe water and sanitation)<br>35. Proportion of bilateral ODA of OECD/DAC donors that is untied |
| | 14. Address the special needs of landlocked countries and small island developing states (through the Program of Action for the Sustainable Development of Small Island Developing States and the outcome of the 22nd special session of the General Assembly) | 36. ODA received in landlocked countries as proportion of their GNIs<br>37. ODA received in small island developing states as proportion of their GNIs |
| | | *Market Access* |
| | 15. Deal comprehensively with the debt of developing countries through national and international measures in order to make debt sustainable in the long term | 38. Proportion of total developed country imports (by value and excluding arms) from developing countries and from LDCs, admitted free of duties<br>39. Average tariffs imposed by developing countries on agricultural products and textiles and clothing from developing countries |

| GOAL | TARGETS | INDICATORS |
|---|---|---|
| 8. Develop a Global Partnership for Development, *cont'd.* | 15. Deal comprehensively with the debt of developing countries through national and international measures in order to make debt sustainable in the long term, *cont'd.* | *Market Access, cont'd.*<br>40. Agricultural support estimate for OECD countries as percentage of their GDP<br>41. Proportion of ODA provided to help build trade capacity<br>*Debt Sustainability*<br>42. Total number of countries that have reached their HIPC decision points and number that have reached their HIPC completion points (cumulative)<br>43. Debt relief committed under HIPC initiative, in US dollars<br>44. Debt service as a percentage of exports of goods and services |
| | 16. In cooperation with developing countries, develop and implement strategies for decent and productive work for youth | 45. Unemployment rate of fifteen- to twenty-four-year-olds, each sex and total |
| | 17. In cooperation with pharmaceutical companies, provide access to affordable, essential drugs in developing countries | 46. Proportion of population with access to affordable essential drugs on a sustainable basis |
| | 18. In cooperation with the private sector, make available the benefits of new technologies, especially information and communications | 47. Telephone lines and cellular subscribers per 100 population<br>48. Personal computers in use per 100 population and Internet users per 100 population |

Table B

## THE MANDATE FOR A GLOBAL DEVELOPMENT ORGANIZATION

### PURPOSE

To advocate for global action on human development; to be the lead scientific and technical agency for development; to coordinate bilateral and multilateral development programs; and to set standards for development work.

### FUNCTIONS

- To make globalization work for sustainable human development
- To achieve the Millennium Development Goals
- To systematically collect evidence about the theories and practices of development work
- To collaborate with governments to build institutions and systems to address economic, environmental, and epidemiological threats
- To create partnerships to help finance development
- To disseminate information about best practice to partner agencies
- To initiate a long-term research program into development issues
- To strengthen information and communication technologies and information capacity in developing countries

# REVISED REPUTATIONS

# 6

# VACCINE MYTHS

IMAGINE THAT YOU are a country doctor with an idea for an experiment. Your only difficulty is finding a suitable person to experiment on. This obstacle faces all would-be investigators: willing human participants are hard to come by. But a neighbor of yours owns his own business, and one of his employees—Phipps—has a healthy eight-year-old son called James. You ask this boy's father if you can experiment on him. The father agrees. After all, you are a respected figure.

Your experiment goes something like this. A young girl, Sarah Nelmes, is a patient of yours and is known to be infected with the human immunodeficiency virus (HIV). You draw a syringe full of blood from her arm and go back to James Phipps to make two superficial cuts in his skin, each about half an inch long. You dip a needle into the serum of Sarah Nelmes's blood and gently place the infected fluid into the incisions on the boy's arm. You wait. Although James is unwell for a few days with a fever, he recovers. You return to Sarah Nelmes and take another blood sample, but this time you inject the blood directly into a vein in the boy's arm. This experiment, which seems so brutal, and is obviously unethical by modern standards, is the equivalent of Edward Jenner's first trials of vaccination. In May 1796, he took material from a pustule on the hand of Sarah Nelmes, a dairymaid who had cowpox, and placed that fluid on incisions made in the arm of James Phipps. A later attempt to infect Phipps with smallpox failed.

The comparison with HIV is not as ludicrous as it may at first appear. American researchers once suggested the existence of strains of HIV that do not lead to AIDS. Blood taken from an individual thought to have been infected with this benign form of HIV for over ten years was injected into eleven HIV-infected patients whose disease had not responded to drug treatment. The American team noted a clinical benefit in four patients. This experiment was condemned by some as "unethical, unscientific, and dangerous," but it is, in essence, identical to Jenner's. Similar objections have been raised against the work of the French immunologist Daniel Zagury, who claimed he had developed an AIDS vaccine that he gave to uninfected individuals, including himself. Concerns over his work led to a protracted inquiry and to a ban on his work by the French government. Even today, the methods Jenner adopted are able to stimulate ill-tempered debate among members of a normally reticent scientific community.

Born on May 17, 1749, Jenner was the second son of the marriage between the vicar of Berkeley, Gloucestershire, and the daughter of a former vicar of the same parish. Orphaned at the age of five, he attended grammar school and soon became an apprentice to a local surgeon. At twenty-one he moved to London to continue his medical studies as anatomical assistant to John Hunter at St. George's Hospital. Although Jenner returned to his Berkeley medical practice in 1773, Hunter had recognized Jenner's scientific prowess and encouraged him in his research. "Why think—why not try the experiment," he wrote in 1775. Hunter's patronage led to Jenner's renowned work on the breeding habits of the cuckoo, published in the *Philosophical Transactions* of the Royal Society in 1788. Jenner observed that the cuckoo is reared in the nest of another bird such as the hedge-sparrow, and that the natural offspring of the cuckoo's foster parents were frequently ejected. He noted that the cuckoo was responsible for this eviction, and described a depression in the cuckoo's wing, which he claimed assisted the bird in shouldering his foster brothers out of the nest. On the strength of this work, he was elected a Fellow of the Royal Society in 1779.

Jenner was a sympathetic physician, a scientist who keenly observed the natural world around him, and a man who moved in influential political and social circles. And, of course, he "discovered" vaccination. That his life deserves attention is endorsed by the countless number of studies—105 secondary sources are listed in one recent and comprehensive account—that already exist. His most recent biographer, Richard Fisher, a Yale history graduate, is a "full-time writer" who has "found time to take an M.S. in brain sciences." In *Edward Jenner, 1749–1823*, he turns his subject's life into a hagiographic fairy tale.[1] Until now, Fisher's literary efforts have largely been directed toward a prodigious output of dictionaries. Drugs, mental health, slimming, body chemistry, symptoms, and diseases have all come in for his A-to-Z treatment. Perhaps this explains why he produced such a turgid and unbalanced account of Jenner. "Lord Bacon complains of biographical literature of his day. He says that actions both great and small, public and private, sho'd be so blended together as to secure that genuine nature and lively representation, which forms the peculiar excellence and use of biography." Fisher quotes these wise words of Jenner's, but then goes on to ignore them. Church records have been analyzed, Gloucestershire villages visited, graveyards picked through, and adulatory opinions of Jenner accepted uncritically. The desire to catalog assiduously, so important to the compiler of dictionaries, is not an attribute that serves the potential biographer well. Amid all its impressive detail, there is only the one frayed thread to hold the story together: its concern with Jenner as heroic scientist. An alternative view of the life emerges if one takes a more critical look at the factual evidence available. Fisher makes no attempt to analyze how Jenner maneuvered himself through potentially adverse circumstances to a position of maximum advantage, and reveals himself as a sophist of some excellence in his assessment of a Dorset farmer, Benjamin Jesty.

Two years after the experiments on James Phipps in 1796, Jenner published his classic description of vaccination, *An Inquiry into the Causes and Effects of the Variolae Vaccinae*, which gave sketchy details of at least ten other cases in support of his main thesis. His decision to publish this work at his own expense followed advice from senior colleagues at the Royal Society who judged his flimsy evidence insufficient to merit publication in *Philosophical Transactions*. After the *Inquiry* had appeared, Jenner returned to Gloucestershire. There was little response to it until Henry Cline, another pupil of Hunter's, repeated Jenner's experiments and confirmed his result.

The first published comment on the *Inquiry* came from George Pearson, who verified the efficacy of vaccination from his own collaborative work with William Woodville at the Smallpox Hospital in London. Woodville went on to describe over five hundred individuals who had received vaccinations, and his work lent credibility to Jenner's preliminary observations. Although the initial discovery of vaccination was attributed to Jenner, it was Benjamin Jesty who deserves priority as the first known vaccinator.

Benjamin and Elizabeth Jesty lived with their three children in Yetminster, North Dorset. In 1774, it was commonly believed that milkmaids were protected from smallpox because of previous exposure to the cowpox virus. Traditionally, milkmaids were thought to be fair and attractive because of their smooth skins, which had been spared the unsightly pits usually left by the smallpox virus. The Jesty family employed two milkmaids, Ann Notley and Mary Reade, who had both nursed relatives with smallpox and yet had not contracted the disease. The average life expectancy one could hope for in the mid-eighteenth century was little more than forty years and smallpox killed one in three of those it infected. This poor outlook (his wife was already fifty) led Benjamin, who was afflicted with cowpox as a young man, to persuade his wife that she and their two sons should be infected with cowpox as protection. He found a cow with "mature" pox and, with the point of a stocking needle, transferred matter from a pustule on the cow to a scratch that he had made on his wife's arm. He repeated the procedure on the two boys. These inoculations were the first recorded vaccinations.

The rudimentary and unhygienic procedure that Jesty applied was not without its complications. Although his sons had a mild illness and recovered quickly, his wife became very sick. On hearing of Jesty's "bold" actions, those living in his village reacted angrily. Benjamin was "hooted at, reviled and pelted whenever he attended markets in the neighbourhood. He remained however undaunted and never failed from this cause to attend to his duties." His wife recovered and lived until she was eighty-four. Although Fisher mentions Jesty's experiment, he avoids any comment on the likely authenticity of this work that might detract from Jenner's supposedly central position in the history of vaccination.

Jenner's experiments were completed twenty-two years after Jesty's first vaccination, but because he was both (to quote Fisher) "a successful doctor with landed interests which assured his status as a member of the ruling English gentry" and already recognized as an experimentalist of some distinction, Jenner was in a position to capitalize on this discovery. He deserves credit for recognizing the public health importance of his work and he worked tirelessly to disseminate his findings. Both Thomas Jefferson and Napoleon promoted vaccination vigorously among their respective compatriots. There is no doubt that Jenner was unaware of Benjamin Jesty's work when he completed his first experiments in 1796. However, Jenner's subsequent actions expose both his ruthless ambition and his ability to manipulate his peers for financial gain.

After Woodville's publication of his 510 cases in *Reports of a*

*Series of Inoculations for the Variolae Vaccinae or Cowpox* in 1799, both Woodville and Pearson in London and Jenner in Gloucestershire worked closely together to secure the place of vaccination in the fight against smallpox. But their partnership was soon to show signs of strain. In an exchange in the *Medical and Physical Journal* in 1800, Pearson noted that some of his patients experienced a generalized eruption of pustules after cowpox vaccination. Normally this reaction was seen with smallpox; cowpox usually led to pustules only at the site of inoculation. Jenner replied in the same issue that "I very much suspect, that where variolous pustules have appeared, variolous matter has occasioned them," implying that Pearson's vaccine was contaminated with smallpox, a claim that suggested grave negligence on the part of the London physicians. Moreover, in December 1799 Pearson had set up the Institution for the Inoculation of the Vaccine-Pock. The patron was the Duke of York, and the director and chief physician Pearson himself. Jenner was offered the position of "extra-corresponding physician," which he judged an insult. He proposed the formation of the Jenner Society and sought a meeting with the Duke of York to persuade him to withdraw his patronage from Pearson's institution. Jenner was successful and, together with the support of the Duke of Bedford, Admiral Berkeley, and the Lord Mayor of London, he established the Royal Jennerian Society in 1802 to promote vaccination and "put an end to smallpox." Pearson had been trounced both by Jenner and by his aristocratic supporters.

Jenner's inability to accept criticism eventually led to the collapse of his own society in 1808. It insisted on examining claims that vaccination might not give lifetime protection against smallpox infection, one of the cornerstones of Jenner's theory. Despite his initial intransigence, Jenner was forced to admit that vaccine failures could occur. He had also become concerned that his part in the discovery of vaccination might be devalued as the technique was taken up across the country. He persuaded his friends to petition Parliament, on his behalf, for official recognition of his work and for financial reward. A committee was formed in 1802 under the chairmanship of Admiral Berkeley. One can imagine Jenner's delight at the Admiral's appointment, for he was now assured of a favorable hearing. The Jenner family had close associations with the Berkeley estate. Edward's brother, Stephen, was a tutor to the son of the Earl of Berkeley, the Admiral's brother. The Earl had a reputation for ruining one young woman after another, but his affections finally settled on a sixteen-year-old domestic servant called Mary Cole. Although he took her for his wife, no marriage followed. The Earl made an unsuccessful attempt to forge an entry in the local church marriage register, but later had to marry her in London. At that point, his wife was four months pregnant and Jenner, who had been a loyal and unquestioning family physician during these times, attended her throughout a difficult pregnancy. The Berkeley family owed Edward Jenner a sizable debt.

Jenner wrote a defense of his priority, *The Origin of the Vaccine Inoculation*, which he submitted as evidence to Parliament. He began his statement with the surprisingly forthright comment that "my inquiry commenced upwards of twenty-five years ago." This takes the origin of vaccination back not to 1796 and James Phipps, but to the mid-1770s, exactly the time when Jesty had vaccinated his family. The work of the Dorset farmer came to light in a paper written by Pearson in 1797. Clearly, Jenner felt vulnerable to the accusation that Jesty's work may have predated his own. Pearson repeated his claims to the House of Commons committee, but vigorous lobbying by Jenner's supporters led Parliament by a narrow margin (59 votes for, 56 against) to award him £10,000.

In 1805, Benjamin Jesty was invited to London to sit for a portrait. He was feted by Pearson's Vaccine-Pock Institute and was presented with two gold-mounted lancets and a document attesting to his discovery of vaccination. Jenner sought further money from Parliament in 1806 and, despite the restatement of Jesty's case for priority, Jenner was awarded a further £20,000 so that he could enjoy "a state of ease, affluence and independence for the remainder of his days."

Jenner refused to accept the claims made by others on behalf of Jesty. He was especially contemptuous of George Pearson and "his treatment of me before the committee of the House of Commons, the portrait of the farmer from the Isle of Purbeck with the farmer's claim to reward as the discoverer [of vaccination] at the foot of it, with a thousand minor tricks." Nevertheless, Pearson's claims had been occasioned by the testimonies of four independent witnesses—Mr. Dolling, Dr. Pulteney, Dr. Drewe, and Dr. Bell—who confirmed Jesty's work and his priority over Jenner. Jenner's attempt to personalize the debate about his priority by pointing to previous disagreements with Pearson, which would have cast doubt on Pearson's motivation, was a blatant attempt to obfuscate the truth. Jenner probably believed that a simple farmer could not have had the intelligence to make the connection between cowpox and protection against smallpox. In an essay published in the *Artist* in 1807, while he was awaiting Parliament's decision on his second claim for financial support, Jenner outlined a sevenfold classification of the human intellect. He described the Idiot, a vegetative being; the Dolt, a weak and poor creature; Mediocrity, most of mankind; Mental Perfection; Eccentricity; Insanity; and the Maniac. Jenner believed this essay to be of sufficient merit to have it reprinted in 1820. Fisher comments that this work was "a fair summary of the common eighteenth-century wisdom on mental attributes, elevated slightly by being ordered into classes." One wonders where Jenner would have placed Jesty and himself in his classification.

To reduce a scientific discovery to the activities of a single person is to misunderstand the process of scientific achievement. If it had not been for country folklore, neither Jesty nor Jenner would have had the idea for their experiments. The work of Cline, Pearson, and Woodville corroborated Jenner's observations and brought them to greater public attention. The ultimate explanation of why the name of Jenner is attached to the discovery of vaccination was stated simply by John Fosbroke in 1829: "Had he not both fortune, fame and high alliance, his merit would have been crushed or faintly supported."

In 1967, the World Health Organization stated its wish to eradicate smallpox. The estimated number of cases in the world at that time was over ten million. And yet, ten years later, WHO was able to announce that endemic smallpox had indeed been extinguished. But who now remembers the inscription on the tombstone of Benjamin Jesty in Worth Matravus Church in Dorset: "an upright honest man particularly noted for having been the first person (known) that introduced the cowpox by inoculation, and who from his great strength of mind, made the experiment"?

"Doctors' Dilemma: Damned If They Publish, Damned If They Don't." So ran the headline on Friday, February 27, 1998, in a leading British newspaper,[2] after *The Lancet* published an extraordinary study linking the widely used measles, mumps, and rubella (MMR) vaccine with a previously undescribed syndrome of autism and bowel disease. The acrimonious debate that has raged in the UK ever since has cost governments millions of pounds to shore up damaged vaccination campaigns, harmed the reputations and careers of several highly respected physicians and scientists, pitted anxious parents against their confused doctors, and provoked a backlash of vicious opprobrium against a few individuals deemed culpable for their reckless endangerment of the public's health (I was enthusiastically thrown into this last category by some of the great and the good of British medicine).

Today vaccines are largely an untouchable subject, their benefits too obvious to be questioned. Any hint of dissent concerning their clinical effectiveness and all-around social value is met with bitter rebuttal and resentment. Peter Lachmann, now Sir Peter and the former president of the UK Academy of Medical Sciences, once telephoned me in a fury and threatened to get me sacked for publishing work that raised questions about the MMR vaccine (and, to make matters worse in his mind, genetically modified foods). I also well remember a question barked at me at a dinner party almost five years after we had published this controversial research. "Will you *ever* be forgiven?" spat the partner of a government vaccine specialist. Forgiven for what, I wondered?

Yet, in a sense, the newspaper headline did capture one aspect of *The Lancet*'s (and my) difficulty when Dr. Andrew Wakefield and his colleagues sent their manuscript to the journal for publication in 1997. Their main goal was to report twelve children with an intriguing new syndrome. When parents were asked if they had noticed any event prior to the onset of symptoms, two said none, one reported an ear infection, another thought of measles, and eight said the MMR vaccine. "We did not prove an association," Wakefield wrote.[3] As is usual for any research paper, it was sent for peer review to experts in the field of study. In the case of the Wakefield paper, four reviewers made favorable comments, although questions about the methods used and interpretations drawn were raised—and justifiable concern was expressed about the impact of the findings on the public's confidence in a very important vaccine. The paper was revised and edited to make sure it was clear to readers that absolutely no proof existed that the MMR vaccine had caused this strange syndrome. We highlighted the preliminary nature of these findings by finally publishing the article under the heading "Early Report."

We also tried to remind readers of the benefits of measles vaccination. We reported figures showing that existing measles vaccines had reduced the number of cases of infection by almost 100 percent, and cut the annual number in the US alone from 900,000 in 1941 to just 135 in 1997. While two respected vaccine experts, Robert T. Chen and Frank DeStefano from the US Centers for Disease Control and Prevention, invited readers to examine the Wakefield data "with an open mind," they obviously doubted the veracity of the alleged association themselves. Proof would have to await "critical virological studies." They ruefully pointed out that vaccine scares tended to occur when vaccines were at their most effective: once the realities of the disease being prevented have been forgotten, low-grade risks assume a disproportionate significance in the public's mind.[4] According to the latest data from WHO, 745,000 people died of measles in 2001.[5] Chen and DeStefano warned that reports such as Wakefield's "may snowball into societal tragedies when the media and the public confuse association with causality and shun immunisation." Despite our best efforts as editors, a snowballing effect is exactly what happened. I take responsibility for all subsequent events, since there is no doubt that by being published in *The Lancet* this work was given more credibility than it deserved as evidence of a link between the MMR vaccine and the new syndrome.

Some of the research team decided to hold a press conference to announce their findings. This gave them an opportunity to stress the benefits of the MMR vaccine and the inconclusive nature of their findings with respect to the link between the syndrome and the vaccine. But even though the event was chaired by Arie Zuckerman, dean of the medical school where Wakefield worked and a noted vaccine expert himself, the press conference did far more harm than good. Instead of avoiding any unfounded recommendations about the safety of the triple vaccine, the team's press release said:

> The majority opinion among the researchers involved in this study supports the continuation of MMR vaccination. Dr. Wakefield feels that vaccination against the measles, mumps, and rubella infections should undoubtedly continue but until this issue is resolved by further research there is a case for separating the three vaccines into separate measles, mumps, and rubella components and giving them individually spaced by at least 1 year.

An accompanying Royal Free Hospital video news release opened with a child being vaccinated. Since the vaccine's three separate components were not available separately in the UK, Wakefield's advice at the press conference was taken, for all practical purposes, as a recommendation to parents not to have their children vaccinated at all. Despite the clear caveats in the research paper, Wakefield and the Royal Free Hospital implied that the link between the MMR vaccine and the new syndrome was far stronger than it really was. I am not passing the blame here. There would have been no press conference or press release, video or otherwise, if *The Lancet* had not published the study in the first place. But the additional later twists to a message that we had carefully tried to craft on paper certainly did not assist the gentle landing that I had hoped for in the media.

The Wakefield findings eventually found their way to the US Congress, when Representative Dan Burton, chairman of the Committee on Government Reform, launched an investigation into rising rates of autism in America.[6] Burton's inquiry was triggered by his own experiences as the grandfather of a child who later developed autism. He opened his hearing, which included then-unpublished evidence presented by Wakefield, with a story explaining his own personal interest in this issue:

> I don't have to read a letter to experience the heartbreak. I see it in my own family. My grandson Christian was born healthy. He was beautiful and tall. We were already planning his NBA career. Then, his mother took him for his routine immunizations and all of that changed. He was given what so many children were given—DTP, OPV, Haemophilis, hepatitis B, and MMR—all at one office visit. That night Christian had a slight fever and he slept for long periods of time.... When he was awake he would scream for hours.... Over the week-and-a-half after the vaccinations, Christian would stare into space and act like he

> was deaf. He would hit himself and others.... He would shake his head from side to side as fast as he could. He lost all language. Unfortunately, what happened to Christian is not a rare isolated event. I am not against vaccinations, and I don't think that *every* autistic child acquires autism after receiving childhood immunizations. However, there is enough evidence emerging of some kind of a connection for some children that we can't close our eyes to it.

Six families then gave evidence linking the MMR vaccine to their child's illness. Experts followed these parents, but their testimonies were conflicting—and ultimately inconclusive. Nevertheless, Burton has continued his campaign. In November 2002, he wrote to President Bush inviting him to host a White House conference on autism and to ask why the condition had reached epidemic proportions—up from one in 10,000 in the 1980s to one in 250 today.

Meanwhile, the reaction to Wakefield's 1998 research was immediate and intense. Experts from WHO argued that the *Lancet* paper "fails at every level to make a causal association." They questioned the merit of publishing these findings, describing the event as "tragic." Other critics bemoaned the public concern generated by widespread and alarmist reporting in the mass media, which was "out of proportion to the strength of evidence presented,"[7] and thought that controversial and newsworthy work should carry health warnings.[8] Correspondents emphasized not only the speculative nature of the research but also the likelihood of a "public health disaster." Criticism was sometimes highly (and, for a scientific debate, unusually) personal: "I think you [the editor of *The Lancet*] will bear a heavy responsibility for acting against the public health interest which you usually aim to promote. Moreover, you will only increase the anguish of the parents of the sick children with whom all doctors will sympathise."

Since a split among the scientific team had opened up at the Royal

Free press conference, replies to these critics came from two distinct camps. Andrew Wakefield emphasized his duty to his patients, who were coming to him with an illness that had to be explained. This duty came before his responsibility to the entire health of the public, he seemed to be saying. He wrote: "The approach of the clinical scientists should reflect the first and most important lesson learnt as a medical student—to listen to the patient or the patient's parent, and they will tell you the truth.... This is a lesson in humility that, as doctors, we ignore at our peril."

By contrast, the specialists in intestinal diseases of children replied separately. They were led by Professor John Walker-Smith, a distinguished pediatric scientist. He argued that it was right to publish these findings, given the consistency of observations in the gut of affected children. The debate about the MMR vaccine as the cause of these intestinal abnormalities had been "emotionally charged," but, he and his colleagues believed, "notably balanced."

There was heavy lobbying against me in private as well as in public. A former director of the UK's Public Health Laboratory Service, who had also been a member of the government's Joint Committee on Vaccination and Immunisation for seventeen years, wrote confidentially to the chairman of *The Lancet*'s editorial board in April 1998 to express his dismay about my decision to publish Wakefield's findings. He accused me of responding defensively and of failing to repair the damage already done to the public health or to *The Lancet*'s reputation for sound judgment in its publication policy. He suggested, on what grounds he did not make clear, that the paper had not been peer-reviewed. And he argued that I should not have published such a preliminary report in a journal with *The Lancet*'s reputation and readership. He chose not to write to me directly and presumably did not want me to know that he had written at all. There is no chairman of *The Lancet*'s editorial board, and so his letter did come to me. I replied, probably defensively, but did not hear from him again.

Other critics claimed that my motivation was one of pure self-interest. Simon Fradd, a senior figure in the British Medical Association, wrote in the UK newspaper *Doctor* that "the process of peer review in accepting this paper for publication in a high-profile medical magazine needs examining. Does the paper stand up to professional scrutiny or is there an element of recognising the effect of the resulting publicity on circulation?" If he is suggesting that we select research papers for publication because we think readers of *The Lancet* might be interested in reading them, then he is obviously correct. It would be a strange journal indeed if we chose work designed to make readers turn the page in boredom. But our efforts to put the work in context did fail.

Although I knew that this paper would be controversial, I did not expect the level of vituperative attack and personal rebuke that followed. I was terribly and, looking back now, embarrassingly naive. I should have met with the Royal Free team before they held their press conference. I should have at least tried to persuade Andrew Wakefield not to recommend splitting the vaccine. I should have seen the Royal Free's video and stopped their overzealous publicity office from drawing attention to vaccination. All in all, my attitude was far too laissez-faire. If this is what critics meant—and still mean—by reckless, then I am guilty of that charge. I failed to do enough to manage the media reaction to this work. Until the Wakefield paper, I had not seen this media management role as one for a scientific medical journal editor. I now see it as one of my main responsibilities.

But I do not regret publishing the original Wakefield paper. Progress in medicine depends on the free expression of new ideas. In science, it was only this commitment to free expression that shook free the tight grip of religion on the way human beings understood their world. Sometimes the ideas proposed will be unpalatable. Nobody wanted to believe the existence of the first few cases of AIDS in the early 1980s. Nobody wanted to believe that bovine spongiform encephalopathy

(BSE) would somehow jump species to cause variant Creutzfeldt-Jakob disease among humans. In that instance, it was the suppression of concerns about this possibility that led to massive public fear and anger when the first cases were confirmed. Whenever new ideas are reported, they must be subsequently tested to check their reproducibility and validity. Verification is the right test of new thinking, not censorship. Debate since publication of the Wakefield paper has established that his work opened up an important new field of science—the relation between the brain and the intestine in the etiology of autism.[9]

There was also an unpleasant whiff of arrogance in this whole debate. Can the public not be trusted with a controversial hypothesis? Must people be protected from information judged too sensitive for their consumption by a scientific elite? The view that the public cannot interpret uncertainty indicates an old-fashioned paternalism at work. But one could argue that believing in unfettered open debate, while intellectually credible (that is, the public is entitled to know as much as possible), ignores the brutal realities of the disease. The fall in rates of MMR vaccination after publication of the Wakefield paper was striking. In the UK, MMR vaccine coverage in children over two years of age was above 90 percent in the pre-Wakefield era. One year later, rates had fallen to 87.6 percent, a small but significant drop. The rate had dropped still further, to 83.8 percent, by July 2002. Measles outbreaks occurred in poorly protected communities. Creating the conditions for a resurgence of measles is bad medicine. Or is it? Good medicine, by this definition, means forcing families to immunize their children with the MMR vaccine. Fortunately, we do not yet live in a police state where public health doctors dictate what we can do (exercise and eat fruit) and what we cannot (smoke and eat burgers), even if their advice is wise and reasonable. If one of the results of freedom of choice is an adverse outcome for the public's health, that is a regrettable but necessary consequence of our democracy. The responsibility rests with public health experts to educate and to persuade with understanding and compassion—not to berate with anger and frustration. And medical journals are not instruments of the public health service. Medical journals are simply highly specialized newspapers. We publish what is new and newsworthy in medicine and we do our best to publish work that is true. But only time, sometimes a long time, will tell if we have chosen well.

Another argument that is harder to refute concerns the rights of the child (and I write here as the father of a two-year-old girl who has had the MMR vaccine). If the balance of medical opinion is that the MMR vaccine is safe, which is indeed the case, do parents have the right to deny their children the vaccine, a denial that could, in rare circumstances, lead to the death not only of their child but also of other children? Is such a denial even a form of child abuse? As a father and a doctor, I can see that it may well be so. But most parents I know have agonized deeply over whether to give their children MMR. Certainly I have. These parents are not neglectful or irresponsible. They are not abusing their children. They are simply and genuinely uncertain about what to do. And events such as the BSE crisis have made them mistrustful of what government scientists tell them. Doctors cannot condemn families, as some have, for being skeptical of experts. On many occasions—BSE is one good example—we should have been *more* skeptical. And doctors are not without their own mercenary motivations for encouraging vaccination. In the UK, doctors are paid extra money for reaching certain vaccination targets. The MMR debate threatened those targets. One primary care physician wrote to me: "Thanks to your publication of insubstantial erroneous so-called research you are single-handedly reducing my income by £2–3000." In February 2003 *The Times* reported that because of this financial penalty doctors were refusing to register children onto their patient lists if parents refused the MMR vaccine. This practice was widespread, said general practitioners. Hypocrisy surrounds the whole MMR debacle.

Since 1998, Andrew Wakefield has published extensively about the risks of the MMR vaccine and measles infection. And Prime Minister Tony Blair caused thousands of parents to waver once again over vaccinating their children when he refused to disclose whether his own son had received the MMR vaccine. But others have convincingly refuted any association between the vaccine and autism in large studies across different populations. Scientific committees have studied these data and found no support for Wakefield's views. Not one person or group has confirmed the original finding published in *The Lancet*. On balance, there is no substantiated evidence that the MMR vaccine causes an autism-like syndrome, although the possibility of a rare idiosyncratic reaction to the vaccine cannot be completely ruled out. For Wakefield, the past five years have seen the collapse of his career at a leading London teaching hospital. I worked at the Royal Free from 1988 to 1990 and met him on many occasions. He is a committed, engaging, and charismatic clinician and scientist. He asks big questions about diseases—what are their ultimate causes?—and his ambition often brings quick and impressive results. But his findings sometimes have limited staying power, and are overturned or substantially modified by less iconoclastic colleagues. His reputation unfairly in tatters, Wakefield resigned from the Royal Free Hospital, realizing that he had no future there and that he would be virtually unemployable in the work that he wanted to do anywhere else in the UK. There were rumors, not denied, that he was put under pressure by university authorities to leave. His colleagues, once so eager to pursue their careers on his coattails, mostly abandoned him. He now divides his time between the US and UK, running a research program on autism in Florida.

Professor John Walker-Smith, the senior pediatric gastroenterologist who looked after the Royal Free children described in the first *Lancet* report, has only recently given his side of this desperately unhappy story.[10] Walker-Smith was "shocked to see the autistic children with very severely disturbed and often destructive behaviour."

He was and remains skeptical of a direct link with the MMR vaccine, but he believes "that there appears to be a small highly selected group of children where there is a risk." While Walker-Smith refused to attend the 1998 press conference, an event he describes as "a great mistake," he sees Wakefield as "a man of utter sincerity and honesty." For his loyalty and commitment to the children under his care, Walker-Smith received hate mail from medical colleagues. He will be called to give evidence in MMR vaccine litigation planned for 2004.

What are the lessons of this sad affair? First, the debate took place because there were almost no safety data about the MMR vaccine to draw on when serious questions were initially posed. This absence of evidence was pointed out by Dr. Thomas Jefferson, head of the vaccine research group of the Cochrane Collaboration, a network of independent investigators who review evidence about important questions in medicine. Jefferson found that the existing research about MMR vaccine safety was poor, although there was no evidence to indicate that the vaccine was dangerous.[11] Second, the way the Wakefield paper was received and discussed in public showed a misunderstanding about the nature of the research process by doctors and journalists alike. A research paper published in a medical journal is not the last word on a subject, an event to be reported on its own. A new finding is simply work in progress, part of a continuous process of advance and retreat in our knowledge about disease. Third, I learned to be a more engaged editor when it came to the media. The MMR vaccine story taught me that science is no different from politics in this respect. Splits, rows, and dissent from orthodoxy all make news. There was no point in being reticent about taking part in a wider public debate if one was going to start it in the first place. Finally, the style of the debate about the MMR vaccine showed how far we are from what Clifford Geertz once identified as the goal of anthropology as a science, a goal that applies to other disciplines: "[Its] progress is marked less by a perfection of consensus than a refinement of debate. What gets better is the precision with which we vex each other."[12] The MMR vaccine has certainly vexed a great many people. But a refined debate? It seems that none of us are quite ready for that just yet.

* * *

I arrived at the University of Birmingham as an eighteen-year-old medical student in 1980. The atmosphere was gray and somber. That summer, a highly critical report into a smallpox outbreak at the medical school was published.[13] Birmingham became a much-reviled institution. Thanks to abysmally lax safety procedures, smallpox had escaped from a laboratory and infected a medical photographer named Janet Parker. A previously healthy forty-year-old woman, she fell ill, but not very ill at first, on August 11, 1978. The characteristic rash of fluid-filled vesicles erupted a week later. She died on September 11, despite having been vaccinated against smallpox some twelve years earlier. Her death caused panic across Britain and the rest of the world. WHO was about to pronounce smallpox completely eradicated. This would have been the agency's greatest triumph, and a landmark in the history of human disease. The last known natural case of smallpox had been reported in a Somalian hospital cook, Ali Maow Maalin, in October 1977. Unlike Mrs. Parker, he lived.

The case was a double tragedy. The man in charge of Birmingham's smallpox laboratory was Henry Bedson, a brilliant and much-respected scientist who had played an important part in the effort to eradicate the disease. Bedson had ambitions of making his laboratory a collaborating center of WHO, which would have catapulted him and his team to a far higher level of international recognition than had hitherto been possible. But his application had failed, meaning he would have to close his research program within a year or so. This was a great personal and professional setback for him—a "bombshell," as he described it. It was Bedson who diagnosed Janet Parker's illness—variola major, the more severe form of smallpox. But before she died, he committed suicide by taking a knife to his throat at home on the day the government announced an official inquiry into the Birmingham outbreak. He was forty-nine years old. Another Birmingham professor also attempted suicide. He lived, and I remember him as an aloof, muttering figure, nervously wandering the corridors of the medical school. As a result of Janet Parker's infection, over three hundred people in Birmingham were quarantined, and travelers abroad had to undergo smallpox vaccination at short notice to prevent the theoretical but potentially catastrophic risk of spread to the European continent.

The government inquiry into the Birmingham smallpox "occurrence" was scathing about the university's safety procedures. Practices had been dangerous, multiple new smallpox strains were imported into the laboratory without notification of the statutory authority, and the staff, especially Professor Bedson, were so overburdened with other duties that they were distracted from what should have been their main task—namely, to monitor closely a lethal virus being manipulated in an insecure laboratory. What safety procedures did exist were poorly implemented and improperly evaluated. WHO had also expressed its dissatisfaction about procedures in Birmingham. Despite repeated warnings, Bedson had done nothing to tighten laboratory safety. Indeed, he had accelerated the pace and volume of his team's work on smallpox. The causes of his suicide were all too clear.

Smallpox has done much to shape human history. The disease weakened Roman armies, thus weakening the Roman state. It may have caused the decline of the Aztec empire in the sixteenth century. Smallpox seems to have been a "blessing in disguise," according to Myles Standish, for the first settlers in America. Once it had killed most of the Native American population living along what is now the New England coastline, the settlers were free to make their homes among the debris of another people. And a massive smallpox epidemic, triggered by the Franco-Prussian War in 1870, killed half a million people across Europe. Even in the 1950s, smallpox infected 50 million people each year, killing every fourth victim it struck. Eventually, the disease was rolled back by vaccination. Members of the Global Commission for the Certification of Smallpox Eradication signed the declaration confirming the virus's demise on December 9, 1979. This final statement of eradication is the most important public health document ever written.

But smallpox has come back to pose another threat—as a bioweapon. The original plan to destroy the last remaining stocks of the virus was halted after 9/11. In a dramatic reversal, WHO decided that security demands—research to develop new vaccines, for example—outweighed the public health goal of total eradication. In 1999, D. A. Henderson, the man who led the smallpox eradication campaign, had argued that "in the US, there is no reason to pursue a vaccine research agenda." Smallpox now exists in only two known locations—the Centers for Disease Control in the US and the Center for Research on Virology and Biotechnology in Koltsovo, Russia, but nobody can be sure that stocks do not exist elsewhere. Yet smallpox would be an inefficient bioweapon. It is best spread face-to-face, unlike anthrax. And it is much less robust, dying when exposed to the air. However, evidence published in 2002 suggests that techniques are now available to aerosolize smallpox for distribution by wind over great distances.

Fear is a much more potent force than evidence in influencing government policy. In the UK, Dr. Ian Gibson, the chairman of Parliament's Science and Technology Committee, has called for the entire population to be immunized against smallpox. Is the threat of smallpox that great? The British government argues that vaccination would probably kill more people—about one or two per million, together with up to a thousand severe adverse reactions per million—than any outbreak of smallpox.[14] Instead, protecting the civilian population against a smallpox attack depends on rapid diagnosis, quarantining those exposed, and targeting vaccination to health workers and those immediately exposed to the disease.

Given the risks of smallpox and the very real dangers of the vaccine, there remains a furious political debate about the merits of targeted versus mass vaccination. The best way to end this uncertainty is to test each approach in the midst of an epidemic. But this solution is obviously impossible—and unreasonable, even if possible. Computer modeling offers one way to answer the question. The difficulty is, as one might expect, that there is more than one model of a smallpox outbreak. Each model can be used to support either a targeted or a mass-vaccination approach.[15] Because of this uncertainty, no one can be sure that President Bush's policy, announced on December 13, 2002, is the right one. After meeting with senior public health officials, who all lined up against mass vaccinations, Bush's team decided to opt for a compromise—to immunize half a million military personnel and offer the vaccine on a voluntary basis to health workers and first-responders (that is, those at highest risk of coming into contact with the virus). After these people have been vaccinated, by the summer of 2003, the vaccine will be offered to other essential personnel, perhaps as many as ten million police, firefighters, and others. This cautious policy goes against the instincts of those who believe that it is an individual citizen's right, and not the government's, to decide whether to have the vaccine. But with the first report in February 2003 of a severe reaction to the smallpox vaccine in a Florida nurse, this cautious attitude seems to have been vindicated. In the UK, the policy is "search and contain." Twelve rapid-response groups are being set up around the country to enable prompt isolation of confirmed or suspected cases of smallpox. Vaccine stocks are being strengthened. Key staff are being immunized and trained.

An additional problem facing politicians and public health specialists is the level of public awareness and knowledge about smallpox. A disease that was eradicated a generation ago and lives on only as an imaginary terrorist threat is ripe for misunderstanding. A study of over a thousand American adults by the Harvard School of Public

Health provides a disturbing insight into public perceptions of smallpox. Over 60 percent thought it somewhat or very likely that a smallpox attack would take place in the event of military action against Iraq. Almost two thirds believed there had been cases of smallpox somewhere in the world during the past five years; 30 percent thought that there had been cases in America too; 78 percent believed that there is an effective treatment (there is not). Most people said that they would survive if they caught the infection. A quarter of people surveyed thought death likely if they were vaccinated. Sixty-one percent would choose vaccination if it were offered as a precaution against a terrorist attack.[16] As the authors of this study rather modestly conclude, there is "substantial misinformation among Americans about smallpox and smallpox vaccination." The public is also at odds with experts over access to the vaccine: more want it, and they seem to want it now.

The Monterey Institute of International Studies identifies Algeria, Cuba, India, Russia, Sudan, and Taiwan as probably or possibly having research programs in bioweapons; and China, Egypt, Iran, Iraq, Israel, Libya, North Korea, Pakistan, and Syria as having offensive programs and likely or possible bioweapon production facilities. And their analysis does not take account of the threat posed by al-Qaeda. The public would be right to seek preventive reassurance, whether it is at the end of a needle or otherwise.

But the signs are that despite the political rhetoric of a smallpox risk, the launch of a preemptive war with Iraq, and a genuine public fear of bioterrorism, most Americans are skeptical about the value of vaccination in the face of an only theoretical threat. In January 2003 Bush called for half a million volunteer health workers to be immunized against smallpox. Tommy Thompson, his secretary for health and human services, pledged to achieve this target within a month. But by March the program had stalled, with only a few thousand people stepping forward to receive the vaccine. Many hospitals and public health departments declined to take part in the government's campaign—health workers judged that the risks easily outweighed the benefits. What they demanded was proof of a credible threat. That proof was not forthcoming. It seemed that, as with MMR, the public was displaying a need to see the evidence for itself. Passing that evidence through an expert or a political leader and relying on their authority to trigger public action was no longer sufficient.

MMR and smallpox are low-risk, high-emotion issues. They occupy the public and media imaginations about vaccines almost to the exclusion of all else. But the greatest protectors of human survival will be vaccines against HIV, malaria, and tuberculosis. And here the news is grim.

Every AIDS vaccine produced so far has failed. Worse still, there is no prospect that an effective AIDS vaccine will be available anytime soon, and certainly not within the next five years. A serious misstep took place in February 2002, when the internationally respected HIV Vaccine Trials Network announced that two promising candidates were, for all practical clinical purposes, inactive. The US National Institute of Allergy and Infectious Diseases, together with two manufacturers, Aventis Pasteur and VaxGen, had hoped to test this regimen in an $80 million clinical trial involving 12,000 people. Although the two vaccines caused no adverse effects, they were so weak that testing them in further trials would have been "scientifically inappropriate." Sugar was sprinkled liberally over this bitter news. Larry Corey, the principal scientist involved in the study, pledged to continue working with these vaccines at different doses and in different populations. But the fact was that another vaccine trial had ended in disappointment, and a once hopeful line of research was extinguished.

A further, but not unexpected, blow came in 2003, when the results of a three-year-long trial to test AIDSVAX, also made by VaxGen, drew a blank. The active component of AIDSVAX is a protein that sits on the surface of HIV, called gp120. The driving force behind this VaxGen study was the $18 million that Genentech demanded before giving away the patents to the vaccine. Two clinical trials were simply pegs on which to hang a justification for a new biotechnology company. The first study (a second is taking place in Thailand) found no variations in HIV infection among five thousand volunteers. However, VaxGen made much of a statistically significant but biologically implausible reduction in HIV rates among African-Americans and other ethnic minorities. Philip Berman, VaxGen's senior vice-president of research and development, made the surprising claim that "this is the first time we have specific numbers to suggest that a vaccine has prevented HIV infection in humans." Other scientists were more cautious, calling the company's spin misleading and premature. The fact is that AIDSVAX will not save one life.

The contrast with treatment could not be more striking. Since the introduction of highly active drugs directed against HIV in 1996, many of the illnesses associated with AIDS have declined in incidence by over 90 percent. Death rates have also fallen. In Europe, before 1995, for example, over a third of HIV-positive patients would have received no drug treatment. By 1999, almost 80 percent were receiving triple drug therapy, and only one in twenty were taking no medications at all. Globally, the most pressing issue is access to these effective medicines. Progress in vaccines is a long way behind.

Yet today, the rhetoric of AIDS vaccines is almost universally upbeat. It has to be. At the end of 2002, 42 million people were living with HIV. A third of this number are between fifteen and twenty-four years old. Almost two thirds live in sub-Saharan Africa, where there is no reliable access to treatment or prevention services. AIDS has become the world's fourth-biggest killer, with 16,000 new infections daily. The political response to AIDS has been strong, and rightly so, but commitments to controlling the virus are hopelessly unrealistic. In one of those desperate acts of hand-wringing that serve mostly to absolve politicians of their global guilt, a United Nations General Assembly Special Session in June 2001 made 2005 the target for reducing HIV infection among that group of fifteen- to twenty-four-year-olds by a quarter. Without a vaccine, this figure will never be met. Inevitably, therefore, another target will be missed, further hand-wringing will take place, and still more improbable goals will be set at grand gatherings of world leaders. The cycles of empty propaganda will continue to turn.

Yet there is an AIDS vaccine strategy that deserves careful scrutiny. The HIV Vaccine Trials Network is the largest international grouping of scientists working on an AIDS vaccine. The network aims to produce a regimen "with more than 95 per cent protection from acquisition [of HIV], for all persons in all regions of the world." But over thirty candidate vaccines have come and gone since volunteers were first enrolled into trials in 1988. Rarely has science failed so spectacularly.

Incredibly, there is still no agreement about what a vaccine must do to protect human beings from infection. HIV exists as genetically distinct subtypes, called clades, and the commonest subtype of HIV worldwide is clade C. Most vaccine candidates currently being studied are clade B—the subtype most often found in the US and Europe, where there are the fewest number of infections. Not one of nine candidates currently undergoing trials is directed toward Africa, where the body count from AIDS makes a vaccine an urgent priority. Of nineteen further vaccines in development, only five include clade C. AIDS vaccine manufacturers have pursued a program driven by profit, not human need.

The HIV Vaccine Trials Network has become part of the profit-driven culture. It describes itself as a hybrid body, having "an organisational structure closer to that of a commercial vaccine company." The network depends on "strong collaborations" with vaccine developers. These "partnerships" between publicly funded research centers and commercial companies are a significant departure from the norms of academic research. When a new drug is developed, a company will sponsor scientists to test the drug's safety and efficacy among patients.

But in the best trials—those that lead to the drug being approved for widespread use—the sponsor is kept at arm's length from the scientists and their work. This standard of rigorous scientific independence protects patients from undue commercial pressure on the doctors responsible for their care; but the principle has been sacrificed in HIV vaccine research, in order to induce large companies to invest in a disease that largely affects the developing world. The policy of the US vaccine network allows manufacturers to have access to the once independent scientific apparatus of study design, data analysis, and safety monitoring. In drug trials, such transgressions into the scientific process would be regarded as highly improper conflicts of interest. Yet they are becoming the new norm in HIV vaccine studies.

The intricate biology of HIV has made a vaccine unusually elusive. Part of the difficulty rests within ourselves, as well as with the virus. We humans have two very different arms to our immune systems, and it seems that both must be activated to counter the threat of HIV. One arm is well known: it produces antibodies to neutralize invading proteins. But antibodies alone cannot quell HIV. Instead, immune protection mediated by cells rather than antibodies seems necessary. Newer HIV vaccine candidates now aim to activate both antibody and cell-mediated immunity. Work on laboratory animals indicates that blood cells called cytotoxic T lymphocytes, commonly known as killer T cells, can protect against new HIV infections by killing other cells infected with HIV. Encouraging these cells to line up in our defense now dominates thinking among HIV vaccine researchers.

The most tantalizing vaccine work so far relies on a small group of sex workers in Nairobi, Kenya. They have been exposed to large quantities of HIV—six clients a day for up to fifteen years—but they have not become infected. Their protection correlates with the activity of killer T cells specific to HIV. Protection is not permanent. If the woman's exposure to HIV declines, so does her protection. Perversely, perhaps, continued exposure to HIV seems necessary for continued protection.

Given the potency of the virus to elicit immunity in some circumstances, is a live but attenuated version of HIV a vaccine possibility? This strategy worked for Albert Sabin's oral polio vaccine. But the dangers are immense. While experiments in monkeys indicated that a live attenuated virus could protect against subsequent infection, an observation that sent waves of premature excitement through the AIDS vaccine community, it is also now clear that HIV eventually breaks through this early immunity. A vaccine that in the long run causes AIDS is a frightful thought. Still, a new trial of an HIV vaccine, based on DNA from the virus itself, began in Uganda in 2003. The origins of the idea for this vaccine came from the sex workers of Nairobi. Results from a safety study of this experimental vaccine are expected in 2005.

The reality of designing a vaccine against HIV is that no single agent will ever protect all people all of the time. Combinations of vaccines are a more likely solution. Even then, the chances that a vaccine will be 95 percent effective are low; HIV will behave more like influenza, for which vaccines are only 40 to 80 percent effective. But even with this variable efficacy, in high-prevalence areas a vaccine offering, say, 50 percent protection could be valuable. Were such a vaccine to be produced, however, the barriers to its introduction would still be formidable.

The first trial of an HIV vaccine in Africa raised many practical difficulties. Misperceptions about the vaccine (that it would somehow protect against unsafe sex) and the study (that volunteers would be exposed to HIV deliberately) were common. Approval of the trial became a complex political process, requiring parliamentary debate and the support of the president of Uganda. Implementation of the study demanded a rethinking of consent procedures—words such as "placebo" were unknown in the local language and had to be rendered differently ("placebo" became "air supply"). Newspaper reports stirred up concern about the vaccine's safety, fueled by jealous disagreements among scientists. The purely scientific challenges of engineering a vaccine are only a small part of the difficulties facing countries burdened with HIV.

In a perfect world, an HIV vaccine should be 100 percent safe, 100 percent effective, produce long-lasting protection, be easy to administer, and cheap. None of these ideals will be met. But opinions about the future prospects for a vaccine are surprisingly diverse. Writing in the journal *Vaccine* in 2001, Michael Klein, a scientist from Aventis Pasteur, found "reason for optimism." In the same journal, also in 2001, Veljko Veljkovic and his colleagues argued "the urgent requirement for a moratorium" on vaccine research "to protect potentially hazardous health risks for vaccinees."

Two years ago, at a dinner at the British ambassador's residence in Addis Ababa, I sat next to an irascible French diplomat who became even more choleric when I asked him about the world's policies toward the millions of people dying from HIV/AIDS in Africa. "There is no hope," he told me. "We must simply draw a line between their lives and the future." He had nothing but contempt for the collectively furrowed brows of political elites. He believed that, with respect to HIV/AIDS, there was little the rich could offer the poor. Even if drugs and a vaccine did become available, it would be too late for most Africans. Although brutally put, there was a kernel of truth in what he said; and despite the vast efforts of many, together with the trenchant idealism of a few, there is truth in it today. As far as a vaccine is concerned, he will be right for many years to come.

Many of the same difficulties, especially lack of commercial interest or incentive, apply to vaccines for tuberculosis and malaria. Helen L. Collins and Stefan H.E. Kaufmann, reviewing the prospects for a tuberculosis vaccine, concluded that "to our knowledge there is currently no new vaccine candidate scheduled for clinical trials in human beings."[17] For a bacterium that infects eight million new people each year, and kills two million, that surreal state of neglect is utterly shameful.

In WHO's summary of the state of the world's vaccines,[18] homage is rightly paid to the near eradication of polio. But WHO also points to gross inequalities in access to vaccines. Thirty-seven million children globally do not receive routine immunizations. In Somalia, for example, fewer than one in five children are vaccinated against diphtheria, tetanus, and pertussis. A new grouping was launched in 2000 to realize the right of every child to immunization against major infectious diseases. The Global Alliance for Vaccines and Immunisation (GAVI) started with an initial grant of $750 million over five years from the Bill and Melinda Gates Foundation. GAVI brings together WHO, UNICEF, the World Bank, and governments—all with the goal of expanding coverage and fostering research into new vaccines. The task is enormous.[19] Many good vaccines are underused—for example, those for hepatitis B and yellow fever. And, in addition to HIV, TB, and malaria, vaccines are desperately needed for diarrheal diseases, bacterial pneumonia, meningitis, dengue, leishmaniasis, and schistosomiasis.

The future for vaccines became a little brighter in 2003. GAVI announced two $30 million grants to the Johns Hopkins School of Public Health to ensure that vaccines against rotavirus and pneumococcus would be available quickly to those most in need once they were licensed. Rotavirus is an important cause of diarrheal disease and a vaccine is expected to be available in 2005. Pneumococcus causes meningitis and pneumonia; a vaccine to protect against strains prevalent in developing countries is expected by 2007.

Vaccines have been one of the great success stories of human scientific ingenuity—and one of the most degrading examples of man's selfishness and greed. At last this paradox is being resolved.

# 7

## AN AUTOPSY OF DR. OSLER

IN THE EARLY summer of 1885, a thirty-six-year-old professor of medicine at the University of Pennsylvania crossed the Delaware River to visit an elderly man with a "transient indisposition." When William Osler walked into a front room on the ground floor of 328 Mickle Street, Camden, New Jersey, Walt Whitman—his new patient—was sitting in a corner. Over thirty years later, Osler, who was by then an immensely influential professor of medicine, recalled the moment:

> With a large frame, and well shaped, well poised head, covered with a profusion of snow-white hair, which mingled on the cheeks with a heavy long beard and moustache, Walt Whitman in his 65th year was a fine figure of a man who had aged beautifully, or more properly speaking majestically. The eyebrows were thick and shaggy and the man seemed lost in a hirsute canopy....

The scene astonished Osler. "The magazines and newspapers, piled higher than the desk, covered the floor so completely that I had to pick my way by the side of the wall of the room to get to the desk." After his house call, Osler began to read *Leaves of Grass* for the first time. The result was not pleasing to him: "Whether the meat was too strong, or whether it was the style of cooking—'twas not for my pampered palate, accustomed to Plato and Shakespeare and Shelley and Keats."

Whitman's view of Osler was similarly ambivalent. A man who was frequently pessimistic and bad-tempered about his own physical state, Whitman wrote, in 1888, that "Osler made light of my condition. I don't like his pooh-poohs: the professional air of a doctor grates on me." When, for example, Osler recommended that he "never let his bowels be closed more than two days," Whitman replied, "I will 'let': it's not a question of 'letting': if that was all there was about it, the matter could easily be settled." And Osler's incessant cheerfulness sometimes produced the opposite result of that intended: "I confess I do not wholly like or credit what he says—I do not fancy the jaunty way in which he seems inclined to dismiss the troubles."

Despite these complaints, Whitman concluded that Osler was "very 'cute, a natural physician, rather optimistic, but best so"; that "he is relieving me: no doctor could do more"; that "he is a great man—one of the rare men: I should be much surprised if he didn't soar way way up—get very famous at his trade—some day: he has the air of the thing about him—of achievement." Osler, he wrote, "is fine looking: examined, he gains on you: you realize him: his forehead is beautiful."

Whitman had good reason to be an accurate judge of his doctor. In *Specimen Days* he had chronicled a period during the American Civil War when he assisted wounded soldiers in a Washington hospital by tending their injuries, arranging for food and reading matter to be delivered to them, giving out small sums of money, writing their letters home, or simply keeping them company. Whitman testified to the "professional spirit and capacity generally prevailing among the surgeons, many of them young men, in the hospitals and the army." If Osler was aware of his new patient's war work among the sick, there is no record of it.

Osler's initial distaste for Whitman's writing was to soften later in life. Osler was invited to give "An Anniversary Address with Personal Reminiscences" about Whitman to Walter Raleigh's Oxford English literature class in 1919. Seven and a half pages of only partly published notes survive.[1] In his extensive research for the lecture, Osler described Whitman as a "patient and friend." And in a letter to *The Times* on May 31, 1919, he noted that Whitman was "possessed in rare degree of the Greek combination of the love of humanity with the love of a craft." Osler died on December 29, 1919, with his lecture unfinished.

There is a strange parallel between the lives of the poet and the doctor. Osler had been introduced to Whitman by their mutual friend and colleague Dr. Maurice Burke. Osler described Burke as a "hero-worshipper," a man who displayed "absolute idolatry" of Whitman. Where Osler "saw only a fine old man, full of common sense and kindly feelings," Burke claimed that Whitman was "one of the world's great prophets." Osler was intrigued by the influence that Whitman cast over other men; he described "a cult of a type such as no other literary man of our generation has been the object." Toward the end of his lecture notes, Osler underlines this view: "Whitman's greatness is in no way more clearly demonstrated than in his ability to survive the megalomaniac exaggerations of a cult."

In *William Osler: A Life in Medicine*, Michael Bliss draws on the Whitman connection to assist his own dissection of the present-day Osler cult.[2] Bliss gives a well-paced and intellectually fascinating account of Osler's life. He pins down the significant moments in a spectacularly diverse career as a physician and teacher of medicine who did original research on, among other subjects, the components of blood, and wrote in 1892 *The Principles and Practice of Medicine*,[3] perhaps the most widely read and admired medical textbook of its time. He sets Osler's scholarly achievements against the background of the usually neglected hinterland of his family affairs. Bliss quotes

Whitman approvingly on the work of a poet who "drags the dead out of their coffins and stands them again on their feet." But even for Bliss, an experienced biographer, the exaggerations that have grown around Osler's life prove hard to strip away.

Osler's upbringing gave little hint that he would eventually dominate Anglo-American medicine for thirty years. His family emigrated from England to Canada in 1837 and his father—Featherstone, a well-read clergyman—hoped that his eighth child would follow him into the Anglican ministry. William was a bright student at a Toronto private school, prone to pranks that led not only to expulsion (for shouting abuse at a teacher) but also, Bliss hints, to a few days in prison for cruelly persecuting an unpopular matron. The turning point in his school life came during a spell of illness, when he developed a passion for natural history and learned microscopy from his inspiring school warden, the Reverend William Arthur Johnson.

Still destined for clerical studies, Osler's mind was finally diverted to medicine by James Bovell, an eccentric Toronto physician infamous for transfusing milk into the arteries of patients with cholera. While studying medicine at McGill University, Osler was taken under the wing of another appreciative mentor, Palmer Howard, a physician with an interest in the new European sciences who helped Osler gain a precocious reputation for research.

Medicine was not a safe career in the 1870s, even for such a talented student as Osler. In 1872, he moved to London for what was the equivalent of medical finishing school. After declining an offer to become professor of botany at McGill, he traveled to Berlin and Vienna to study pathology in the great institutions led by Rudolf Virchow and Karl Rokitansky. Two years later he returned to a lectureship in McGill's medical faculty. Bliss describes Osler's difficult early career by charting his meager income as a Canadian tutor. In 1874, for example, he earned $1,129, and his salary had risen only a few hundred dollars by the end of the decade. This precarious situation forced Osler to develop a flourishing clinical practice to secure his finances. He also began to treat smallpox among the down and outs of Montreal, a gruesome task he carried out successfully. He threw himself into autopsy work, completing a thousand postmortems in the style of Virchow[4]; and he gave a hundred lectures in an exhausting first year at McGill. He was also beginning a successful research career, being one of the first scientists to describe a new type of blood cell that later came to be called the platelet.

Osler's time at McGill was not wholly orthodox. He took an unexpected excursion into criminology. In 1879, Moritz Benedikt claimed that "the brains of criminals exhibit a deviation from the normal type." Osler sought out the brains of two Canadian murderers and refuted Benedikt's anatomical findings.[5] Harvey Cushing, Osler's previous biographer, concluded that this odd "episode is important only in showing Osler's eagerness in the pursuit of knowledge and his outspokenness of opinion." Bliss goes beyond this bare interpretation by placing Osler's investigation in a new philosophical setting. He cites this 1882 paper as the first in which "Osler wrote on an issue involving the divide between science and liberal thought." This subject became a persistent and important theme in Osler's later writing.

His reputation was growing and his ambitions too. In 1885, he was invited to deliver the prestigious Gulstonian lectures at the Royal College of Physicians in London. This international honor made him an ideal candidate for a vacancy that had just arisen at the University of Pennsylvania, America's oldest medical school. In Philadelphia he quickly expanded his research interests across a vast range of subjects —he wrote about pneumonia, endocarditis, typhoid fever, duodenal ulcers, cerebral aneurysms, cholera, blood cells, and epilepsy, although his "deep conservatism," as Bliss calls the Osler family nature, led him to cling to vestigial techniques such as bloodletting and leeches.

Philadelphia could not contain Osler for long. The establishment of Johns Hopkins Hospital in Baltimore on May 7, 1889, marked an irreversible shift in academic leadership from the old European medical centers to the modern schools of America. Osler became chief physician at Johns Hopkins and in 1890 wrote: "I have everything I could desire and more than I could deserve." His research continued to extend even farther across the human corpus—heart, aorta, gut, blood, liver, brain, and thyroid. But he also had the task of creating a new medical school. Osler was now able to import the principles he had first observed in Europe—namely, clinical apprenticeships on the hospital wards rather than dry instruction confined to the lecture theater. "The student begins," he wrote, "with the patient, continues with the patient, and ends his studies with the patient, using books and lectures as tools, as means to an end."

But Osler's greatest achievement in Baltimore was his textbook, *The Principles and Practice of Medicine*. The book was dedicated to his three mentors—Johnson, Bovell, and Howard. Bliss calls Osler's *Principles* "one of the great books in the history of medical education and publishing." Indeed, it solidified America's new place in world medicine. Bliss describes the conditions in which Osler produced the 1,079-page text—"in his shirtsleeves, surrounded by books in time-honored and Whitmanesque authorial style, dictating to his stenographer"—and its success (14,000 copies sold in its first two years).

Although *Principles* is "a book of diseases and how to treat them," it was far more than that. It combined an account of the natural history and science of disease with observations on the impact of those diseases on society. Bliss traces Osler's widening interest in public health to the late 1890s. But *Principles* offered Osler an earlier forum to develop his ideas on the social aspects of disease. For typhoid, Osler reports results from Munich which showed how the prevalence of the disease "is directly proportionate to the inefficiency of the drainage and the water supply." "There is," he concludes, "no truer indication of the sanitary condition of a town than the returns of the number of cases of this disease." He emphasized the importance of disinfecting ports to drive out yellow fever and he insisted, as Bliss acknowledges, that accessible sanitariums be provided for patients with tuberculosis.

But Osler's most original comments were reserved for syphilis. He begins his discussion of preventing the disease by admitting that "irregular intercourse has existed from the beginning of recorded history, and unless man's nature wholly changes—and of this we can have no hope—will continue."[5] Osler identifies two preventive measures. First, that of "personal purity," which can be achieved only through "hard work of body and hard work of mind," since "idleness is the mother of lechery." Second, and here one must recall that Osler is writing in the conservative climate of the late nineteenth century, "a rigid and systematic regulation of prostitution." Although he agrees that public sentiment of the time opposed such a policy, "the choice lies between two evils—licensing, even imperfectly carried out, or wide-spread disease and misery." Even today, a century later, licensing prostitutes to curb sexually transmissible disease remains an impossibly controversial matter in many countries.

Research, teaching, autopsies, university administration, publishing academic papers, and writing a textbook—there could hardly have been time for much else in Osler's life. Yet during his period at Hopkins he also became an influential essayist. His first volume, *Aequanimitas*, collects his most important speeches from 1889 to 1905. The title, and most famous, essay discussed two virtues of the successful doctor. The first was imperturbability—"coolness and presence of mind under all circumstances"—a "quality which is most appreciated by the laity though often misunderstood [as] hardness." In a paternalistic style at odds with today's attitudes, Osler advocates not only coolness but "a callousness which thinks only of the good to be effected, and goes ahead regardless of smaller considerations." Other virtues were equanimity, "an infinite patience," and "an ever-tender charity."

Essays such as these turned Osler into America's foremost physician. Bliss attributes a not altogether complimentary self-awareness to Osler's writing: "He begins to see himself as an elder statesman, or a high priest or bishop of a profession he constantly compares to the clergy." In effect, Bliss concludes, he is preaching, but often entertainingly so. In one of his final addresses to Johns Hopkins in 1905, Osler spoke about "the fixed period." He began by wondering if professors outstayed their welcome through long uninterrupted periods of rule at one institution. He thinks they often do, thereby suffering from the twin diseases of "intellectual infantilism" ("the mind too long fed on the same diet in one place") and "progeria" (in which the mind "is sterile, with the mental horizon narrowed, and quite incapable of assimilating the new thoughts of his day and generation"). Osler went on to disclose two of his "harmless obsessions." First, the "comparative uselessness" of men when they reach about forty years of age. Second, the unqualified "uselessness" of men over sixty. The logic of his argument was that "the teacher's life should have three periods, study until twenty-five, investigation until forty, profession until sixty, at which age I would have him retired on a double allowance."

To promote his vision, Osler suggested euthanasia with chloroform for his older colleagues. Of that idea, he said he had "become a little dubious, as my own time is getting so short." The American press took up Osler's "useless at forty" claim. Studious news reports, humorous columns, and sarcastic editorials and cartoons filled the newspapers. Osler was stung and he had to give a series of interviews to clarify his remarks. His serious attempt to launch a debate about the need for older professors to give way to their younger, more creative colleagues was lost amid the hullabaloo.[6] The controversy dogged him for the rest of his life.

In 1898 he reached the official peak of his career, becoming a Fellow of Britain's Royal Society and dean of Johns Hopkins. His salary continued to rise, reaching $23,440 in 1897 (about $700,000 today, according to Bliss), and $47,280 in 1903. Osler was rapidly heading for burnout. In the fall of 1898 he developed pneumonia and after weeks of illness resigned his deanship. By 1902, as other work crowded into his schedule, he cut back ward rounds and classes, and canceled holidays to catch up on his writing. The astonishing pace of this period seemed to foster recurrent chest infections and "sub-sternal tension, a warning," he thought, "of too high pressure." He simply could not continue to work at such a rate.

Osler was only second choice for the Regius Professor of Medicine at Oxford—a largely honorific position founded in 1546 by King Henry VIII—but that did not make him less keen to escape Johns Hopkins. He considered that the move to Oxford in 1905 was tantamount to a "retirement."[7] Bliss quotes Harvey Cushing: Oxford would be "a synecure—no work big salary—nothing to do but give one lecture a year and drink port." True enough. Oxford life provided a butler and maids for his young family. (He had married Grace Linzee Revere, a descendant of Paul Revere, in 1892, and their son, Revere, was aged nine when they emigrated.) Bliss assembles a list of Osler's duties and preferments in England: college dinners, aristocratic receptions, membership of the Athenaeum, and a baronetcy in 1911. Little has changed.

Osler immersed himself in family life, and Bliss shares the general view that Osler used Oxford as a means to indulge his love of old medical books (his library of eight thousand titles is now at McGill), periodicals (he founded the *Quarterly Journal of Medicine* in 1907), classical literature (he was president of the Classical Association in 1918), and the brotherhood of his fellow doctors (he co-founded the Association of Physicians of Great Britain and Ireland). This standard presentation of Osler's final fourteen years is, I think, a serious, although common, misinterpretation. For Osler's lighter clinical workload allowed him to pursue two interests—philosophy and public health—that had emerged earlier in his life, but had remained peripheral to his inescapable university obligations.

Bliss duly records some of the lectures and essays that set out Osler's views on these matters, but he underplays their importance. Emphasizing the historical aspects of Osler's interests rather than their philosophical implications, he fails to stress the coherence of Osler's last intellectual efforts, and he does not explore the depth and originality of the arguments Osler develops.

First, Osler was concerned with the epistemology of medicine. His interest in philosophical matters began early in his research career when he wrote about the link between the minds and brains of criminals, challenging claims of inherited criminal tendencies. In that 1882 paper he had posed the question of how the child of a philosopher might fare among bushmen, and his essay raises important issues concerning free will and determinism. He returned to philosophy in a later study of John Locke. After a diligent review of all available primary manuscripts, Osler showed how Locke worked closely with the physician Thomas Sydenham to refine the basis of seventeenth-century medical thought—namely, "to return to Hippocratic methods of careful observation and study." Locke criticized doctors of his time for trying to fit observations to "their own fancies." He argued that "this is beginning at the wrong end," and commented, "I see it is more easy and more natural for men to build castles in the air of their own than to survey well those that are on the ground." Locke wrote an introduction to a treatise on the philosophy of medicine (*Ars Medica*), and Osler reports that "one cannot read the fragment without feelings of deep regret that the design was not carried out."

Philosophical issues became a central concern again in 1906, when Osler delivered the Harveian Oration at the Royal College of Physicians of London. His subject was "the growth of truth, as illustrated in the discovery of the circulation of the blood." In this essay, Osler argues, contrary to his times, a strong relativist position on knowledge: "All scientific truth," he said, "is conditioned by the state of knowledge at the time of its announcement." Although Osler roots his belief in Plato's *Theaetetus*, describing "the states of knowledge" as "acquisition, latent possession, and conscious possession," his point of departure is not Plato but, once again, Locke, who wrote that "truth scarce ever yet carried it by vote anywhere at its first appearance." The "final struggle for acceptance" was the real challenge in achieving knowledge, and Osler doubted whether doctors of his time were more receptive than their predecessors centuries ago.[8]

The example he chooses to prove the "iron yoke of conformity" is William Harvey, who waited in fear for twelve years before publishing his 1616 lecture outlining a new theory on the general circulation of the blood. When Harvey challenged the still-prevailing doctrines of the second-century physician Galen, his views were received with disdain by most of his contemporaries—Osler calls Harvey's opponents "intellectual Philistines," who were guilty of "mental blindness." In France, official recognition of Harvey's discovery came only in 1673. The reason, Osler suggests, was neither the prejudice of physicians wishing to defend Galenic doctrines nor the narrow-mindedness of scientists who could not follow Harvey's experimental logic. Although Harvey's discovery certainly did mark the beginning of experimental medicine, Osler wrote,

> even when full grown in the conscious stage truth may remain sterile without influence or progress upon any aspects of human activity.... The special distinction which divides modern from ancient science is its fruitful application to human needs.... In making knowledge effective we have succeeded where our masters failed. But this last and final stage, always of slow and painful consummation, is evolved directly from truths which cannot be translated into terms intelligible to ordinary minds.... [Despite]

> Harvey's triumph . . . there was nothing in it which could be converted immediately into practical benefit.

The technical complexity of Harvey's new discovery, together with its apparently limited practical application, buried his findings for much of the seventeenth century. The new scientific methods that Harvey developed seemed to render science obscure and practical knowledge elusive; this had troubling implications that remain with us today. The impenetrability that affects so much of modern science—from particle physics to post-genomic biology—has diminished its public understanding and therefore has often produced confusion about its implications for public policy. The difficulties faced by science reporters trying to cover the subject of genetically modified food is a modern case in point.

Osler's second preoccupation was public health. His early interest in syphilis continued at Oxford. In addition to a campaign of education and treatment, Osler advocated confidential notification of cases and compulsory drug therapy. He drew attention to the deep stigma associated with the disease, the "ghastly failure" of "the preaching of chastity," and the fact that "for the aggressive harlotage that still disgraces our streets man is primarily responsible." Osler also developed a new concern with tropical diseases. The acquisition of an empire brought with it responsibilities, he wrote, "to give to the inhabitants of the dependencies, Europeans or natives, good health—a freedom from plague, pestilence, and famine."

However, it was World War I that did the most to shape Osler's later contributions to public health. When conflict broke out, he was almost complacent in his view about the likely course of war. In a letter to *The New York Times* on October 21, 1914, he wrote, "I think this war will set a new record for low mortality among the wounded." But he soon began to report in the *Journal of the American Medical Association* how frostbite, cerebrospinal fever, poison gas, and shell shock were affecting soldiers in France and Belgium. His interest at first was wholly scientific: "It is intensely interesting to see a set of severe cases some weeks after their admission." In September 1915, Osler visited a Canadian General Hospital Unit at Camiers, where he saw "everywhere great squares of graves—marked with the names of the men of the Regiments."

On his return, he traveled to Leeds to give an address at the opening of the medical school. He could no longer remain a detached observer. In his essay "Science and War,"[9] Osler displays to the full his skill as a writer, but it remains his least convincing performance as an orator. He begins by calling attention to the fact that "the pride, pomp, and circumstance of war have so captivated the human mind that its horrors are deliberately minimised." He goes on to discuss the impact of science on methods of warfare:

> In three directions science has scored in a mission of destruction. What a marvellous adaptation of physics, pneumatics, and mechanics is displayed in a submarine, with which the highest standard of wholescale destruction is reached.... And the new guns and modern explosives! Chemistry, electricity, physics, optics, mathematics, every aspect of the subtlest human study has contributed to their perfection.... Every device of science has been pressed into use....

Osler tries to balance his argument by emphasizing that science can also be a "beneficent force." But in reading his essay today, one cannot help feeling, with Bliss, that his effort to cast science for, and not against, humanity is "flat" and "forced."

Worse was to come for Osler personally. Revere Osler was sent to the front in October 1916. Meanwhile, his father had launched himself into war work, helping to organize military care in Oxford and attending wounded soldiers returning from the battlefield. In

Belgium, Revere survived poison gas, but near Ypres he was hit by shrapnel. He died the following morning—August 30, 1917—with Harvey Cushing at his side. When the news reached Oxford, the usually imperturbable Osler collapsed, and Grace wrote to a friend of her husband "sobbing hour after hour."

Bliss asks: "Was William Osler the greatest doctor in the history of the world?" Two recently published reviews of his biography reflect the long-established divided opinion on this question. Sherwin B. Nuland, a surgeon and medical historian, claims that Osler "really was a kind of medical saint."[10] He argues that

> Osler is a fascinating man whom we need nowadays. In this time of cynicism, it is good to know that the earth can be inherited by those who have faith and trust in the improvability if not the perfectibility of humankind; in this time of bioethical conundrums, it is good to know that patience, good will, and personal morality will untie far more intellectual knots than the disarray of rancour, conflict, and special interests....

By contrast, the historian W. F. Bynum writes,

> The wonder is that, during Osler's life and after, so much fuss was made about a man who did not discover anything of much importance...Bliss succumbs to the Osler magic.... [He] reinforces rather than displaces the received image of Saint William.[11]

Bliss seems caught between these two extreme views. One can sense his uncertainty about which interpretation to follow. He acknowledges that Osler's essays are "dated" and that "he charged high fees, came to be chauffeured around in a flashy car, and regretted that champagne did not agree with him." The mystique of Osler does indeed look a rather shabby affair today. But Bliss also concludes that Osler "may never be surpassed as English-speaking medicine's most inspirational father-figure, mentor, and role model." Bliss does not hide his difficulties as Osler's biographer:

> His was a life that stands up almost too well to critical dissection, even microscopic scrutiny. In an age when biographers make their reputation by claiming to have discovered hidden internal derangements in their subjects, this project has been an unusual intellectual autopsy, at times something of a modern biographer's nightmare. Try as I might, I could not find a cause to justify the death of Osler's reputation.

Efforts to canonize Osler fill the medical literature to this day.[12] The embalming process began early with the tremendous success of *Principles*. His textbook became standard for at least two generations of doctors. His speeches and essays bestowed a reflective scholarship and sense of identity—"The unity of knowledge, its orderly continuity and its steady progress throughout the ages," according to one critic—on a profession challenged by the new science of the nineteenth century. And when Osler died, he quickly became a legendary figure. An editorial in the medical press began, "William Osler was the greatest personality in the medical world at the time of his death." His obituary in *The Lancet* commented,

> The medical profession has lost in Sir William Osler an acknowledged head; the east and west of Anglo-Saxon worlds have been deprived of their firmest common friend; and the individuals who mourn him today stand in every class not only in this country and in America, but throughout our Dependencies and the Continent of Europe.

Public meetings were held and permanent memorials planned. But it was the success of Cushing's biography that provided the strongest historical foundation for Oslerian legend, which has undergone a spirited revival during the past decade or so. The rebirth of Osler's reputation parallels another period of turmoil for medicine, although this time not from the creative energies of science but from the exigencies of health economics. Here are the titles of just a few papers invoking Osler's memory, all published in the 1990s: "Clinical Education: The Legacy of Osler Revisited," "Osler and His Thoughts for Us in 1991," "Osler's Changing Influence," "What Is the Oslerian Tradition?," "William Osler and *The Fixed Period*: Conflicting Medical and Popular Ideas about Old Age," and "William Osler: A Model for the 21st Century?" (to which the answer was yes).

These eulogies are puzzling, since Osler himself cheerfully acknowledged his own personal failings, especially his brusque egotism. (He wanted his brain preserved for study and posterity in the Wistar Institute in Philadelphia.) A further contradiction to his sacred contemporary image is supplied by one of his mentors, W. A. Johnson. In a letter to his son, Johnson wrote, "I am not surprised at your not taking up with Professor Osler. He is an Osler and there is that in him, unless I am much mistaken, which you must never admire." Johnson recognizes Osler's application but he cannot discern "any talent . . . or any high principle of action. Simply great application, and, probably, the motive is money making."[13]

A more insistent question that emerges from Osler's life—one that Bliss, Bynum, and Nuland avoid—is why a few doctors have expended so much energy during the past century in creating a cult around this man. I write "a few" because most doctors could not give a hoot about Osler, or any other doctor beyond their immediate experience. Many of us will have had mentors whom we admire, perhaps even revere. But veneration of the medical dead is unusual. So why Osler?

The fact is that original scientists are more likely to be remembered and celebrated than medical doctors. Those engaged in ordinary medical practice and teaching commonly lack not only the elusive spark that leads to significant advances in science or treatment but also the glamour that invites public applause. Here perhaps lies the reason for Osler's extraordinary reputation. Doctors who are simply doctors, and who are not famous researchers, have had few heroes since the days of Hippocrates. In any professional order of merit the science of experimental medicine has eclipsed the skill of the clinical practitioner. Doctors are less esteemed than they once were. Their authority has been eroded and their traditional influence heavily circumscribed.

A once-prized clinical freedom to practice and prescribe as one wished has now, thankfully for patients, evaporated. Doctors are rightly, but unusually when one looks back across the history of medicine, expected to adhere to evidence, applying the findings of clinical research to their patients in a more ordered way. This approach, by which doctors must follow guidelines, has been exploited by public and private health providers as a perverse means to limit care by imposing spurious restrictions on cost. A consequence of this distorted market is that medicine is becoming dramatically deprofessionalized. To celebrate the life of Osler is, for some, to recall a different and better time for medicine, when an intelligent and devoted physician could expect to become a respected specialist or perhaps even, for those with less self-effacing desires, a public hero.

Here lies an obvious danger. There is much in Osler's life to study with modern advantage. His achievements are a remarkable testament to professional ideals that deserve discussion and reinterpretation among every new generation of medical practitioners. But to sustain the Osler myth, as doctors and medical historians have done, serves only to promote a version of medicine that is disengaged both from contemporary clinical inquiry and the difficult political discussions that affect the future of health care. Those inquiries and debates need fresh thinking, not curatorial reverence.

# 8

# TRUTH AND HERESY ABOUT AIDS

AFTER MORE THAN two decades of intensive medical research into AIDS, energetic international public health campaigns, and the emergence of a vast academic and commercial industry built around human immunodeficiency virus (HIV), the confident observer might dismiss the following proposition:

> Despite enormous efforts, over 100,000 papers and over $35 billion spent by the US tax payer alone, the HIV-AIDS hypothesis has failed to produce any public health benefits: no vaccine, no effective drug, no prevention, no cure, not a single life saved.

The scientist who made this statement is not an obscure crank. He is Peter Duesberg, a professor of molecular and cell biology at the University of California at Berkeley, a brilliant virologist, and the recipient of an award for outstanding investigative research from the National Institutes of Health (NIH). Duesberg discovered the first cancer-related gene in 1970. Yet in the 1990s he became perhaps the most vilified scientist alive. His work inspired excoriating attacks. In a review of *Inventing the AIDS Virus*,[1] published in the scientific journal *Nature*, John Moore, who works at the Aaron Diamond AIDS Research Center in New York, concluded:

> Duesberg wraps together his twisted facts and illogical lines of argument to create a tangled web to trap the unwary, desperate or gullible. But however much he attempts to gild his writings with philosophies of scientific truth, the reality is that his premises are based not on facts but on faith: faith that he is right, and everyone else is wrong.... How sad, and how ultimately pathetic.[2]

What extraordinary course of events had led him to be dismissed by his peers and ridiculed by his colleagues? This is a story that shows not only the limits of scientific tolerance but also the forces that shape the way science does business in the public arena.

Duesberg made two astonishing claims. First, that HIV is not the cause of AIDS. And, second, that since AIDS cannot be understood as a single disease, it must have different causes depending on which group of people—hemophiliacs or homosexual men, for example—one studies. The case against HIV was made by Duesberg in fifteen articles, in *Infectious AIDS: Have We Been Misled?*[3] and in *AIDS: Virus- or Drug-Induced?*[4] Three years after its first announcement, and three publishers and five editors later, his most recent book, *Inventing the AIDS Virus*, drew together these arguments into a historically and logically coherent tale. In describing AIDS as "a fabricated epidemic," he recounted the scandals of misleading research, the accusations of fraud leveled against scientists such as the co-discoverer of HIV, Robert Gallo, and the hyperbole of early estimates predicting huge epidemic proportions of AIDS. And in an unusual aside, the publisher, Regnery, declared that "if Duesberg is right in what he says about AIDS, and we think he is, he documents one of the great science scandals of the century."

On the basis of thirty years of research experience into the group of viruses known as retroviruses, he acquitted HIV as the cause of AIDS. He showed how dissidents who shared his view had been snubbed by most other scientists. They were forced to organize their activities into small covens, of which one was the Group for the Scientific Reappraisal of the HIV-AIDS Hypothesis. He recounted how scientists who had flirted with dissident views, such as Luc Montagnier, who, with Gallo, identified HIV, were dissuaded from pursuing their alternative theories. He used the examples of scurvy, beriberi, and pellagra to show how infectious agents had been blamed as causes of common diseases only to be cleared years later when it was admitted that scientific evidence failed to satisfy hastily constructed theories. He argued that diabetes, multiple sclerosis, and many other diseases had been falsely attributed to infectious causes. The same, he believed, was true of AIDS.

Duesberg did not substantiate his argument with new data. Rather, he believed that "the answers will instead be found by reinterpreting existing information . . . [in order] to make sense of the data already in hand." His close reading of published research aimed to provide detailed refutations of every assumption and every piece of evidence involved in creating the HIV/AIDS theory. But the core of his case rested on two propositions. Existing theories about the cause of AIDS were based on circumstantial—namely, epidemiological—evidence and not direct scientific proof. The epidemiological evidence was that HIV had been found in all persons who had AIDS. The orthodox view was best summarized by the American AIDS epidemiologist William Blattner and his colleagues:

> The strongest evidence that HIV causes AIDS comes from prospective epidemiological studies that document the absolute requirement for HIV infection for the development of AIDS.

Duesberg constantly warned against such epidemiological inferences because of their inherent uncertainty. In 1988, he argued that an "epidemiological correlation"

> is insufficient because such evidence cannot distinguish between HIV and other causes, unless there is also evidence for biochemical activity of HIV in AIDS.

In 1993, he elaborated further:

> Because of its descriptive nature, epidemiological search for an infectious pathogen is restricted to correlations.... Epidemiology can...never prove that an infectious agent causes a disease.

In addition to this failure to prove causality, Duesberg contended that AIDS is not an infectious disorder. In supporting this view, he challenged the efforts to implicate other viruses as causes of human diseases. He cast doubt on the alleged associations reported between the human papilloma virus and cervical cancer, between hepatitis B and liver cancer, and hepatitis C virus and hepatitis, together with the viruses allegedly linked to various lymphomas and leukemias. Citing evidence suggesting that HIV infection was present in the 1960s and 1970s, he also asserted that HIV is not a new virus.

If AIDS was caused by an infectious agent, Duesberg claimed, one would expect it would have five specific characteristics: (1) it would spread randomly between the sexes; (2) the disease would rapidly appear—at least within months; (3) it would be possible to identify "active and abundant [HIV] microbes in all cases"; (4) cells would die or be impaired, beyond the ability of the body to replace them; and (5) we would see the development of a consistent pattern of symptoms in those infected. None of these expectations has been met. In the US and Europe, men are affected far more commonly than women; the onset of clinical disease takes a median of ten years; the complete virus particle is difficult to isolate in patients with AIDS. Nor are the direct effects of the virus on one group of target cells, called CD4 lymphocytes, believed to be responsible for the observed immunodeficiency.

And the symptoms vary strikingly (for example, between Africa and America), although they have a supposedly common infectious origin.

Arguments such as these have persuaded respected scientists to express their skepticism that HIV is the cause of AIDS. Kary Mullis, who won the Nobel Prize for chemistry in 1993, wrote in his foreword to *Inventing the AIDS Virus*:

> I like and respect Peter Duesberg. I don't think he knows necessarily what causes AIDS; we have disagreements about that. But we're both certain about what doesn't cause AIDS.
>
> We have not been able to discover any good reasons why most of the people on earth believe that AIDS is a disease caused by a virus called HIV. There is simply no scientific evidence demonstrating that this is true.

Is AIDS a single disease? No, said Duesberg. HIV is present in different population groups: homosexual men and women, heterosexual men and women, injecting drug users, hemophiliacs, and children (who are infected during pregnancy, at birth, or from breast-feeding). And the differences in the symptoms of AIDS among these groups proved, Duesberg believed, that HIV could not be the common cause for such geographically and demographically divergent clinical events: Kaposi's sarcoma is more common among homosexual men; infection in Africa is associated with wasting diseases, which cause drastic reductions in weight, whereas in Europe and the US infections like Pneumocystis pneumonia are more common. In Duesberg's view, the Western form of AIDS is caused by long-term recreational use of drugs, such as cocaine, nitrites, amphetamines, or drugs used to treat AIDS itself—AZT, for instance. (The evidence from surveys that many homosexuals in fact take nitrites to enhance sexual experience or take other drugs such as amphetamines and cocaine is central to this argument.)

The hypothesis linking AIDS and drugs, Duesberg believed, resolved several longstanding paradoxes about the AIDS pandemic. American AIDS was new not because of HIV, which is an old infection, but because drug use had spiraled during the past twenty years, especially in men below the age of forty. Many diseases associated with AIDS, such as dementia, do not depend on a state of immunodeficiency. If the drug hypothesis was correct, diseases in developing countries that were "associated" with HIV infection would no longer be forced to fit into the invented category of AIDS, thereby creating a syndrome with a pattern entirely different from its Western counterpart. What Duesberg calls the "drug-AIDS hypothesis" would lead us to conclude that many of the diseases now defined as AIDS in the developing countries are old diseases—tuberculosis and salmonella infection among them—and occur equally between the sexes. Any evidence of HIV infection was an irrelevant coincidence. In all settings, Duesberg wrote, HIV is a harmless "passenger" and does not cause disease.

Where does this radical argument take us? Duesberg noted that

> The drug-AIDS hypothesis predicts that the AIDS diseases of the behavioral AIDS-risk groups in the US and Europe can be prevented by controlling the consumption of recreational and anti-HIV drugs, but not by "safe sex" and "clean injection equipment" for unsterile(!) street drugs.

Here his arguments took him into dangerous territory. For if HIV was not the cause of AIDS, then every public health injunction about the need for safer sex became meaningless; every call to offer clean needles to injecting drug users may have been unnecessary—or worse. Duesberg noted that "the clean-needle program of the AIDS-establishment would appear to encourage rather than discourage intravenous drug use." And, he wrote, most remarkably of all, that "screening of blood for antibodies to HIV is superfluous, if not harmful, in view of the anxiety that a positive test generates." In his opinion "AZT is AIDS by prescription"; this drug should "be banned immediately."

How could so many scientists have got it all so badly wrong?

The thesis that HIV is the cause of AIDS is undisputed by most other researchers. Duesberg accepted that epidemiological investigations find an association between the virus and the syndrome. His tactic was to argue that HIV is merely what scientists call a "confounding variable": that is, its presence is explained by its relation with the much more significant history of drug use. HIV and AIDS-related diseases, such as Kaposi's sarcoma, were for Duesberg all simply the results of drug use, the true cause of AIDS. To be sure, one task of AIDS research has been to convert statistical associations into clear statements about physical factors that seem likely to increase the risk of immunodeficiency. There is now substantial evidence—the life cycle of HIV, the events surrounding early infection, and the damage to the immune system as the disease progresses—to show how HIV might lead to a state in which the immune system fails to function. Duesberg recognized the importance of this evidence. He wrote, however, that "even a perfect correlation with HIV does not prove causation without functional evidence." That "functional evidence" is now accumulating rapidly. However, researchers readily admit that there are huge gaps in our understanding. In one authoritative account of the time, *The Molecular Biology of HIV/AIDS*, edited by A. M. L. Lever, scientists wrote:

> Despite knowing so much about the molecular biology of HIV we still have little understanding of how HIV causes AIDS and why progression to disease can take a long and variable time.

> It still remains to be established precisely how viral replication and viral gene expression are regulated and how they influence progression to clinically significant immunodeficiency.

> The cell type which is first infected following HIV transmission has still not been defined.[5]

These uncertainties did not mean that HIV was not the cause of AIDS. Here was an important distinction that Duesberg ignored. Though we may not have understood exactly how HIV causes AIDS, we had a large, most scientists would say overwhelming, mass of evidence linking HIV to this form of acquired immunodeficiency. HIV had been shown to be a necessary factor for the occurrence of AIDS. Whether it was sufficient remained open. The likelihood was that there are genetic, constitutional, and environmental influences, all of which modify the effect of HIV on its human host, some accelerating the emergence of the disease, some perhaps even preventing HIV infection. For example, William Paxton[6] has reported immunological differences—such as increased release of certain active substances, called chemokines, from CD4 cells—that produced resistance to HIV infection in twenty-five people who had "multiple high-risk sexual exposures" to HIV (that is, people who had unprotected receptive sex with partners who subsequently died of AIDS). Paxton had yet to find a full explanation for such resistance but speculated that it might account for the variable rates of the progression of the disease seen in those with HIV infection.[7]

Moreover, that HIV infection could be exacerbated or retarded by other factors—"cofactors"—had long been recognized as important. The unpredictable course of illness raised the possibility that other microorganisms might be candidates affecting the pathogenicity of HIV. In addition, as yet unidentified viruses might be involved in causing the diseases that are now considered integral parts of AIDS. One such virus, a new herpes virus, was reported to be the cause of Kaposi's sarcoma, once classed as a disease that defined AIDS and therefore also HIV.[8]

Could drugs have been an additional cofactor? Duesberg wrote that there are high rates of drug use among AIDS patients, and he correlated drug use "epidemiologically and chronologically" with the AIDS epidemic in both the US and Europe. He cited studies showing that 96 percent of representative groups of male homosexuals had used nitrite inhalants, up to 70 percent had used amphetamines, and up to 60 percent cocaine or LSD. His uncompromising rejection of the causal power of epidemiological evidence was temporarily set aside when he dogmatically affirmed that

> distinct AIDS diseases occur in distinct risk group[s]—because they use distinct drugs (e.g., users of nitrites get Kaposi's sarcoma, users of intravenous drugs get tuberculosis, and users of AZT get leukopenia and anemia).... The duration and toxicity of drug consumption and individual threshholds for disease determine when AIDS occurs, irrespective of when and whether HIV infects.

Here Duesberg abandoned his skepticism about epidemiology, which he deployed so tenaciously in his criticisms of HIV causality. In fact, the issues he raised had been tackled by researchers. Well-designed studies cited in Lever's book showed that

> the annual probability of developing AIDS does not differ significantly between haemophiliacs infected via factor VIII [that is, a clotting protein, whose absence leads to bleeding], homosexuals infected sexually and those who acquired HIV as a consequence of intravenous drug use. These findings provide presumptive evidence against a role for bacterial infections or for drug and alcohol use, all of which are more common in intravenous drug users, in disease progression.[9]

Duesberg's inconsistent use of language also betrayed his lack of objectivity. He argued that some infections—"old parasitic" diseases, such as tuberculosis—and other noninfectious and cancerous conditions associated with AIDS were "indicators of an acquired immunodeficiency." The error in this argument should by now be clear. The plethora of conditions that are associated with AIDS reflect those diseases present in the local environment and are consequences of HIV-induced damage to the immune system; they are not simply "indicators" of a newly invented syndrome.

The AIDS pandemic in sub-Saharan Africa, driven mainly by heterosexual transmission, provided Duesberg with an opportunity to stretch his theory beyond the bounds of all reasonable belief. He called it a "myth" and repeated the argument that "none of the African AIDS diseases is new." The facts are these: the World Health Organization estimates that, up to the end of 2002, there were 30 million Africans living with HIV. In Uganda, adult infection rates range from 1 percent to as high as 30 percent in some villages. In a belt of countries beginning in the Central African Republic and sweeping eastward and then south, urban rates of HIV infection are nearly 25 percent. In Musuka district, in southwest Uganda, if you are an HIV-positive adult you are twenty times more likely to die than if you are HIV-negative. To claim that HIV is not causally associated with immunodeficiency-related diseases is to ignore the evidence of tens of thousands of deaths.

Another crucial, and decisive, line of evidence refuting Duesberg came from the hemophiliac population.[10] The British researcher Sarah C. Darby has reported on deaths among the UK population of hemophiliacs between 1977 and 1991. Between 1977 and 1984, the annual death rate among patients with severe hemophilia was 8 per 1,000. Between 1985 and 1992, this rate remained identical among HIV-negative hemophiliacs but increased to 81 per 1,000 in 1991–1992 in those with HIV infection. Moreover, interruption of the spread of HIV clearly prevents the occurrence of AIDS. Contrary to Duesberg's hypothesis, preventing HIV transmission prevents AIDS.

* * *

How might HIV cause AIDS? HIV is a retrovirus and exists as two distinct species: HIV-1 and HIV-2. HIV-2 is found in West Africa and is less pathogenic than HIV-1. HIV is composed of a spherical protein case containing two identical pieces of genetic material (ribonucleic acid, or RNA), and it is coated by a membrane through which point seventy-two surface projections. These projections are called gp120/gp41 and are collectively known as gp160; they bind the virus to human cells. The core of the virus also contains three enzymes—reverse transcriptase (RT), integrase, and protease. In total, the genome of HIV contains the code responsible for making at least seventeen proteins, many of which have important regulatory roles, such as one called Nef.

The life cycle of HIV begins when gp120 binds to a molecule called CD4 on the surface of the blood cells known as macrophages and lymphocytes. Coreceptors for HIV-1 must also be present on target cells to assist HIV entry. CCR5 is a coreceptor for strains of HIV that prefer macrophages. CXCR4 has a similar function for lymphocytes. HIV then enters the cell: the next step is critical. The unique feature of a retrovirus is its ability to take over the machinery of the cell by converting its RNA to DNA, using the enzyme RT to do so. (Drugs such as AZT, didanosine, and zalcitabine are used against AIDS because they inhibit the effects of RT.) RT makes mistakes and the result is mutation. The enormous diversity of HIV types that is a consequence of this high mutation rate allows HIV to escape human defenses. HIV is very hard indeed to pin down. At any rate, viral DNA is then permanently integrated into the host cell's own total complement of genetic material, or genome. Subsequent viral replication is helped by several factors, but the most powerful are viral proteins called Tat and Rev. If either of these proteins fails to function, HIV becomes noninfectious. Finally, assembly of the complete virus requires the enzyme protease. Therefore Tat, Rev, protease, and Nef are all potential targets for anti-HIV therapy.

HIV can be transmitted sexually. It can also be transmitted before, during, and after birth. It can also be transmitted occupationally (through needle-stick injuries), as well as through unsterilized blood products or contaminated equipment (needles and syringes). It was formerly thought that the virus, once integrated in a host cell, existed in a latent phase. Duesberg makes much of this belief. In 1995 he wrote that

> HIV is latent, and neither chemically nor clinically detectable in "HIV antibody-positives" [that is, people with HIV] with and without AIDS.

This is not so. Soon after it is assembled, HIV undergoes tremendous replicative activity and a high level of virus can be found in the blood. Although the virus is then cleared from the blood, replication continues apace throughout the body's lymphoid tissue, which is the main repository of our immune system. This continued and damaging activity over the long term leads to immunodeficiency, leaving the infected individual susceptible to infections, such as Pneumocystis, and cancers, such as lymphoma. One long-running dispute has concerned the way that HIV destroys immune cells. Duesberg argued that HIV could not possibly kill CD4-bearing cells directly. In 1987 he wrote that HIV is "not directly cytocidal"—that is, does not kill cells directly. Again, this is not so.

Once infection has taken place, the disease is clinically latent—that is, usually it is not expressed in AIDS symptoms for some years, even though the viruses are replicating. Martin E. Schechter has shown, however, that cases of AIDS developing in a group of gay men occur only in those with pre-existing HIV infection.[11] The reasons for the variable rate at which the immune system declines remain unclear. It may be that drugs, such as nitrites, interact with HIV in some unknown way to influence the progression of the disease. Such a finding would not affect the conclusion that HIV is the cause of AIDS, but it would throw light on the confusing evidence about the variable course the disease takes. In any case, what is clear is that (1) during clinical latency, HIV is present in abundant quantities in lymphoid tissue and, (2) as the clinically latent interval becomes longer and as lymphoid tissue is gradually damaged, there is a corresponding increase in the viral load in the blood. The eventual disruption and degeneration of the immune system produces a significant immunodeficiency: AIDS.

At the time that Duesberg was developing his anti-HIV arguments advances in treatment had been disappointing. Duesberg interprets those genuine frustrations as proof that "the war on AIDS has been a colossal failure." It is true that several key questions remained unanswered. The most alarming uncertainty was that no one quite knew the best time to begin treatment with antiretroviral drugs. Still, by sharp contrast with Duesberg's view, most scientists agreed that treatment directed against the virus had the best hope of success. In the words of a leading AIDS researcher, David D. Ho of the Aaron Diamond AIDS Research Center, it was "time to hit HIV, early and hard."[12] How justified was this belief?

On purely biological grounds, such a conclusion was perfectly reasonable. Following infection, millions of new virus particles are produced each day. Early treatment to inactivate these viruses before long-term damage to the immune system takes place makes good sense. Modern cocktails of highly active antiretroviral therapy have had astonishingly beneficial effects, substantially reducing the risk of an HIV-infected person progressing to AIDS.[13] However, in their early enthusiasm for such tantalizing advances, many AIDS researchers forget that the key question for the patient is whether a new treatment will prolong life or improve its quality. An exclusive focus on the virus beyond all else, even the patient, has produced some plainly absurd claims. At one international conference on AIDS, held in Yokohama, Japan, in 1994, the World Health Organization's Joep Lange said, almost incomprehensibly, that "the virus is the real thing. Clinical end points [that is, relieving symptoms and prolonging survival] are the surrogates."[14]

Aside from programs to educate people about limiting their risk of exposure to HIV and to develop new drugs, the search for vaccines to prevent either infection or disease is also part of national AIDS strategies. Early predictions about developing an antiviral vaccine were hopelessly overoptimistic. In April 1984, when Margaret Heckler, then US secretary of health and human services, and Robert Gallo announced at a press conference that HIV was the "probable cause of AIDS," she predicted a vaccine within two years. Duesberg was scornful of the notion that a vaccine will have any benefit: "The [HIV] hypothesis has failed to generate the promised vaccine" and anyway "vaccination is not likely to benefit virus carriers with or without AIDS."

Duesberg was, of course, correct in pointing to the failure to produce a vaccine. But he and many other researchers also failed to predict the huge difficulties that face vaccine designers. Since there are few people with HIV infection who have been able to control the progress of their disease, there are no clear indications about what factors might influence protection against illness. Moreover, there have been many impediments to vaccine development. They include the high degree of variation in the structure of HIV; the latent infection within infected cells; the lack of a suitable animal model to investigate candidate vaccines;[15] and the transmission of the virus mainly across vulnerable tissues—for example, the vagina and rectum. By striking contrast, successful vaccines to date have been developed for infections where integration into the genome is unusual and structural variation in the virus is limited. HIV does not play by the old rules. Despite these serious difficulties, several candidate vaccines are under investigation, though all initial studies have been disappointing.

Duesberg also fails to acknowledge the important safety and ethical issues underlying vaccine development. Many of the most effective vaccines available today are preparations of inactivated whole viruses or live, attenuated viruses. The risk from introducing viable HIV into uninfected people, thereby producing a potentially terminal infection, or enabling transmission of a potentially virulent virus particle to a partner, are obvious concerns.

The standoff between Duesberg and the AIDS establishment became increasingly embittered and ugly. The professional science journals, such as *Nature* and *Science*, which represent the majority opinion of researchers, displayed an alarmingly uneven attitude during this dispute. In 1993 *Nature*'s then editor, John Maddox, denied Duesberg the right of reply to a paper purportedly showing that AIDS was not linked to drug use:

> The truth is that a person's "right of reply" may conflict with a journal's obligations to its readers to provide them with authentic information. Whatever Duesberg's friends say, the right of reply must be modulated by its content.[16]

Two years later, Maddox relented—at least in principle. By then, he was forced to admit that Duesberg had drawn several important and correct conclusions about the paradoxes of linking HIV to AIDS. With the publication of new evidence that addressed many of these paradoxes, he could no longer deny Duesberg a voice in his journal. The details of the exchange between Maddox and Duesberg are recounted in documents published in both *Infectious AIDS* and *AIDS: Virus- or Drug-Induced?* Duesberg's response to new evidence describing early and dramatic viral replication after infection was a long rebuttal paper that was accepted in principle—"We shall publish the essence of what you have to say"—but deemed too long by Maddox, who offered Duesberg five hundred words to make his case. Duesberg wrote a letter of complaint, which was published, but he was denied a full opportunity to counter the new data despite Maddox's initial open invitation without strings attached.[17] Other journals, admittedly less prominent than *Nature*, have adopted a very different approach, their editors believing that dissent is a sign of healthy and vigorous scientific debate. For example, the editor of the *American Journal of Continuing Education in Nursing* chose to give space to Duesberg on the grounds that "we are in the middle of a major scientific controversy about the treatment of AIDS."[18]

Parts of the lay press also adopted a highly partisan position in the Duesberg controversy. In the UK, Rupert Murdoch's *Sunday Times* took a wholly uncritical pro-Duesberg position during the early 1990s, much to the irritation of Maddox. And Simon Watney, director of a UK AIDS charity, wrote:

> Duesberg is able to pass himself off as a beleaguered, isolated radical, struggling against a monolithic scientific establishment that refuses to listen. The truth is quite the reverse. Duesberg has had vast amounts of media coverage, largely because the mass media is only too happy to promote the view that AIDS is caused by deviant lifestyles rather than an infectious agent.[19]

June E. Osborn, a former chairperson of the US National Commission on AIDS, commented that "for the thousands who are suffering from AIDS or trying to cope with the escalating demands of treating this deadly illness, Mr. Duesberg's suggestion that nothing new is happening is as outrageous as it is insulting."[20] Scientists have expressed not entirely unjustified anxiety that a free and open debate about the cause of AIDS might dilute the public messages concerning safer sex and needle-exchange programs.

But there seem other reasons for the science establishment's wish to gag Duesberg and to deny him opportunities to conduct research. Elinor Burkett, in her polemic *The Gravest Show on Earth*, commented:

> Dissidents insist that the HIV-as-the-sole-cause-of-AIDS crowd has no choice but to call them names because leading proponents are so enmeshed in their dogma—professionally, emotionally and financially—that they cannot allow any honest discourse.[21]

She continued, "The scientists involved have been guided by the same force that has driven research into every other public health concern, from heart disease to cancer: the bottom line." In 1984, when Samuel Broder, the now retired director of the National Cancer Institute, wanted to find potential drugs to combat HIV, he turned to the pharmaceutical industry. He soon persuaded Burroughs-Wellcome to look again at AZT, a cancer treatment that had been discarded because it was too toxic. By 1987, the American researcher Margaret Fischl had published a landmark paper on the efficacy of AZT. In 1989, early reports suggesting AZT's success in treating patients who did not yet have AIDS symptoms led Burroughs-Wellcome stock to rise by 33 percent. Burkett chronicled in almost obsessive detail the "gravy train" that has become, and still is, AIDS, Inc.

I remember clearly the press conference called by the Wellcome Institute in London at the time of one study's publication. The gathering was not intended, as one might imagine, to explain to medical journalists the intricacies of the research and how it might be interpreted. The room was, instead, packed with financial reporters who were there to hear of the resolve of the company officials to destroy the credibility of a new study that they had helped to design and analyze, but which had gone against their product.

Apparently under pressure from the company, two co-authors of the study withdrew their support from the clear implication of the trial that AZT was ineffective in otherwise healthy HIV-positive individuals. At the same time, in the final trial report published in *The Lancet*, it was noted that "representatives of the Wellcome Foundation, who were also members of the Coordinating Committee... declined to endorse this report."[22] An open debate with Duesberg would likely have had grave commercial consequences.

The Duesberg controversy also reflects a deep philosophical division within biomedicine, the recent historical roots of which have been underlined by J. Rosser Matthews in his 1995 account of the evolution of medical statistics and the clinical trial during the past two centuries.[23] Two traditions have consistently fought for epistemological authority in medicine: one with roots in the basic laboratory clinical sciences—biochemistry, physiology, molecular biology—and another, broadly falling under the heading of epidemiology, which relies on surveys of disease in populations of actual patients. Duesberg shows his skepticism, as an unapologetic empiricist, at the statistical manipulations and, he would say, falsehoods that emerge from epidemiological research supporting the notion that HIV is the cause of AIDS.

The intellectual lineage of Duesberg's view can be traced back to the early part of the twentieth century and the birth of medical statistics as an independent discipline. For example, Matthews quotes the scientific writer W. P. Harvey in 1909:

> Much misunderstanding seems to exist as to the relationship which should hold between the statistician, anxious to scrutinise the validity of inferences drawn from observations, and the observer of the facts. The latter looks with suspicion on the former and is inclined to doubt whether the intrusion of his fellow scientist into his domain is for any more worthy purpose than simply to show that he is totally wrong in his conclusions.

This can be read as an uncannily precise summary of Duesberg's position as an "observer of the facts." Duesberg has centered his life's work on studying retroviruses, which he concludes are harmless, and he is now being asked to accept a view by scientist-statisticians who do not, in his view, understand his "domain." For Duesberg laboratory-based experimentation must take precedence as the foundation for scientific reasoning, while others are content to rely on epidemiological correlations. NIH has traditionally favored laboratory work, but it has come under sustained attack in recent years for its bias against research based on patients.[24] The debate remains an active one. Matthews emphasizes this dichotomy by asking,

> Do medicine's "scientific" credentials derive from the use of laboratory techniques in such fields as physiology or bacteriology, or from more novel techniques of mathematical statistical inference as used in epidemiology?

This debate still rages now in the highly polarized discussions over the validity of evidence on which clinical decisions are to be based.[25] Duesberg's dispute with the AIDS establishment was one extreme example of this deepening rift within biomedicine.

Yet another part of the current medical landscape that the Duesberg affair illuminated was political and ideological. What should the orthodox scientific establishment do to a scientist whose work and views are out of step with majority opinion? Apparently, in some cases, cut off his funding.

The prevailing "peer pressure of scientific consensus," as Duesberg characterized it, strangles scientific innovation. The usual, and much-vaunted, process of peer review can be crippling. "Under this review system," Duesberg wrote, "a scientist's access to funding, promotions, publication in journals, ability to win prizes, and invitations to conferences are entirely controlled by his peers." As a result, "few scientists are any longer willing to question, even privately, the consensus views in any field." An editorial in *Nature* argued that

> there may come a point at which dissenters forfeit the right to

> make claims on other peoples' time and trouble by the poverty of their arguments and the exasperation they have caused.[26]

And this view was confirmed by US government officials. Donna Shalala wrote that "to deviate funds from scientifically sound findings to those that lack evidence would be unconscionable."

One of the most disturbing aspects of the dispute between Duesberg and the AIDS establishment was the way in which Duesberg was denied the opportunity to test his hypothesis. In a discipline governed by empirical claims to truth, experimental evidence would seem the obvious way to confirm or refute Duesberg's claims. But Duesberg has found the doors of the scientific establishment closed to his frequent calls for tests. To begin with, the grant he was awarded in 1985 to support his work on cancer was not renewed despite an appeal supported by the administration of the University of California at Berkeley. The experimental virology study section of NIH wrote that Duesberg was an "applicant whose productivity has recently diminished both in quantity and most disturbingly in quality." Between May 1993 and December 1994, six further grants to Duesberg to fund cancer research were rejected. In AIDS research, between February 1993 and August 1994, Duesberg tried to secure funding to investigate his hypothesis (which has with time hardened into more of a belief) that nitrite inhalants were a cause of AIDS. These applications were made to the university-wide AIDS Research Program at the University of California and twice to the National Institute of Drug Abuse. His two grant applications to NIDA—both entitled "Animal tests of the AIDS risks of nitrite inhalants"—were supported by letters from Daniel E. Koshland, then editor of *Science*. All three applications were rejected.

This issue is examined in detail by Serge Lang of the Department of Mathematics at Yale in *AIDS: Virus- or Drug-Induced?* His review of the NIDA grant applications is revealing. Duesberg set out his objectives very clearly without much of the exaggeration that pervades his other writing. For example,

> The proposed research would clarify whether immunosuppression and/or Kaposi's sarcoma can result from long-term exposure to nitrite inhalants. Public health efforts aimed at AIDS prevention might increase their effectiveness by discouraging the recreational use of nitrites and other psychoactive drugs, thereby lowering the aids risk even of those already infected with HIV.

In a letter dated August 26, 1993, Daniel Koshland wrote:

> Given the critical information that would be generated by such a study, regardless of its outcome, I believe the time has come for this experiment to be performed.

Although NIDA rejected the application, Lang pursued the issue with *Science* by inviting a member of its staff, Jon Cohen, to consider writing a story about Duesberg's failure to get funded, especially in view of the involvement of *Science*'s editor. Cohen sent the Duesberg proposal to six researchers. After making several criticisms, one wrote that "I think a version of the grant could well be fundable." A second reviewer concluded that "the overall content is very meagre." A third referee commented that he "would not have gone that far," that is, he would not have rejected the proposal so unequivocally. Following the suggestion of the first reviewer, Duesberg submitted a revised application. That, too, was rejected, despite Robert Gallo's support of Duesberg's proposal, subject to a satisfactorily detailed application being submitted. Lang's point is that there had been consistent resistance to funding Duesberg's research proposal. In *Inventing the AIDS Virus*, Duesberg also pointed to what he considered censorship and biased coverage in newspapers and television and in professional journals.

Although an overwhelming body of evidence now exists to confirm the causal association between HIV and AIDS, the principle that original experimental investigation should be given primary importance in science supports the argument that proposals made by serious scientists with proven records of high-quality research deserve careful consideration. This would have been especially true in the early 1990s, given the then widely acknowledged uncertainty about the origins and mechanisms of HIV disease. It is not only Duesberg who pointed to this uncertainty. Michael S. Ascher and his colleagues at Berkeley wrote in 1995 that

> those who would see AIDS as a more-or-less conventional viral infection have consistently refused to recognize the paradoxes that are clearly evident in the experimental data—the problem continues.[27]

And Jon Cohen commented in *Science* that

> no treatment, to date, has had much success. And unless that bleak reality changes, alternative thinkers will likely keep needling their establishment colleagues and urging them to rethink their basic understanding of the disease.[28]

But how far could this rethinking be allowed to proceed? Duesberg, for his part, not only failed to understand the strengths and weaknesses of the epidemiological method; he also, as has been seen, recklessly deployed ill-thought-out epidemiological arguments to support his own drug-AIDS point of view. Nevertheless, as a retrovirologist, Duesberg deserved to be heard, and the ideological assassination that he underwent will remain an embarrassing testament to the reactionary tendencies of modern science. Irrespective of one's views about the validity of some of Duesberg's arguments, one is forced to ask: At a time when fresh ideas and new paths of investigation were so desperately being sought, how could the AIDS community afford not to fund Duesberg's research?

Since 1996, Duesberg has continued his campaign against HIV as the cause of AIDS, but the pace has slowed. His Web site—www.duesberg.com—quotes Einstein: "The important thing is to not stop questioning." And on the site are collected historical summaries, articles, viewpoints, examples of media coverage, and frequently asked questions. He reports that his site had 383,000 visitors between July 2000 and October 2002. A clickable button takes the user from this home page to a place where a "tax deductible donation to help support Prof. Duesberg's lab" can be made. But I could find no new papers on his contrarian HIV hypothesis after 1998. The story seemed to end there.

Duesberg lives an intriguing double life. He also has a cancer Web site (http://mcb.berkeley.edu/labs/duesberg/) where he lists his research interests as carcinogenesis and virology. Since 2000, Duesberg's work has focused on a phenomenon called aneuploidy, a term that means an abnormal balance of chromosomes—and therefore genes—in cancers. An example of aneuploidy in a noncancerous condition is Down's Syndrome, in which cells have an extra copy of chromosome 21. Duesberg has proposed that aneuploidies can cause cancer, and that cancer prevention might depend on avoiding chemicals (in food, for example) that promote aneuploidy. He has published these ideas in reputable journals, such as the *Proceedings of the National Academy of Sciences*. Duesberg's theory contradicts the orthodox view held by most cancer specialists—namely, that mutations in genes are the main cause of cancer. Put simply, instead of a small number of mutated genes having a large increase in their expression, Duesberg suggests that there might be a large number of genes displaying a small increase in expression. But, as with his views about HIV and AIDS, Duesberg has been unable to secure funding to test his ideas, despite, in the case of aneuploidy, considerable support from fellow cancer scientists.[29]

Duesberg will one day be remembered both for his highly original work in cancer and for his dissident views on AIDS. In both fields, he did what scientists are expected to do—develop testable ideas and argue their merits. Some of these ideas were acceptable to the international community of physicians and medical researchers, while others were not. The story of Peter Duesberg puts a lie to any claim that science is free of the ordinary prejudices that influence all other spheres of human activity. Science is politics, writ small.

The argument about the relation between HIV and AIDS has been unusually personal. Two years after an earlier version of this essay was published, the Yale mathematician Serge Lang published a book in which he wrote, "I accuse you, Richard Horton, of scientific and journalistic irresponsibility."[30] Lang had spent the intervening period circulating letters to scientists and journalists advancing Duesberg's point of view and criticizing those, like myself, who disagreed with his claims. Lang wrote that the multiple footnotes in my *New York Review* article gave "a false impression of scientific scholarship." My analysis of Duesberg unfairly isolated him, and I failed to provide examples of the support he had received from other scientists; I aimed my criticisms at Duesberg and did not address the precise issues and questions he was raising. I was "spreading misinformation uncritically," and indulging in ad hominem attacks against Duesberg. Or so went Lang's argument. Meanwhile, a far more insidious consequence of the Duesberg thesis was being played out on the continent where AIDS had taken, and continues to take, its greatest toll.

In his novel *Deadly Profit*—a medical thriller on prominent display in bookshops during the 2000 World AIDS Conference in Durban, South Africa—Patrice Matchaba tells a wholly unbelievable story. A small biotechnology company has discovered a vaccine to prevent HIV infection. The fictional vaccine, which luckily also protects the recipient against tuberculosis, is being tested in South Africa, Zimbabwe, and Thailand, countries where the epidemic is at its worst and yet to peak. Early results from the South African arm of the study indicate that the vaccine is a long-term success. But far from producing international gratitude, this result creates stock market chaos. For a vaccine threatens to destroy the $30 billion pharmaceutical industry feeding off the unquenchable need for expensive antiviral drugs to control the course of an incurable disease. A trail of assassination, corporate malfeasance, and personal tragedy is left behind, with a bizarre attempted suicide and reconciliation between an altruistic physician and a benevolent businesswoman providing an even more unlikely finale.

What lingers in the mind after reading this tale are various asides that Matchaba gives his characters about the predicament Africa faces from HIV/AIDS. In one conversation with a traveling American, Matchaba's hero-doctor comments, "I disliked people like him who saw only AIDS, hunger, corruption and civil war each time they talked about Africa. To make it worse, jerks like him always thought they knew what was right for you and your country." The same protagonist notes acidly that existing drug regimens are completely unaffordable, and therefore of little use to most Africans. Toward the end of his book, Matchaba reflects on why Africa has been hit so hard by HIV/AIDS. He writes,

> In all the developing world [HIV] almost had an affinity for the most oppressed members of society, the women and children.... If poverty and malnutrition were rife, even a small virus like HIV would run riot.... I always argued that the real problem was poverty and malnutrition. Perhaps if people were healthy, they could easily fight this virus off naturally.

Such remarks in Matchaba's otherwise improbable story shed some light on an especially macabre political consequence of the Duesberg campaign against HIV as the cause of AIDS. Placing AIDS in the larger context of African history and the continent's present development challenges is a theme that has been taken up with impressive energy by South Africa's president, Thabo Mbeki. In a letter several years ago to the government's opposition leader, Tony Leon, Mbeki asked that the observers of the AIDS emergency in Africa

> might care to consider what it is that distinguishes Africa from the United States, as a consequence of which millions in sub-Saharan Africa allegedly become HIV positive as a result of heterosexual sexual intercourse, while, to all intents and purposes, there is a zero possibility of this happening in the US.

Leon described Mbeki's "tone and content [as] unhelpful." The cause of this tense public exchange of views was Mbeki's cruel decision to deny rape victims access to a drug used against HIV, on grounds of lack of scientific evidence. He also took issue with the opinion of Charlene Smith, a white woman who had not only been raped herself but also had claimed that "rape is endemic" in South African society. Mbeki called this comment a "deeply offensive statement" given by a woman either "brave, or blinded by racist rage." She replied that he was refusing "to accept causal issues around HIV or sexual violence" and that "his problems are more serious than the criticisms of one small blonde." This demeaning squabble was emblematic of the fact that Mbeki was steering his government through its biggest crisis since democracy was first established in 1994. He had become embroiled in a debate about the origins and cause of AIDS, and was perhaps the only world leader in recent times to have jeopardized his personal reputation over a matter of scientific epistemology.

Mbeki's questioning of the orthodoxy surrounding HIV/AIDS,

prompted by reading Duesberg, has been portrayed by scientists, doctors, and activists in the field as at best an indulgent intellectual distraction, at worst a grotesque betrayal of his own people, one in five of whom is infected with the virus. Certainly, the bar talk among 12,000 delegates in Durban back in 2000 took place against a torrent of incredulity that he could have been taken in by AIDS "dissidents" long ago expelled from the scientific salons in the North. This frustration, loudly expressed, is understandable, even honorable. But it is also crudely misplaced, and lends evidence to the anxiety revealed in Matchaba's parenthetical remarks about Western condescension in matters African.

The approach Mbeki has taken to African politics, from his earliest days as a speech-writer for leaders of the African National Congress to his election as president of the republic in 1999, has never been populist. He has been a key policy strategist for the ANC, having trained as an economist at the University of Sussex in the UK. He worked as Oliver Tambo's political secretary, and he headed the ANC's international affairs department. He has none of Nelson Mandela's charisma, and perhaps lacks a politician's instinct for advantage and opportunism. He also reads. And he is an enthusiastic surfer of the Internet; it was here that he stumbled across alternative views concerning HIV/AIDS. In general, Mbeki takes the long view of South Africa's problems, and he seems to try to fit each issue he confronts into an overarching, coherent, and logical framework for his country's and his continent's progress.

One such long-term vision is that of an African Renaissance, first expressed by Mbeki, I think, in a speech given in April 1997, in the US: "It is this generation whose sense of rage guarantees Africa's advance towards its renaissance.... Africa's time has come." This immensely powerful image is now a dominant political idea in the speeches of many African leaders. It is the principle against which most decisions about Africa by the international community are judged.

In speech after speech during the 1990s Mbeki's diagnosis of what holds back the African Renaissance was the same—poverty. In a statement made on South African television in August 1998, he asked, "Where are Africa's intellectuals today?" He called on "African physicists, engineers, doctors, business managers, and economists" to return from the North: "Africa's renewal demands that her intelligentsia must immerse itself in the titanic and all-round struggle to end poverty, ignorance, disease, and backwardness." The alleviation of poverty is not merely political rhetoric. Since 1994, this goal has been a foundation of the new democracy's Reconstruction and Development Program. Indeed, some early gains were made. Infant mortality rates fell from 51 per 1,000 in 1994 to 40 per 1,000 in 1996.

Here seems to be the key to understanding Mbeki's contrarian attitude toward AIDS. In his opening address to an audience of scientists longing for the South African President to end his flirtation with AIDS dissidents and commit himself to purchasing drugs not only to treat people with HIV but also to prevent transmission of the virus from mother to child, Mbeki instead rededicated himself to the struggle against poverty, "the world's biggest killer and the greatest cause of ill health and suffering across the globe." This message was interpreted as a desperate failure of leadership by most AIDS experts in Durban, even those who live in South Africa. Despite this palpably hostile reception, Mbeki chided those visitors who might, he said, take away from Durban a view of Africa as a rapidly developing region of the world. "You will not see," he told us, "the South African and African world of the poverty in which AIDS thrives—a partner with poverty, suffering, social disadvantage, and inequity."

Meanwhile, South Africa's minister of health, Manto Tshabalala-Msimang, reflected the dismay of many in Mbeki's government who felt that they were being bullied into following a Western prescription to an African problem. In a speech full of emotion, in which she spoke of the ANC's long fight against apartheid, "sometimes to the death, to bring liberty and a better quality of life to all of our people," she asked why, given that history, "would we now turn aside in the face of their impending deaths?" Her government's only wish, she insisted, was to seek "African solutions to the problem."

Jacob Zuma, Mbeki's deputy president, explained his government's difficulty: it simply cannot afford the drugs that have worked well in richer countries. South Africa has "gone on to question whether there exist other ways to deal with the epidemic that would work better given our situation." In Kwazulu-Natal newspapers, for example, the government emphasizes in its health messages the complexity of the challenges in its campaign against AIDS. These challenges are listed, in a brutally honest display of South Africa's weaknesses, as equity (meeting basic needs), human rights (the position of women), poverty (unemployment and illiteracy), lack of resources (financial, material and human), poor infrastructure (access to health services), and changing attitudes (a patriarchal society and traditional cultural and religious beliefs). Maybe, therefore, it is not surprising when a ministerial eyebrow is raised at the swooping in and out of Hollywood personalities, such as Danny Glover, who came to sign his name on an AIDS conference "Love Train."

The response of scientists in Durban, concerned as they were not to dilute the message about the dangers of HIV, was to issue a "Durban Declaration." Five thousand people, including twelve Nobel laureates, signed a statement that aimed to end the debate about what causes AIDS, to "understand that HIV is the enemy... the sole cause of the AIDS epidemic"—not poverty.

Controversy over AIDS in Africa has not receded. In his own way, Dr. David Gisselquist, who works in Hershey, Pennsylvania, reignited a debate in 2003 that many had thought was laid to rest. In a series of research and discussion papers,[31] Gisselquist and his colleagues presented reanalyses of old data on HIV in Africa which caused a reaction of Duesbergian proportions. He argued that the African HIV epidemic was not driven mainly by heterosexual spread of the virus (most experts judge that sexual transmission is responsible for 90 percent of adult HIV disease in Africa). Instead, he claimed that HIV had infiltrated the population thanks largely to exposures in the setting of health care delivery—notably from medical injections. He concluded that "tangential, opportunistic, and irrational considerations may have contributed to ignoring and misinterpreting" important evidence. WHO and UNAIDS swung into action immediately by calling together an expert group which "reaffirmed that unsafe sexual practices are responsible for the vast majority of HIV infections in sub-Saharan Africa." The AIDS establishment seemed to have little tolerance for even mild dissent from the prevailing orthodoxy.

As a moving and yet dissonant counterpoint to Mbeki's opening address to the Durban AIDS conference, Nelson Mandela spoke its final words. Mandela underscored Mbeki's "great intellect." His successor as South Africa's president apparently "takes scientific thinking very seriously and he leads a government that I know to be committed to those principles of science and reason." But Mandela also hinted that Mbeki's intellectual approach, weighing evenly the arguments of orthodox and dissident scientists alike, had produced a paralysis of sorts, and equivocation at a time when "action at an unprecedented intensity and scale" was needed. Mandela was greeted in Durban with joy and respect. He left with adulation and the admiring relief of thousands.

But as I took my flight from Durban to Johannesburg and on to London, happy that the conference had ended with a crusading and inspiring call to arms, I knew that I was leaving behind a country for which neither sentiment nor drugs alone would solve the problems of AIDS. No treatment that presently exists is potent enough to eradicate the virus from the human body. Drugs can suppress HIV, but they cannot destroy it completely. And while the virus remains resolute, sub-Saharan Africa holds three quarters of the world's HIV-positive people.

By 2003, Mbeki still resisted acknowledging the devastating tragedy unfolding in South Africa. After years of cajoling by statesmen and activists alike, one would have expected him to shed his stubbornness. Not a bit of it. In his state of the union address to South Africa's parliament, he devoted just one paragraph to the virus that infects five million of his people, and kills six hundred daily. He refuses to widen access to antiretroviral drugs, despite street protests by many of his own supporters. In an uncomfortably loud echo of the apartheid era, marches against the government have taken place in Sharpeville, the township where sixty-nine apartheid protesters were killed in 1960. Thabo Mbeki, who once had so much to offer his country and Africa, has successfully transformed principle into cruelty. His political and personal failure to balance the evidence before him explains, at least in part, why reasonable dissent in other areas of AIDS policy is now so poorly tolerated.

# 9

## A FATAL EROSION OF INTEGRITY

"WE WILL NEVER accept a world with thalidomide in it," wrote Randolph Warren on July 17, 1998, the day after the US Food and Drug Administration licensed a chemical that had, between 1956 and 1962, caused birth defects in as many as 12,000 children. Warren heads the Thalidomide Victims Association of Canada. He was born with lower-body phocomelia after his mother was given thalidomide for nausea during pregnancy: the bones of his legs failed to develop, leaving his feet to articulate directly with his pelvis. His arms are shorter than usual, and each of his hands has only four fingers. Randolph Warren describes himself as a thalidomider.

The drug was rehabilitated in 1998 to treat a rare but serious condition called erythema nodosum leprosum (ENL), a complication of Hansen's disease (also known as leprosy). No more than one hundred new cases are diagnosed each year in the US. But in making their intensely controversial decision, FDA regulators were in effect also saying that thalidomide could now be prescribed for unapproved use in many other diseases as a drug of last resort. Endorsement by a US government agency appeared like a betrayal to many thalidomiders. For while other countries had suffered epidemics of birth defects some forty years before, the US had uniquely protected itself from harm through the stubborn integrity of a legendary FDA official,

Dr. Frances O. Kelsey, who in the 1960s prevented the FDA from approving the drug.

Yet it was the FDA itself which, in 1995, invited the manufacturers of thalidomide to look again at a drug that had, in their words, "the capacity to cure."[1] By 1996, an advisory committee set up by the FDA was reconsidering thalidomide's capacity to cause birth defects. It concluded that if thalidomide was to be licensed, the FDA somehow had to "ensure that no pregnancy occurs while a patient is taking the drug." In September 1997, the FDA, together with the National Institutes of Health and Centers for Disease Control and Prevention, convened a public workshop to discuss the evidence for and against thalidomide. Randy Warren was an invited speaker, along with Frances Kelsey.

The renewed use of thalidomide was based on the drug's encouraging effects on patients with AIDS, various cancers, and diseases in which the body's immune system attacks its own tissues. At the conference Kelsey set out the history of drug regulation in the US, and the way in which the thalidomide scandal helped to bring about more stringent rules for evaluating drugs. Warren spoke about the difficult balance between thalidomiders' twin fears of unregulated access to the drug and the wider use that would inevitably follow its regulated availability. In his view, the first fear outweighed the second. He supported temporary approval of thalidomide but with several stipulations. The word "thalidomide" should always be used next to any other name for the drug. Patients must be fully informed about side effects. Doctors who prescribed thalidomide must be certified to do so. Research should seek to find safe alternatives. And "someone must be accountable for dealing with any new victims."

In July 1998, Janet Woodcock, a director of the FDA's Center for Drug Evaluation and Research, completed her supervisory review of New Drug Application 20-785 submitted by the Celgene Corporation. She described evidence, some of which was over twenty-five years old, from clinical trials examining thalidomide's efficacy in treating ENL. Her findings were unambiguous: thalidomide consistently and rapidly improved symptoms for most patients with ENL. She also set out proposed "extraordinary restrictions" on the distribution of thalidomide.

These unprecedented measures included a System for Thalidomide Education and Prescribing Safety (STEPS); fully informed patient consent; creation of a mandatory registry of those taking thalidomide; monthly surveys to detect toxicity; a ban on sharing medications and on blood or sperm donation; agreement by women taking the drug to use two methods of birth control and by men to use barrier contraception; regular pregnancy testing; and limiting drug prescriptions to no more than twenty-eight-day supplies. The aim of these conditions was to "deter any prescribing that is not carefully considered."

Still, Woodcock concluded that "the Celgene application meets the standard for demonstrating effectiveness of the drug for the intended use." The first US new drug application for thalidomide was withdrawn on March 8, 1962. This same teratogenic poison was now given official government blessing for clinical use. "The goal," according to Celgene, was "zero defects."

Medical journals in the late 1950s did much to create widespread clinical enthusiasm for thalidomide. On November 22, 1958, *The Lancet* ran an advertisement claiming that Distaval—the UK trade name for thalidomide—had "no known toxicity" and was "free from untoward side-effects." This strong and unqualified statement came at a time when doctors were increasingly worried about the dangers of barbiturates as sedative agents. Thalidomide was, according to the advertiser's copy, a sedative "particularly suitable for children."

The hyperbole adopted by Distillers, the company that made Distaval, would eventually have a grotesque irony. In 1960 and 1961, *The Lancet* published advertisements depicting an inquisitive blond child playing with open medicine bottles. The headline asserted that "this child's life may depend on the safety of 'Distaval,'" and the company went on to claim that "there is no case on record in which even gross over-dosage with 'Distaval' had harmful results." The drug was, Distillers said, "outstandingly *safe*."

In *Dark Remedy: The Impact of Thalidomide and Its Revival as a Vital Medicine*,[2] their thoughtful account of the rise, fall, and subsequent rise again of thalidomide's fortunes, Trent Stephens and Rock Brynner place the origins of this confidence firmly within prevailing 1950s naiveté about science. The introduction of thalidomide became the single most important event in ending the postwar mirage of an impending technological utopia. Its consequences were deep and long-lasting—yet they are in danger of being forgotten.

Thalidomide was inadvertently stumbled across in a series of experiments aimed at developing new antibiotics. The man who led this work was Wilhelm Kunz, chief of chemical research at the German pharmaceutical house Chemie Grünenthal. Company executives puzzled over what to do with this substance which did not kill bacteria and had the tantalizing quality of seeming unusually safe. They pushed hard to find a disease for thalidomide to treat since no matter how high the dose given, laboratory animals would not die from it. Thalidomide was tested without success as a treatment for, among other complaints, constipation, seizures, and influenza. Eventually, in 1957, after observing the drug's calming effects, Chemie Grünenthal decided to market thalidomide as a sedative. Distillers signed up as UK distributors the following year, avoiding any further human trials to check either safety or efficacy. Thalidomide would eventually be sold, usually without prescription, in forty-six countries.

Early experience with the drug proved promising. Doctors reported a surprising lack of toxicity despite accidental overdoses. Such anecdotal observations were confirmed by Distillers in the laboratory. Experiments on mice and rats showed that thalidomide caused far fewer adverse effects than a barbiturate.[3] But by the end of 1960, questions were being asked about the drug's safety. In the *British Medical Journal*, Dr. A. Leslie Florence described four patients who developed nerve and muscle disorders while taking thalidomide. Distillers played down this report by labeling the reaction "rare." But further cases of neuropathy were described the following year. The typically wry British conclusion was merely that "the perfect hypnotic has not yet been discovered."[4]

A gruesome twist came in December 1961, when Distillers first alerted doctors to thalidomide's "harmful effects on the fetus in early pregnancy." They withdrew the drug from the UK market immediately, a few days after it had been withdrawn in Germany.[5] Two weeks later, on December 16, Dr. William G. McBride, an obstetrician working in New South Wales, Australia, reported in a letter to *The Lancet* severe congenital abnormalities in a fifth of women taking thalidomide during pregnancy.[6] In his brief one-hundred-word letter, McBride described the beginning of a tragedy that continues today in the lives of approximately five thousand thalidomide survivors.[7]

Looking through the weekly scientific correspondence in medical journals during 1962 detailing thalidomide's devastating toxicity, we can relive the panic of the time. Distillers made pleas for calm. Researchers undertook desperate efforts to find other causes for the reported birth defects. All those trying to secure more certain information about the evolving disaster were in a state of despair. The overriding impression left by these publications is one of the incomparable fragility of human embryonic development, a process that we usually take for granted. Otherwise spare scientific prose is punctuated with photographs of infants displaying thalidomide-induced deformities. Sometimes these newborn babies are screaming into the camera lens, their contracted limbs bent into seemingly impossible angles. Or else they are looking away, eyes fixed on a doctor perhaps, their gaze trusting. Occasionally, faces of children are blanked out, rightly to preserve privacy, but in a way that erases the human reality—and cost—of thalidomide's legacy.

Stephens and Brynner justly credit an often forgotten German pediatrician, Dr. Widukind Lenz, as being the first to tie thalidomide publicly to human malformations at a conference in November 1961. Lenz mixed a passion for astute observation and inquiry with a desire to hold accountable those ultimately responsible for harming so many children. When Distillers urged that "the problem [of thalidomide] can be solved without emotion and alarm," Lenz shot back, "I can hardly imagine that any person will be able to face the facts without emotion and alarm."

When a criminal trial began in 1968 against executives of Chemie Grünenthal, Lenz was a key prosecution witness. But the German courts deemed his testimony unduly biased in favor of the thalidomide children, and his evidence was held to be inadmissible. Lenz's response was quietly implacable: "I decided to take it as a compliment to my moral engagement, rather than an offense to my scientific honesty."

After initial clinical reports by Lenz, McBride, and others, belated experiments investigating thalidomide's toxicity showed that the drug could harm mouse, rabbit, chicken, and monkey (but not rat) embryos; any of these experiments, if performed earlier, might have alerted doctors to the risks of the drug in pregnant women. Indeed, it was the same G. F. Somers of Distillers, the person who had earlier praised thalidomide's limitless safety, who later described multiple deformities in rabbits "remarkably similar to those seen in humans."[8]

The debate quickly moved on from whether or not thalidomide was a teratogen—an agent that causes malformation of the fetus—to what should be done for the children and families affected. Terrible parental distress, stigma, and the child's personal and medical needs all became pressing concerns. In a rush to make amends for this iatrogenic epidemic of disability, surgeons took knives to limbs with often damaging effect. Prostheses were forced on children when they had little use for them. And providing children with ridiculously complex (and wholly unworkable) power-assisted arms simply reinforced their feelings of physical inadequacy. Worst of all, many hospital staff members, themselves unable to confront such extreme deformities, provided little comfort. One mother wrote:

> The staff at the hospital had not met such a situation as ours and, I think, were at a loss to know what to do. They did not tell me; and, although I didn't know quite what was wrong, I was sure that I had done something horrible. Had I been told at once that, although my baby was unusual, he was still just a baby I would have accepted it more easily. . . .[9]

Thalidomide soon began its slow return to respectability. Only three months after McBride's letter was published, Gerard Rogerson, a doctor from Shropshire, England, wondered

> whether this drug, which seems to have such remarkable inhibitory powers on growing tissues in certain cases, is being investigated for possible anti-carcinogenic properties.[10]

By 1965, preliminary studies with thalidomide had revealed its potent effects on ENL. The thalidomide story then divided into two separate histories, one concerning the drug's obscure mechanism of action, the other exploring its extraordinary therapeutic range. *Dark Remedy* unites both histories in an unusual way.

Stephens is a professor of anatomy and embryology at Idaho State University. He has devoted his career to the question of how an organism comes to be the particular shape it is, and his research has concentrated on the development of limbs. Thalidomide proved an important experimental tool for studying this delicate system.

Stephens is also a Mormon bishop. In his book *Evolution and Mormonism*,[11] he argues, together with two Mormon biologist colleagues, that it is satisfying for them as scientists to believe that God created the processes by which life is formed rather than individual organisms themselves. Last year he published a detailed theory, which owed nothing explicitly to Mormonism, concerning the process by which thalidomide exerts its effects on the developing embryo.[12] Brynner, by contrast, is a historian who contracted a disease—pyoderma gangrenosum—that could only be treated with thalidomide. Thanks to the FDA's license, he was able to take the drug and made a good recovery, although he has suffered nerve damage in his fingers and toes. Both Brynner and Stephens have become captivated by thalidomide's possibilities. And with good reason.

Following Rogerson's hunch, Robert J. D'Amato and his colleagues at Harvard Medical School discovered that thalidomide could stop the growth of new blood vessels critical to tumor formation.[13] Early work indicates that thalidomide produces encouraging results when used against some types of brain cancer; it has had variable effects on Kaposi's sarcoma, leukemia, and kidney, prostate, colorectal, and liver cancers. The drug even seems to benefit patients with heart failure.

Thalidomide also influences the body's immune system by switching off a substance—tumor necrosis factor alpha (TNF)—that provokes inflammation. In patients infected with HIV, this switching-off effect can reverse weight loss and wasting, relieve diarrhea, and improve the symptoms of tuberculosis. Results such as these caused those with AIDS to argue, against thalidomiders, that "the real danger is keeping a possible life-saving treatment from people who need it."

But the most striking effects of thalidomide are to be found in patients with multiple myeloma, a cancer affecting bone marrow. When existing drugs fail, thalidomide can produce sustained benefits in some patients with this incurable disease.[14] Results from the Mayo Clinic even indicate that thalidomide may no longer be a drug of last resort. Instead, it seems to be an effective first-line treatment. Since, in the US, 11,000 people die from myeloma each year and 14,000 people are newly diagnosed, the impact of thalidomide, if these preliminary results are confirmed, could be substantial.

This optimism has been largely fostered by Celgene, a New Jersey–based pharmaceutical company that describes thalidomide as its "flagship product." The firm's belief is that thalidomide is a precursor to "new families" of agents that modulate immune responses and selectively inhibit chemicals—cytokines, such as TNF—that do much of the immune system's work. The company's Web site (www.celgene.com) lists over seventy ongoing clinical studies involving thalidomide. In 2002, Celgene made $119 million from sales of thalidomide, well over three quarters of its total revenue and a 45 percent increase on 2001 sales figures. Sol Barer, the company's president, promised in December 2000 that "we will continue to expand our clinical trial programs" with the drug. He planned to submit "a supplemental new drug application to the FDA in 2001" to take thalidomide's license well beyond ENL. Jerome Zeldis, the chief medical officer of Celgene, committed the company to "proceed aggressively" with future clinical trials. In January 2001, Celgene became listed on the Nasdaq biotechnology index. By December, the company won the right to distribute the drug in Europe. The prospects for thalidomide have never seemed brighter. Colgene expects that revenues from thalidomide will increase by 50 percent annually.

But what of thalidomide's toxicity? Few other substances have such a clearly documented record of adverse effects. The most recent reports about thalidomide's effectiveness all repeat the well-known warnings about possible complications of nerve damage, sedation, dizziness, confusion, depression, tremor, headache, nausea, low blood pressure, hypersensitivity, rash, severe skin reactions, paradoxically raised HIV load, constipation, muscle aches, and blood clots. For people taking thalidomide, the burden of toxicity can be high.

As the uses of thalidomide broaden, we can expect that sooner or later another child will be born with an entirely preventable congenital malformation. Stephens and Brynner ask, "Who is responsible if another baby is born with birth defects?" I would replace "if" with "when." Perhaps our consciences are spared if the responsibility is spread among many—government regulators, Celgene executives, advocacy groups, doctors, and scientists. But is the success and stock price of an innovative pharmaceutical company sufficient justification for the FDA to extend its license? For those patients with conditions refractory to existing treatments, perhaps it is. If a patient with resistant myeloma was a member of my family, and thalidomide was the only hope for prolonging length as well as quality of life, I think I would be the first to consider it and call on the FDA to relax its rules. But arguments such as these, although emotionally powerful, are not a good basis for designing national policies on drug regulation. If I became a parent of a thalidomide-damaged child, I might equally recall the searing reports from the early 1960s and the present-day testimonies of thalidomiders. And then ask, why?

If thalidomide is to offer hope that is without undue risk, it can only be through its own chemical offspring—analogues that are more powerful and safer than their parent. Celgene is searching for such analogues. At the 2001 annual meeting of the American Association for Cancer Research, Celgene scientists reported that thalidomide analogues did indeed have "anti-cancer properties." In view of this promising early work, it seems to me that thalidomide's use should continue to be tightly circumscribed.

What are the lessons of thalidomide? Frances Kelsey has emphasized the "profound effect" the tragic use of the drug has had on drug regulation worldwide.[15] Almost at a stroke, the sciences of pharmacology and toxicology assumed central positions in medical practice. Animal testing became a necessary condition for appraisals of safety.

Medical authorities quickly agreed on the need for carefully conducted and reported clinical trials, including a patient's informed consent. Careful monitoring to warn of adverse events was instituted, and information about drug safety was shared internationally. It became clear that the FDA needed to be strengthened through new laws—as it was in the 1962 Kefauver-Harris amendments to the Food, Drug, and Cosmetic Act of 1938—to withstand the severe commercial pressures placed upon it.

Kelsey had an important part in this process. She was honored by the Kennedy administration with a distinguished federal civil service award. On October 7, 2000, she was inducted into the National Women's Hall of Fame. A Canadian by birth, she has a school on Vancouver Island named after her. And most recently her name was appended to an asteroid—minor planet 6260.

The FDA today is proud of its impact on public health. Its statement of its mission places safety before efficacy for foods, drugs, devices, and cosmetics. But this rhetoric conceals a conflict at the heart of the use of pharmaceuticals in medicine. Big pharma is big business, and the politics of drugs brings constant pressure to bear on the FDA to be more favorable to the industry in its deliberations. For example, as Stephens and Brynner point out, it was only in 1996 that the US Senate proposed making it legal for companies to promote the use of drugs for purposes different from those shown on the label. Newt Gingrich called the FDA "the leading job-killer in America." Even Kelsey once admitted there was legitimate debate to be had about whether the FDA "impeded the flow of new and important drugs."

But if the FDA is so conservative and safety-conscious, how could the Lotronex debacle have taken place? Lotronex was the trade name of a drug made by GlaxoWellcome for the treatment of women with irritable bowel syndrome, a non-life-threatening condition that affects as many as one in five adults.

In March 2000, *The Lancet* published the results of a clinical trial reporting that Lotronex "was well tolerated and clinically effective in alleviating pain and bowel-related symptoms" in women with irritable bowel syndrome. Michael Camilleri and his colleagues described their findings as "important."[16] Indeed, irritable bowel syndrome can be severely disabling. The apparent breakthrough generated an explosion of new research interest into this type of bowel disease.

Camilleri also found that one in ten patients taking Lotronex withdrew from the trial because of constipation, but he argued that this symptom was not "perceived as a negative consequence" of treatment. He concluded that "no serious drug-related adverse events or deaths were reported during the study." A single case of ischemic colitis (a complication in which the gut is damaged by a shutdown in its blood supply) was, he wrote, misdiagnosed.

Lotronex was approved by the FDA in February 2000. By November, GlaxoWellcome had voluntarily withdrawn Lotronex from the market. At least five people had died after taking the drug. Yet many within the FDA's leadership quickly wanted to bring Lotronex back. An advisory committee meeting set up to do so was planned for June or July 2001. This story reveals not only dangerous failings in a single drug's review and approval process but also the extent to which the FDA—in particular its Center for Drug Evaluation and Research (CDER)—has become the servant of industry.

New Drug Application 21-107 (Lotronex—alosetron hydrochloride) was submitted to CDER on June 29, 1999, and assigned priority review. Seven months later, Victor Raczkowski, deputy director for the FDA's Office of Drug Evaluation, who was dealing with the drug, wrote to inform GlaxoWellcome that, in the FDA's view, Lotronex was "safe and effective for use as recommended." He also reminded the company of its commitment to "a large, long-term (1 year) population risk trial to assess the incidence of colitis in patients receiving alosetron." The FDA was clearly anxious about the drug's risk profile. The printed information accompanying Lotronex warned about the possibility of acute ischemic colitis but noted that such cases "resolved over several days to weeks without sequelae or complications."

Glossy six-page advertisements in specialist medical journals claimed that Lotronex had "a favourable safety profile and [was] generally well-tolerated." The advertisements did, however, mention the problem of ischemic colitis, although the warning emphasized that a causal connection between the drug and this adverse event was uncertain. By July 2000, concerns about the balance of risk and benefit were being voiced. Between February and June of that year, seven patients had developed serious complications of constipation; three of them required surgery. After eight further cases of ischemic colitis were reported, the FDA had an opportunity to reevaluate its earlier decision. The clinical data confirmed the substantial and potentially life-threatening risks hinted at during preapproval review. But instead of withdrawing Lotronex and calling for more studies, the FDA issued a medication guide designed to warn patients of increased risks, while keeping the drug on the market.

This decision was to prove fatal. On November 28, GlaxoWellcome withdrew Lotronex from the market after the deaths of five patients taking the drug. There had been forty-nine cases of ischemic colitis and twenty-one of severe constipation, including instances of obstructed and ruptured bowels. In addition to the deaths, thirty-four patients had required hospital admission and ten needed surgery. A letter from Janet Woodcock, director of CDER, declared that the "FDA is committed to working with pharmaceutical sponsors to facilitate the development and availability of treatment options for patients with IBS." There was no word of sorrow or regret for the families of those who had died.

The course of these events can be followed through documents posted on the FDA's Web site. But what these press releases, talk papers, and letters do not reveal is the internal struggle and suppression of dissenting opinion that took place within the FDA once reports of serious complications and deaths began to come in. An evaluation of Lotronex's risk profile in the summer of 2000 found that the warning in the proposed medication guide was impracticable. The new guidance would be that women should stop taking Lotronex if they experienced "increasing abdominal discomfort." But since abdominal pain is also a primary symptom of an irritable bowel, FDA scientists argued that it was unreasonable to expect either patients or their physicians to judge pain as an early warning of possibly fatal ischemic colitis. This view was dismissed by FDA officials. The scientists who raised these issues felt intimidated by senior colleagues and were excluded from further discussions about Lotronex's future. Instead, the FDA preferred to support a series of epidemiological studies into ischemic colitis and constipation. An independent review of these research protocols revealed profound flaws in their design. A more rigorous research proposal from one FDA scientist was ignored.

A memorandum dated November 16, 2000, and released through the Freedom of Information Act by Public Citizen's Health Research Group shows the extent of FDA scientists' concern. GlaxoWellcome believed that the risk of Lotronex could be managed safely by looking for warning symptoms. But a note from FDA scientists to Lilia Talarico, director of the Division of Gastrointestinal and Coagulation Drug Products, explains that "early warning of the dire side effects of this drug is clearly not feasible." The scientists state that "the sponsor [GlaxoWellcome] has not identified a subset of women who will respond to Lotronex therapy safely." Moreover, and crucially, given the maneuvers to reintroduce Lotronex, the report states that "a risk management plan cannot be successful that will eliminate deaths, colectomies, ischemic colitis, and complications of treatment that were never seen previously in the management of IBS."

This unambiguous conclusion was blurred by the time of the key November 28, 2000, meeting between GlaxoWellcome and FDA officials. Rather than reject the company's risk-management proposal and withdraw Lotronex, the FDA offered several conciliatory options —for example, voluntary withdrawal of Lotronex, temporary suspension of marketing pending further discussion, and restricted marketing to specialists. Pleased and quite likely surprised by the FDA's desire to bargain over the terms of public access to Lotronex, the company pressed for a new advisory committee hearing and affirmed its view that risk management was feasible. It heavily criticized the FDA's options, deemed the process unfair, and accused FDA scientists of not taking irritable bowel syndrome seriously. There was stalemate, and the company blinked first.

Once GlaxoWellcome had withdrawn Lotronex, recriminations within the FDA began in earnest. In addition, Woodcock was swamped by e-mails from patients asking for the drug to be brought back. The company gave money to support groups for patients with irritable bowel syndrome to assist their research and educational programs, according to Ramona DuBose, a GlaxoSmithKline spokeswoman. The FDA was brought under further pressure when the new Bush administration removed its commissioner, Jane Henney, probably because of her support for the abortion-inducing drug mifepristone.

As arguments about Lotronex intensified, FDA officials took an increasingly hard line toward their own scientists. Yet new data acquired since the November 2000 withdrawal only strengthened the view that Lotronex should not be made widely available again. A further internal review of the incidence of ischemic colitis among women taking Lotronex suggested that the company may have seriously underestimated the hazards of the drug. And additional adverse reports obtained by Public Citizen showed rising numbers of cases of ischemic colitis and severe constipation in women who continued to take Lotronex.

While the FDA held further internal discussions about how to respond to patients' groups and congressional pressure, private communications opened up between Woodcock and senior executives at the newly merged GlaxoSmithKline (GSK). The company was now worried that the open advisory committee meeting it had proposed could produce a media circus, that committee members might disagree with a settlement made via these private communications, and that the entire process might be unduly prolonged. When I called the FDA for a comment in 2001, I was told that the agency was "working with GlaxoSmithKline to discuss issues surrounding Lotronex and we are making progress." It was expected that the company would reluctantly agree to a few conditions for the reapproval of Lotronex—that is, restrictions on which physicians could prescribe the drug and a requirement for signed patient-physician agreements. To ensure that the advisory committee did not overturn this privately determined decision, a senior representative of the company asked the FDA about the composition of the committee. And the FDA undertook to work with the company to set limits to the meeting's agenda and questions.

This two-track process, one official and transparent, one unofficial and covert, is contrary to the FDA's stated policy. According to Crystal Rice, an FDA spokeswoman, the correct procedure is for the company to write officially to the FDA, replying to CDER's concerns and providing new data on safety. A full FDA review should then take place before an advisory committee meeting.

In the case of Lotronex, private communications appear to have subverted official procedures, while suppressed scientific debate prevented a full and open review process. GSK commented that "a team of FDA and GSK scientists have met on several occasions in an attempt to work out a risk management plan that would allow appropriate patients to receive benefit from the medicine while risks can be clearly understood and appropriately managed." The company also denied that there had been a back channel for private communication between CDER officials and the sponsor. This claim was "untrue and very misleading," according to DuBose: "All meetings between GSK and the FDA have occurred primarily at the operational level between scientific teams." The FDA would "not comment on or discuss any details with regards to internal discussions between FDA and sponsors." Lotronex was eventually reapproved for restricted use on June 7, 2002. GSK now admits "the serious gastrointestinal adverse events, some fatal, that have been reported with the use of Lotronex."

A further insight into the FDA's favorable attitude toward industry was provided by a 1998 survey of FDA medical officers. Many of these physicians reported that since the 1992 Prescription Drug User Fee Act (PDUFA), which enabled the FDA via $329 million in direct industry funding to hire almost seven hundred more medical officers to review new products, standards for drug approval have declined. Many officers received inappropriate calls from sponsors about drugs under review; and they believed that the FDA too often interfered on behalf of companies in the drug-approval process. The Lotronex episode may show in microcosm a serious erosion of integrity within the FDA, and in particular the CDER, whose operating budget now depends heavily on industry money.

The public is largely unaware of these dangerous flaws in the world's most important drug regulator. For example, blocking public access to post-marketing requirements for further research into a drug's safety, as laid down in the FDA's own approval letters, is linked to PDUFA funding. Post-marketing study commitments are more than five times more likely to be censored in post-PDUFA approval letters than in letters sent pre-PDUFA. The evidence shows that PDUFA has produced a culture of secrecy within the FDA about safety issues. The public availability of these safety concerns is important since serious adverse drug reactions tend to occur after a drug's approval. A new medicine has to have been on the market for some years before its safety can be assured. Most of the public will assume that safety is a prerequisite for licensing, but this is not the case.

The view that safety concerns are being suppressed is now acknowledged within CDER itself. An internal 2001 inquiry into CDER operations confirmed the oppressive atmosphere within which drug evaluations take place. The investigation, the results of which were posted on CDER's intranet, was undertaken by two experienced CDER reviewers. They surveyed the attitudes of 40 percent of fellow CDER staff. Reviewers complained not only of "editing" of reviews by team leaders, deputy division directors, and division directors, but also of "requests" to change their opinions. Reviewers reported "pressure to favor the desires of sponsors over science and the public health." The inquiry report notes that "one third of our respondents did not feel comfortable expressing their differing scientific opinion." Moreover, reviewers argued that "decisions should be based more on science and less on corporate wishes." Too often, decisions that went against the company "are stigmatized in the Agency." One of the thirteen recommendations in the report is "Encourage freedom of expression of scientific opinion."

When the FDA approved Lotronex, the agency knew about its adverse effects. Why did officers at the FDA not act sooner? The answer is that, even today, the threshold for drug approval in the US is too low. When evidence does point to risk, the FDA often gives the company the benefit of its doubt, with death being the only event that forces regulators to think again. The Lotronex episode might well have been predicted. In 1997, Congress weakened US drug regulation by passing the FDA Modernization Act. One of the act's most important provisions was to reauthorize "user fees," which are paid by companies in order to shorten the average time for the drug review process to be completed. A system of regulation that depends financially on the very entities it is supposed to regulate is ripe for error. User fees invite regulators to take a lax attitude toward safety concerns. After all, it is industry money that pays their salaries. Since PDUFA was enacted, thirteen drugs approved by the FDA have been withdrawn up to 2002. Most of these medicines had safety problems that were known to regulators at the time of their approval. The FDA Modernization Act and

PDUFA have had damaging impacts on the independence of the FDA's safety review practices and standards. But the issue of pharmaceutical power is not confined to drug licensing.

Two tendencies are currently injuring relations between medicine and the drug industry. First, companies frequently manipulate information in a way that goes beyond the bounds of acceptable marketing. Examples are legion.[17] But the pattern is often the same. A new drug is designed and must be tested. A contract is drawn up between the sponsor company and a research team. In return for money to pay for the trial, the investigators will relinquish a degree of control over their findings to the firm. Let us say that the study shows the drug is less effective than the company hoped for. The investigators will still want to publish their results. But often the company will now stall. There are several possible outcomes.

The company's contractual rights—mixed with the threat of litigation—might persuade the investigators to keep quiet. The data could be published, but with a heavy spin in favor of the sponsor's point of view. Or the conflict may escalate until one side or the other blinks. The strategy of suppressing information, promoting disinformation, and sowing confusion is identical to that practiced by Chemie Grünenthal when the first hints of thalidomide toxicity surfaced.

Second, the relationship between many doctors and pharmaceutical companies has now become corrupt. The UK's equivalent of the FDA is called the Committee on Safety of Medicines. Its members review drug applications and decide on new licenses. Whether personally or professionally, they often depend on industry money. Each of the committee's thirty-six members must declare personal and nonpersonal—that is, research—interests in drug and device manufacturers. As of December 2000, twenty-seven members had declared industry interests. These included shareholdings, fees, consultancies, nonexecutive directorships, grants, and financial support to attend meetings. No member with a conflict of interest is allowed to take part in discussions that relate to a product he or she has an interest in. But the culture of the regulatory process is one in which it is acceptable for participants to profit personally from industry. The FDA's rules on conflict of interest are more nuanced than those in the UK. For example, exclusions from reviewing committees are subject, in certain specified circumstances, to waivers. And in response to public criticism, the FDA broadened its disclosure of committee members' conflicts of interest in 2002. But the cultural norm, which is overtly pro-industry, is largely the same.

The research process itself is also immersed in a financial quagmire of conflicts of interest. A recent study at the University of California–San Francisco found that a third of faculty investigators received payments from companies for delivering lectures and accepting consultancies.[18] Ownership of shares in pharmaceutical companies and personal financial ties are common. Prestigious medical conferences organized by some of the world's most respected specialist societies—such as the European Society of Cardiology—are now packed with industry-sponsored symposia promoting a product, a company, or both.

There is, moreover, convincing evidence that in some cases the opinions of medical experts can be bought by the highest bidder. Doctors who take money from drug companies are more likely to sing the company line—hiding anxieties about safety—than those who keep their hands firmly in their pockets.[19] Such is the atrocious venality of modern academic medicine.

The notion of pharmaceutical research as a curiosity-driven enterprise in the service of medicine has become a comforting but erroneous myth. As the cost—and risk—of drug development in a post-genome era soars, and competition between companies intensifies in ever-narrower markets, public health inevitably emerges as the first casualty. How many remember thalidomide now?

# 10

# SECRET SOCIETY

HENRY OLDENBURG IS a forgotten man. His name now means little to most contemporary scientists. But Oldenburg, and the standards for communicating scientific discoveries that he did so much to set, deserves a prominent place in our memory. Why? First, because he was responsible for the birth of science journals, inventing what still remains the principal means of communicating and archiving new research, establishing who did what first, filtering the good science from the bad, and creating a court for settling scientific disputes. Second, and more interestingly, because he had a delightful enthusiasm for causing endless mischief, to largely beneficial effect, among his more conservative scientist colleagues. Against the grain of his time, Oldenburg pitted disagreeing (and often disagreeable) scientists directly against one another, testing the strength of their tentative new hypotheses and teasing out weaknesses in the inferences they drew from frequently serendipitous observations. By creating a climate of fearsome debate, he hoped to reveal the truth or falsehood of each newly reported discovery.

Oldenburg was an outsider in British affairs, and he used this position to advantage.[1] Born in Bremen in 1619, he first took theological training before traveling and teaching across Europe. In 1653, he was given the diplomatic task of persuading Oliver Cromwell that Bremen was a neutral party in the first Anglo-Dutch war. Oldenburg found England a congenial new home, and the acquaintances he made through teaching gave him entry into a small but enlightened scientific circle at Oxford. He soon became a convert to the controversial and much-criticized philosophy of Baconian empiricism, which was starting to oppose the stultifying effects of a still-prevalent Aristotelianism.

Oldenburg's interest in science flourished during further travels in France and Germany. On these visits abroad, he began his habit of persuading otherwise reticent scientists to exchange their ideas. He threw himself into writing letters to friends and colleagues, building up a fledgling network of scientists who were not only desperate to learn of news elsewhere but also anxious to defend vigorously their own points of view.

What had been a rather meandering career quickly turned out to be ideal training for the new life that began when he returned to London in 1660. The Royal Society, which he described as "the new English Academy very recently founded here under the patronage of the king for the advancement of the sciences," was searching for supporters. It found one in Oldenburg. He was appointed to a committee of the new society, regularly attending and contributing to its meetings. Oldenburg's role was further secured in 1662, when he was made "second secretary," a position he held until his death in 1677. During this period, the Royal Society wrested leadership in the natural sciences away from the universities.

From its inception—it received a first royal charter on July 15, 1662, and a second in 1663—the Royal Society saw its function as encouraging scientific communication. Scientific meetings were the core of this work. But the lack of a common international language for science, together with an unreliable postal service, imposed severe limitations on those wishing to extend these early efforts. The most successful method of publication in the mid-seventeenth century was the reprinted and distributed letter. However, this means of communication was inefficient and irregular. Someone was needed to organize the burgeoning correspondence. Oldenburg had both the inclination and the position to do so. He received letters from across England and Europe, transmitted a summary of their contents to competing scientists, and invited replies. Oldenburg thus became the world's first scientific editor, and his approach remains a model for many of his journalistic descendants today.

Nevertheless, his method was, and remains, a cause of much dissent. He angered many scientists by his deliberate attempts to provoke debate. According to Rupert and Marie Boas Hall, who have collated Oldenburg's vast correspondence, the charges against him were that he was "a tiresomely active meddler, far too ready to do justice to the wrong party, the fomenter of disputes." But Oldenburg simply wished to flush out new ideas and observations from sometimes reluctant scientists. The informal exchanges that he incited became so successful that he decided to bring them together in a regular periodical. *Philosophical Transactions*, the first English-language scientific journal, was launched on March 6, 1665. (The French *Journal des Scavans* beat *Philosophical Transactions* to the presses by two months.) The English journal set out to communicate and promote "philosophical Matters." "It is therefore thought fit," Oldenburg wrote in the first issue,

> to employ the Press . . . to the end, that such Productions being clearly and truly communicated, desires after solide and useful knowledge may be further entertained, ingenious Endeavours and undertakings cherished, and invited and encouraged to search, try, and find out new things, impart their knowledge to one another, and contribute what they can to the Grand Design of improving Natural Knowledge, and perfecting all Philosophical Arts, and Sciences.

For this work, in 1669, aged fifty, Oldenburg was granted an annual wage of £40.

The Royal Society of today retains these ideals of what it now calls "excellence in science." But given its extraordinary history of seeking out new research findings, energetically facilitating their presentation and publication, and endeavoring to stimulate debate around them, the controversy concerning the Royal Society and Arpad Pusztai's genetically modified potatoes seems strangely out of character.

On August 10, 1998, with the full support and encouragement of his scientific superiors at the Aberdeen-based Rowett Research Institute, Pusztai claimed in a television documentary (UK Independent Television's *World in Action*) that genetically modified potatoes harmed laboratory rats. For doing so, he was widely condemned by his colleagues for breaking the fundamental scientific rule that scientists should not report the results of their research to the public before those findings have been presented to their peers, either at a scientific meeting or in the pages of a scholarly journal. It seems like a gag clause, and it is. At one level, the rule is well meant: it allows other scientists to pass judgment—in the form of peer review—for or against a piece of work before letting it loose on the public. At another level, the rule imposes a tight constraint on what is deemed acceptable science, how it should be released to the public, and the terms in which it should be discussed.

Peer review acts as a conservative brake on new ideas. For science, that could be an unwelcome hindrance to progress. But in medicine, such a conservative force can be a useful means of preventing either health scares or sudden changes in clinical practice when the evidence to support them is weak. If scientists break this rule, they can cause great confusion. The "discovery" of cold fusion, for instance, was first presented at a press conference in America several years ago. The work was impossible to substantiate and its refutation caused widespread anger about the way in which scientists had exploited an unsuspecting media for their own ends. Stephen Poliakoff explored this particular example, and the motivations that can lead scientists to abandon their usual practices, in his 1996 play, *Blinded by the Sun*.

In the case of genetically modified foods, Pusztai saw dangerous forces at work. Of his decision to appear on television before publishing his work in a peer-reviewed scientific journal, he said, "I knew what the companies were doing and what we were doing and I knew that there was a huge gap between the two. It would have taken the minimum of a year to publish it." He believed that commercial pressures might have prevented his work from being published. Putsztai acted recklessly to circumvent those perceived (but unproven) forces of censorship, and he paid a heavy price for this indiscretion. He lost his job, his research program was stopped, and his data were confiscated.

The public storm that followed these events forced Pusztai to seek formal publication of his findings. In December 1998, he and a pathologist, Stanley Ewen, submitted a research letter, in the style that Oldenburg so encouraged, to *The Lancet*. We sent their letter to six external advisers—a human pathologist, a veterinary pathologist, a nutritionist, a plant molecular biologist, an agricultural geneticist, and a statistician. Four of these peer reviewers recommended publication after clarifications and revisions. Our nutritionist noted that the paper was "seriously flawed." Nonetheless, his judgment was that "I would like to see [the work] published in the public domain so that fellow scientists can judge for themselves. If the paper is not published, it will be claimed there is a conspiracy to suppress information." Our sixth reviewer, an agricultural geneticist, also argued that Pusztai's work was "badly flawed" and that the letter "should be rejected."

We spent eight months seeking four revisions of the original letter submitted to us. Eventually, we were comfortable with a much-strengthened and less speculative manuscript. We decided to go ahead and publish it, and we notified our reviewers of our intentions. But now another bizarre rule of scientific publication was broken, with chaotic consequences. Scientific material submitted for publication is sent to external reviewers on the understanding that editors will protect the confidentiality of those reviewers. In turn, reviewers are asked to protect the confidentiality of what is sent to them. In the case of our Aberdeen potatoes, John Pickett, the agricultural geneticist who recommended outright rejection, went public. On October 11, *The Independent* reported that *The Lancet* planned to publish the work of Pusztai and Ewen, "on the grounds that publication of even flawed research could be in the public interest." This report presented peer review as the gold standard for judging science. Steve Connor, *The Independent*'s science editor, wrote, "The study that sparked the furore over genetically modified food has failed the ultimate test of scientific credibility." By "the ultimate test" he meant peer review. Here was the origin of much subsequent confusion.

The only true test of scientific credibility is for other scientists to repeat the experiments in question. If the initial results are not reproducible, those original findings will quickly and properly be consigned to the waste heap of science. If the data are reproducible, their credibility is likely to be enhanced. Peer review, by contrast, is simply a way to collect opinions from experts in the field. Peer review tells us about the acceptability, not the credibility, of a new finding. Even scientists can misread peer review, in the hope that it can safely arbitrate controversial findings. In his presidential address to the Royal Society, given in November 1999, Sir Aaron Klug argued that peer review was a means of conferring "a degree of authenticity on the published paper." Not so. Peer review can only elicit comments about what is written—the importance of the question being posed; the description of the study's design, execution, and analysis; and the scientists' interpretation of what they have found. It can say nothing about the validity or "authenticity" of the experimental findings themselves. Indeed, peer review is often prejudiced, unjust, incomplete, sycophantic, insulting, ignorant, foolish, and wrong. Still, it remains the best method editors have for judging the enormous amount of research they receive. (*The Lancet* is sent over ten thousand papers each year, of which only five hundred or so are published.)

How, therefore, might one have expected the Royal Society to respond to Pusztai's work? With some enthusiasm, given the Society's past record, to see his findings reach the light of day, so that they could be held up to critical scrutiny. Indeed, in 1981, an entire issue of *Philosophical Transactions* was devoted to genetic modification—*The Manipulation of Genetic Systems in Plant Breeding.*[2] The history of genetic modification in the twentieth century, as summed up in this volume, had been plagued with controversy. According to C. D. Darlington, a Fellow of the Royal Society, "The great pioneers of our subject were tormented by crises of belief and uncertainty, which we need to understand in facing our own problems today. It is only today after seventy years that such understanding is coming within our reach—and may soon slip out of our reach."

This theme of unpredictability was picked up again in a concluding paper by Sir Kenneth Mather, who noted that future prospects for genetic modification would "depend on such things as the requirements, preferences or even idiosyncrasies of the consumer, on economic considerations and on the agronomic needs and practices of the grower." His views were uncannily prescient, and he did "begin to discern, however dimly as yet, the possibility of deliberately manufacturing genes themselves, with properties that we can specify in advance." Given this early interest from the Royal Society's own journal, its subsequent engagement with the Pusztai data was not a surprise, although the form it took certainly was.

In April 1999, a working group was convened to look at "the apparent evidence that genetically modified potatoes adversely affected the health and growth of rats." Earlier, on March 15, Pusztai had been invited to submit his evidence to the Royal Society. In his response, Pusztai emphasized that he was "anxious to co-operate," but that he wanted an assurance that his written and verbal evidence would remain confidential, since premature publication of his findings would jeopardize their "acceptability" for scientific journals. It was unfortunate that he had not adopted such a cautious approach in his interview for *World in Action*. Pusztai also noted that his participation in the Royal Society's inquiry was crucial, since he was "the person who had devised the experiments, overseen their execution and drawn the conclusions from the data." The deadline the Royal Society gave him for submitting evidence was March 30. Pusztai commented that, since he was also expected to provide evidence to the House of Commons Science and Technology Select Committee, this timetable was likely to be unrealistic.

On March 23, the Royal Society agreed that Pusztai's data, if provided, would remain confidential. However, Pusztai failed to meet their deadline. He described the time scale as "impossible," given the amount of detailed information he needed to put together. And he asked, on May 12, for "your written confirmation that in view of the incomplete nature of the information provided to your reviewers their comment so far obtained will be held in suspense and not published." Meanwhile, Ewen offered to present the results of his work with Pusztai to the working group in person. According to Ewen, his proposal was ignored. Both Pusztai and Ewen began to sense that the Royal Society intended to damn their research, regardless of any input they might give.

The working group's final review was published on May 18. It underlined the principle that "scientists should expose new research results to others able to offer informed criticism before releasing them into the public arena." But the working group also found Pusztai and Ewen's work "flawed" and "uninterpretable." Their research had been judged in their absence, breaching the usual rules of due process that apply in peer review. In his 1999 address, Klug argued that "in our work on GMs we are following the tradition of our predecessors."

But it is hard to avoid the conclusion that the Royal Society's inquiry failed Klug's standard. It was hasty, incomplete, and unfair.

The reasons have old origins. After Oldenburg died, his journal suffered from benign neglect. He had not groomed a successor, and no one in the Royal Society had the slightest clue about how to run a journal. In 1752, *Philosophical Transactions* finally became the official periodical of the Royal Society, and it quickly took a conservative turn for the worse. The most famous example of this new cautiousness was the Society's response to Edward Jenner's experiments into vaccination. Jenner submitted an early version of his work to *Philosophical Transactions* in 1797, but his paper was rejected after consultation between a Fellow and the president of the Society. This frustrating experience led Jenner to publish his findings privately in 1798. Peer review had almost killed off a brilliant idea.

The Royal Society of today has turned its conservatism into a strength by making it the cornerstone of a robust corporate image. In the words of the Society, to achieve greater influence it has needed "to work harder at projecting a consistent image" by adopting the usual marketing accoutrements of a "corporate affairs section" for public relations, "an entirely new visual image," and "a new logo." The Royal Society now markets itself to the government as the chief lobbyist for science funding in Britain. It works to emphasize the economic and industrial value of the nation's science base, and it defends its ongoing government support—almost £30 million annually—by publicly demonstrating a strong commitment to this purpose.

Public–private partnerships with industry are being established in all spheres of the Royal Society's work. There are twenty-one industry-sponsored fellowships, and the Royal Society notes in its annual reports that "links between industry and academia are being strengthened" through these schemes. Present corporate partners include BP Amoco (a "flagship £1m programme" to enhance scientific relations with China and to promote science and public awareness), GlaxoWellcome (a "major endowment," together with a research professorship), Rolls-Royce ("a main player"), and National Westminster Bank (bringing "together entrepreneurs, innovators, and venture capitalists to identify, share, and progress common interests and needs"). There is a GlaxoSmithKline prize and a GlaxoSmithKline lecture. Other "important" supporters include GEC, Nycomed Amersham, Esso, Filtronic, Aventis Pharma, and Astra Zeneca. GlaxoSmithKline is also a member of the President's Circle, a group established in 1996 "to recognize the generosity of major benefactors." The Royal Society boasts that "support from private individuals, companies, and trusts makes a significant difference to the work of the Society." The Society and its sponsors aim to "promote shared objectives" and these links are "a priority." In other words, payment brings influence, a fact that sits oddly with the Society's claim to "its unique combination of scientific authority and independence from vested interest."

Similar economic arguments are used to justify the Royal Society's support of genetically modified technologies. Peter Lachmann, like Oldenburg a former secretary of the Royal Society, chaired the Society's working group into genetically modified plants for food use. He wrote in *The Lancet* that the effects of the "campaign of vilification" against this technology on "the science base and the prosperity of the UK may be serious." And instead of welcoming a debate about the science of genetically modified foods once the Pusztai and Ewen data were finally published, the Royal Society issued a press release headed "Royal Society rejects latest claims in *The Lancet* on GM potatoes." The Society was now taking on the role of public relations advocate to support the genetically modified food industry.

These ever-closer connections between the Royal Society and industry have led to concerns in areas far removed from genetically modified foods. For example, a Royal Society report on management of separated plutonium, which considered how plutonium from nuclear reactors might be disposed of, was heavily criticized for paying too little attention to the risks of plutonium as a reactor fuel and its potential for terrorist use. Klug agrees that there is a difficulty for the Society here. He lamented in his 1999 presidential address that "it is getting harder and harder to fill advisory panels with people who are both expert and irrefutably disinterested."

The Royal Society recognizes the tension between its desire to promote free scientific inquiry accountable to a taxpaying public and its own need to pursue a campaign for science funding based on the premise of economic prosperity. In his 1998 presidential address, Klug acknowledged the political link between science and wealth creation. But he spoke of the "burden of economic growth" felt by the scientific community, and the need for government to take a long-term view of its investment. When discussing genetically modified foods he also agreed that "the fears of the public are legitimate" and that only "trials and experiments" will reduce the public's uncertainty. These remarks were entirely contrary to the Society's later response to the work of Pusztai and Ewen, and seemed to reveal a confusion about the Society's own view of its direction and priorities.

To be sure, part of the fear driving the Royal Society's conservatism is the requirement of keeping its business investors happy. But there is also concern about the media's tactics of exaggeration in their reporting of controversial science. After the Pusztai data were published, frenzied and alarmist press reports often did not stress the preliminary nature of this research, the uncertainty over whether it could be extrapolated from rats to humans, and the fact that although the potatoes in question seemed to alter animal tissues, there was no proof that they harmed those tissues or the animals themselves.

Attention was drawn to the low standard of this public debate in a subsequent report from the Economic and Social Research Council. In *The Politics of* GM *Food*, the ESRC argued that "the public are not stupid and ignorant about their approach to risks but have a sophisticated grasp of the main issues." The report insisted that ministers, scientists, and journalists should have a higher regard for the intelligence of their audience, and not be afraid of a more widely informed public. These views were endorsed by Sir Robert May, then the government's chief scientific adviser, and Lord Sainsbury, the science minister, both of whom urged scientists to take more account of public concerns about new technologies and their risks.

A more questioning and skeptical public reflects, as Anthony Giddens has pointed out in *The Consequences of Modernity*, a qualitative shift away from a time when traditional voices of authority were listened to with grateful respect. There have been too many errors—bovine spongiform encephalopathy is one recent example—to rely on trust alone to oversee institutions governing science and medicine. Klug seems to regret this decline in traditional authority. In his 1999 address, he commented, "There is a notion around that, since all men are equal, and all people are entitled to think what they want, all thoughts and value systems are therefore also of equal merit. This of course is not true...." The erosion of science's claim to the one and only truth, he went on, "has opened the door to new sorts of tyrannies such as the coercion of political correctness and the manipulations of some of the single-issue pressure groups." These changes have made life uncomfortable for scientists, many of whom do not relish defending their work in an increasingly toxic public arena. And yet we seem condemned to repeat the same mistakes again and again—the safety of vaccines, beef on the bone, and genetically modified food. Is there not a better way forward?

In the US, when a controversial scientific issue arises—such as research using human embryos—the National Academy of Sciences launches an expert inquiry that includes public meetings across the country. Evidence is taken from scientists and laymen alike. These forums are open to the media, and they encourage a full debate about complex issues over many months.[3] There are no sensationalist news reports, no allegations of unfairness, no easy means of hiding information, and no accusations of industry gerrymandering.

The issue of genetically modified foods has only lately become a matter for national debate in the US. The response? On October 18, 1999, the Food and Drug Administration quickly announced a series of three meetings to seek the public's views about whether existing "policy should be modified and also to comment on appropriate means of providing information to the public about bio-engineered products in the food supply." With over a year to ponder the same matter, the Royal Society preferred a secret indictment to a public investigation.

What would Henry Oldenburg have made of this latest dispute involving his beloved Royal Society? He would, I think, have defended the Society's right to intervene in a scientific debate of such intense public interest. But I suspect he would have shrunk away from the peremptory manner in which the Society dealt with the controversial findings of Pusztai and Ewen. During an angry dispute concerning a bitter review by Robert Hooke of Isaac Newton's 1672 paper on light and color, Oldenburg noted his desire to avoid personal attack and to focus instead on fair and open inquiry. In a letter to Newton, Oldenburg summed up his sentiments about how the Royal Society should conduct its business, sentiments that still have merit today: "Those of the R. Society ought to aim at nothing, but the discovery of truth, and the improvement of knowledge, and not the prostituting of persons for their mis-apprehensions or mistakes."

Lord Robert May of Oxford succeeded Sir Aaron Klug as president of the Royal Society in 2000. His term of office lasts for five years. May, knighted in 1996, was created a baron (a life peer in the House of Lords) in 2001. And he became a member of the Queen's Order of Merit in 2002, one of only twenty-four people, joining such past recipients as Mother Teresa, Winston Churchill, and Nelson Mandela. Born in 1936, May was educated in Sydney, Australia, and at first completed a doctorate in theoretical physics. But midway through his career, he turned to zoology, becoming a professor of biology at Princeton from

1973 to 1988. His books and research papers have been extremely influential in shaping our understanding about infectious diseases. He is also an experienced leader of public institutions, having been president of the British Ecological Society (1992–1993), chairman of the Natural History Museum (1994–1998), and a trustee of the World-Wide Fund for Nature and the Royal Botanic Gardens at Kew.

Despite these layers of establishment encrustation, May has begun a process of slow but perceptible reform at the Royal Society to pull it out of a late-twentieth-century torpor. The society's insularity and resentful attitude when facing a genuinely concerned public has begun to dissolve. In his first presidential address, May announced moves to make elections to the Royal Society more inclusive and diverse. He stressed his desire to give voice to those who dissented from majority scientific opinions and to acknowledge uncertainty where it existed. He argued that decisions about the place of science in society depended on the values and beliefs of all the public—science was simply one among many equal voices in this conversation. And in that new spirit, the Royal Society launched a series of public meetings, where scientists and nonscientists alike met to discuss pressing scientific issues of the day. The first meeting took place in May 2001, in Birmingham. Seven areas of concern were identified, which remain annoying irritants in the way science is discussed by scientists and the public alike. They are the cause of much unnecessary controversy:

- The role of the media: scientists and journalists need more training to minimize the risk of distorting complex issues.
- Poor understanding of science by the public: scientists are often poor communicators.
- The importance of ethics in science: moral issues related to scientific research are too frequently underplayed in public debates.
- Confusion between science and its application: "Science should see itself as the servant of society."

- Poor understanding of risk: science is all about defining the limits of certainty; but very often a blame culture grows around an issue and uncertainty clouds the public need for reassurance.
- Lack of good science education: science is undervalued in schools —and in government.
- Vested interests in science: independent research should be fostered and dissenting opinions embraced.

Meetings elsewhere in the UK have reinforced many of these concerns. In March 2002, the Royal Society held its first National Forum on Science. The top five science issues concerning the British public were biological weapons, global warming, genetic modification of food and animals, BSE and variant Creutzfeldt-Jakob disease, and nuclear power. Indeed, it is those very issues that have done most to damage public confidence in science. Some of the origins of this mistrust were also revealed by the Royal Society's own surveys. People were anxious about the overcommercialization of scientific research; they felt unable to influence the scientific questions being asked; and many felt unhappy about the way in which the media reported science.

This early work by Lord May was a prelude to an important parliamentary inquiry into the workings of British learned societies. The House of Commons Science and Technology Committee, whose report was published in August 2002,[4] concluded that the Royal Society achieved "a great deal." But it called the government's funding arrangements for the Society "haphazard." The committee also argued that the Society's "considerable expertise" was "under-used," that the "number of women among their Fellows is disappointing" (only 3.7 percent of the total Fellowship, although the committee rejected the accusation of sexual discrimination), that there seemed to be a bias against newer scientific fields, and that the "absence of ethnic monitoring [made] it impossible to judge whether [the Royal Society was] representative."

The committee also detected some of the arrogance that May had tried hard to shed. It concluded, for example, that "the Royal Society's confidence in its all-round expertise may be misplaced." It branded Lord May as "presumptuous" in his attempts to define what the committee could ask about (how the Royal Society spends its money) and what it should remain silent on (reasonable questions about how its 1,200 Fellows were elected). The evidence given to the committee by its foreign secretary, Professor Dame Julia Higgins, caused special concern, and one can see why. When asked about the lack of ethnic monitoring at the Royal Society, she replied, "We do, of course, know how many Indian Fellows we have because they are part of the Commonwealth. We actually do rather well on numbers of Indians." The committee drew the conclusion that, given "the current political climate," this sort of view suggested "a head in the sand attitude" toward ethnicity. In its comment on the report, the Royal Society agreed that it needed to look again at its policies for ensuring equal opportunities to those nominated for fellowships. It admitted that it had laid itself open to criticism for not making this a strategic priority in its affairs.

What about genetically modified foods? The larger public issue surrounding genetic modification concerns the validity of the precautionary principle. This principle states that where there are significant risks of damage to the public health we should be prepared to take action to limit those risks, even when scientific knowledge is not conclusive, if the balance of likely costs and benefits justifies it. The precautionary principle offers a useful litmus test for those deciding about what risks are acceptable to pass onto the public. But Klug remarked in his 1999 address that this rule was "no way to deal with uncertainty—it is a recipe for [scientific] stagnation."

Lord May seemed to change tack. By 2002, he had opened the Royal Society's doors to representatives of Greenpeace and Friends of the Earth. The evidence they provided revealed the incredible gulf between a purely scientific appraisal of safety and a larger, almost philosophical response to the question of genetic modification. Here was an exchange between the Royal Society and Greenpeace, as represented by Doug Parr, their chief scientist, and Janet Cotter:

> Q: Suppose you had three new varieties of banana: one produced by conventional breeding, one by GM, and one by irradiation of seed. The genome has been sequenced in all three and shown to be identical. Would you have objections to the GM form?
>
> Parr and Cotter: Yes, we would have a problem if it were produced using recombinant DNA technology. Our objections go beyond the scientific safety assessment and are to do with ethics, respect for nature, and concerns about the release into the natural environment.... We object to any release of GM plants into the environment.

It is this type of argument that so infuriates Richard Lewontin, and rightly so. He points out that insulin, by this definition, is genetically modified and so should be banned, since it too is produced by recombinant DNA technology. Yet no one is suggesting that we should abandon the production of insulin and allow all those people living with diabetes to die.

The Royal Society went further still. In February 2002, it called for improved safety assessments of genetically modified foods before they were declared fit for human consumption. There needed to be far tougher regulations for all new foods, especially taking into account the risk of allergies and their overall nutritional content. The tone of these conclusions was entirely different from that adopted under Klug:

> We fully support the public's right to know that all new foods, regardless of whether they contain GM ingredients, are sub-

> jected to rigorous safety and nutritional checks.... The rather piecemeal approach to the regulation of GM foods in the UK, and European Union in general, means that there may be some important gaps and inconsistencies.

The Royal Society went on to hold public and scientific meetings about the benefits and risks of genetically modified crops in 2003. This push to foster a public debate was triggered by the UK government's chief scientific advisor, Professor David King. In an open letter published in 2002, he wrote,

> The GM science issues that interest and concern the public, and the scientific community, must drive the science review.... This review presents the scientific community with a challenge and I want to stimulate a response from you.... What can science say about public concern over possible unanticipated long-term effects of GM?"

The government Web site for this GM science review—www.gm-sciencedebate.org.uk/—includes many contributions from pro- and anti-genetic-modification groups.

Looking at the landscape of the debate about genetic modification in 2003, the science now seems to be tipping in favor of the safety and effectiveness of genetically modified organisms. Early concerns published in the prestigious journal *Nature*—namely, that genes introduced into crops in Mexico had contaminated nongenetically modified crops[5] —were abandoned by the magazine's editors in an unusual rebuke:

> We [have] received several criticisms of the paper, to which we obtained responses from the authors and consulted referees over the exchanges. In the meantime, the authors agreed to obtain further data, on a timetable agreed with us, that might prove beyond

> reasonable doubt that transgenes have indeed become integrated into the maize genome. The authors have now obtained some additional data, but there is disagreement between them and a referee as to whether these results significantly bolster their argument. In light of these discussions and the diverse advice received, *Nature* has concluded that the evidence available is not sufficient to justify the publication of the original paper. As the authors nevertheless wish to stand by the available evidence for their conclusions, we feel it best simply to make these circumstances clear, to publish the criticisms, the authors' response and new data, and to allow our readers to judge the science for themselves.

*Nature*'s US rival, *Science*, then published the unexpectedly beneficial results of planting genetically modified cotton across 157 farms in India.[6] Cotton yields increased by 80 percent and pesticide use was cut dramatically.

Some scientists do still have concerns. Matin Qaim and David Zilberman, who discovered the enhanced Indian cotton yields following genetic modification, concluded: "Although there is mounting evidence on the benefit side . . . responsible risk management and balanced science communication are prerequisites for overcoming acceptance problems and ensuring sustainable use of GM crops." And Professor Sir Gustav Nossal, chairman of the Strategic Advisory Group of Experts for the Vaccines and Biologicals Program of WHO, together with Professor Ross Coppel, a microbiologist at Monash University in Australia, argued in their book *Reshaping Life* that "this technology has enormous benefits but it can be developed at a studied and leisurely pace."[7] A cautious approach, they believed, would allow for "more stringent controls . . . for transgenic organisms with the capacity to spread widely." A key goal must be to look carefully for unintended effects of genetic modification in settings where spread beyond a particular experiment is impossible.

So does genetic modification offer the prospect of eradicating famine? Is it the only solution to an expanding population that will require ever more efficient food production? There is no consensus on answers to these questions. The US government views transgenic plants as substantially similar to nongenetically modified crops. In Europe, there is far greater skepticism,[8] a squeamishness that has annoyed American trade advocates. Robert Zoellick, a US trade representative, has unhelpfully called the European attitude "immoral."

What the genetically modified food debate has contributed to is nothing less than a major repositioning of science in society, a reevaluation that most scientists have underestimated and still fail to appreciate. Many scientific leaders would prefer to ignore the need for the public accountability of science. In commenting about Andrew Wakefield's work on the MMR vaccine, for example, Professor Patrick Bateson, a vice-president of the Royal Society, noted, "If the MMR paper had been more rigorously peer-reviewed it might never have been published."[9] His argument entirely misses the point. The MMR vaccine paper was published not because peer review indicated that the findings were true—peer review can never prove truth, only indicate acceptability to a few experts, as was indeed the case with Wakefield's findings—but because the issue raised was so important for public health and so in need of urgent verification that not to publish with appropriate caveats would, in my view, have been an outrageous act of censorship.

Lord May might possibly agree. In his 2002 address to the Fellows of the Royal Society, he expressed a radical view about how science needed to renegotiate its contract of trust with the public. He urged scientists to acknowledge that dissident views, especially in the early phase of a scientific debate, often "contained valid elements which, with the wisdom of hindsight, we can now wish had been taken note of." He went on to say: "It is most important that consensus is not reached too early.... I strongly emphasise the need deliberately to seek out and consider dissident opinions." At some point, this questioning—for instance, about whether HIV causes AIDS—becomes unhelpful when it ignores clear and contradictory evidence. But choking off debate too soon damages not only science but also science's covenant with the public.

In Marie Boas Hall's biography of Henry Oldenburg, she argues that he was the pivotal point of contact between the Royal Society and the scholarly scientific world. Oldenburg was important because he brought together an emerging and widely dispersed scientific community. Today, the challenge is different—to bind an increasingly aware, questioning, and even skeptical public with a scientific community often ill-equipped to deal with this newly transparent world. Is Lord May the twenty-first century's Henry Oldenburg?

# 11

## WORLD HEALTH DISORGANIZATION

> Despite its mandate and achievements, WHO has not been able to respond as effectively as necessary to the world's new complexities. The need to improve that response, recognised both inside and outside the organisation, has created a broad constituency for a changed and strengthened WHO.
>
> —Independent Group for Global Health, 1997[1]

CORRUPT, BUREAUCRATIC, INEFFICIENT, unresponsive, unaccountable, overly medical, and far too male. These are some of the more unkind accusations thrown at the World Health Organization, the leading international health agency, during the past decade. WHO's reputation reached a peak in the 1970s with its then director-general Halfdan Mahler's advocacy of Health for All by the Year 2000 and the successful worldwide eradication of smallpox. During the 1980s and 1990s it lost much of its authority. Too easily, the blame was put on one man—Mahler's successor, Dr. Hiroshi Nakajima.[2] But for the first time since its creation in 1948, WHO is now a decisive participant in the global political debate about health and human development. Thanks to partnerships such as Roll Back Malaria (RBM) and StopTB, together with the work of WHO in UNAIDS (the Joint UN Program on

HIV/AIDS), G8 heads of government at their Okinawa 2000 summit set ambitious and optimistic aims for improving world health by 2010: halving the burden of malarial disease, reducing deaths from tuberculosis by 50 percent, and cutting the number of HIV-infected young people by 25 percent. WHO is the agency coordinating efforts to achieve these targets. Much of this reversal of fortune can be attributed to WHO's director-general from 1998 to 2003, Dr. Gro Harlem Brundtland, a former prime minister of Norway who successfully restored WHO's international credibility—an achievement that seemed almost impossible when she took office in July 1998. WHO has become a global agency to be reckoned with.

But WHO remains under scrutiny. I sought the views of several *Lancet* contributors who know it well, working either at country level in WHO programs or in collaboration with one of the departmental "clusters" created by Brundtland when she took office—for example, on evidence and information for policy, on communicable diseases, on noncommunicable disease and mental health, and on sustainable development and healthy environments. Most offered warm praise for the director-general's work. She was described, variously, as having the "right qualities of a leader"; "focusing on a few priorities and pushing them"; and being "honest, committed, energetic, and politically adept." Yet there were serious concerns—for instance, about management style ("dissent is vigorously squashed") and the sense of missed opportunities ("inability to capitalize with the staff on early enthusiasm for her appointment"). WHO itself was also heavily criticized by those same concerned onlookers. Its independence had been compromised. External advisers to the agency had been "told off several times for being critical of the [pharmaceutical] industry." "Spin and image take precedence over evidence and quality," said one. "WHO are reneging on their essential advocacy role, and therefore failing the developing world," reported another. Of senior staff, one clinical scientist working in South Asia said, "Many seem most intent on doing nothing but keeping that Geneva tax-free bank account and the Mercedes with light-blue number plates."

Although one acrimonious departure cannot symbolize the views of all the staff at WHO, the six-page resignation letter by Daphne Fresle, a member of the Essential Drugs and Medicines Policy group, sums up the attitudes of many WHO employees. Her letter, dated December 23, 2001, began with a statement of disappointment that the "high hopes" of Brundtland's election "have not been realized." Her argument then divided into two parts: the first on policy issues, the second on administration and management. Fresle stated that she was "appalled... by WHO's unwillingness to speak with a strong public health voice on issues which are of such vital importance to the developing countries who should be the main concern of this organization." She accused WHO of playing safe in its public statements, and of censorship when criticism was made of the pharmaceutical industry. Of the *World Health Report 2000*,[3] which was devoted to an analysis and ranking of health systems, she voiced the feelings of many I spoke with who felt "embarrassed... to be associated with this highly criticized product." The Commission on Macroeconomics and Health,[4] which was initiated by Brundtland in 1999 and reported its findings in December 2001, was, according to Fresle, "much too favorable to the pharmaceutical industry."

There were common themes among the comments I have heard in Geneva, the arguments in the Fresle letter, and the views of *Lancet* advisers. A picture emerged of independence put at risk, shaky science, and invisible advocacy. But when I listened to Brundtland set out her aims in animated conversation, discussed WHO's direction and policies with several executive directors in Brundtland's Geneva cabinet, and talked with those at the policy end of WHO's work, these criticisms seemed misplaced. To be sure, there are serious issues that the leaders of WHO must address, but one of their most perverse challenges is to explain WHO's new mission to its staff and outside health professionals. Although Brundtland achieved success in the international political arena by building novel alliances, she and her team neglected many within their own public health and clinical communities. By doing so, WHO's leadership has failed to draw on the skills, enthusiasm, and dedication of its most important constituency. And as she hands over the organization to Jong Wook Lee, her successor from South Korea, in July 2003, WHO faces the most serious test of its credibility in its fifty-year history.

Dr. Brundtland has occupied high state offices since 1974, when she was appointed minister of the environment in the Norwegian government. This long experience largely explains her successful early repositioning of WHO's role. In an address to WHO staff in July 1998, she spoke of "making a difference" and promised a substantial "change in focus." Internally, she wanted "one WHO," an agency that was less hierarchical in structure, more open in its decision-making, and driven by results. Externally, she sought new partnerships with government, the private sector, and the research community. She wanted to move WHO from being an agency concentrating exclusively on health to one fashioning "a vital mandate for health and human development." "We were not moving to Health for All when I came in," she told me. "I wanted to bring this issue further from public health, civil society, activists, up to the decision-makers in governments."

To reinvent WHO's role, Brundtland centralized the agency's management and redistributed resources to Africa. Although regional directors in Manila, New Delhi, Harare, Alexandria, Copenhagen, and Washington were still respected, they were marginalized by a new cabinet based around the nine clusters that now oversaw WHO's work. Before taking office, Brundtland launched two projects that defined her approach to policymaking: Roll Back Malaria and the Tobacco Free Initiative. This root-and-branch organizational change indeed focused WHO's work on a few visible priorities, but at the cost of very public failures that wounded WHO's sense of unity—only two of her original nine Geneva cabinet members remained in place until the end of her tenure.

Brundtland's interpretation of WHO's purpose was "gathering, creating, advocating, and spreading the knowledge that is necessary for countries to move towards promoting health and preventing disease, especially for the poor and disadvantaged." This more prosaic summary resisted the attractive, but superficial, label of "Health for All." From 1998 on, Brundtland promoted priorities and policies guided by evidence rather than advocacy; concentrated on delivering better health by measuring—controversially—health care systems within countries (see Chapter 17); and broadened the interest of WHO to include disability, inequalities, and risk factors for disease. Contrary to what her critics claim, she spoke of WHO's "bedrock principle" of securing "universal access to quality care." This new strategy shifted the health debate onto fresh ground. For example, neuropsychiatric disorders and injury rose in WHO's priorities after a study of the global burden of disease revealed their neglected importance.

In sum, Brundtland argued that WHO should become the world's first health knowledge agency, devoted to the production, collection, and distribution of information as a global public good. WHO is, she said, "a repository of public-health knowledge" that is free, can benefit all people equally, and whose use will not diminish its benefit for others. Brundtland's particular contribution was to set WHO's sights on securing political commitment "to put health at the core of the international development agenda." In practice, that meant WHO moving its interest away from ministers of health to finance ministers—even to prime ministers and presidents.

By the end of her time in office, some of Brundtland's initiatives were being judged by donors who had committed substantial resources to her vision for WHO. Roll Back Malaria, for example, has recently been reviewed by the UK's Department for International Development (DFID), the project's largest external donor. When RBM was launched, it was paraded as an example of how diverse parts of the UN family, the public sector, the research community, and non-governmental organizations could work together to pool expertise. The project was "co-owned" by these parties and received support from African as well as G8 leaders. David Alnwick, RBM's project manager, calls their work a "movement" against malaria. But the DFID review, led by Richard Feachem, a former dean of the London School of Hygiene and Tropical Medicine, was harshly critical of RBM's progress. Feachem's team found fault with the World Bank for its lending strategies, UNICEF for paying insufficient attention to malaria, and the partnership itself for poor governance. WHO has contested Feachem's conclusions, arguing that what he sees as weaknesses are actually RBM's strengths. But clearly this "pathfinder" initiative, as Brundtland once called it, tried to satisfy the irreconcilable interests of too many parties, while failing to deliver on the aims set by G8 leaders in Okinawa. In trying to be all things to all people, the partnership fostered paralysis.

Access to medicines has become the test above all others by which the rich world will be judged in its dealings with the poor. The excuse that without a proven primary health care system distribution of drugs would not only be chaotic but also dangerous has been shown to be a myth.[5] In 1999, Médecins Sans Frontières (MSF) launched a radical and highly successful campaign for access to essential medicines. Their advocacy is built on three goals: overcoming access barriers (for example, lending support to health ministries unable to acquire drugs), challenging trade restrictions, and stimulating new research into neglected diseases. MSF is leading the debate about how to translate the November 2001 Doha Declaration into a practical plan for drug availability. The Doha Declaration states:

> We recognise that under WTO [World Trade Organization] rules no country should be prevented from taking measures for the protection of human, animal, or plant life or health.... We stress the importance we attach to implementation and interpretation of the Agreement on Trade-Related Aspects of Intellectual Property Rights (TRIPS Agreement) in a manner supportive of public health, by promoting both access to existing medicines and research and development into new medicines.

The TRIPS council was charged with finding a solution to the difficulty of access to medicines for those countries with no manufacturing capacity by the end of 2002. Thanks to a veto by the US government in December 2002, no agreement was reached. The US argued that although it could tolerate access to medicines for diseases such as AIDS, TB, and malaria, it could not resist the demands of its domestic pharmaceutical industry to block access to drugs for noninfectious diseases, such as diabetes and high blood pressure. Public health arguments cut no ice with the US trade delegation, despite Doha. A deal will eventually be made—it is a legal requirement—but, once again, access to vital drugs to treat health emergencies among those living in poverty will be restricted solely to protect profit. And WHO has nothing to say on this issue.

Organizations such as MSF have replaced WHO at the leading edge of policy development. So what is the position of WHO on access to essential medicines? I met with senior members of the Essential Drugs and Medicines Policy group in Geneva. At the time of our meeting, Fresle was still part of this program and there had clearly been substantial and unresolved disagreement over the direction WHO policy was taking. The impression that I took away was that a large proportion of this group would like to be given greater freedom to advance WHO's role in this sensitive political area. However, as an intergovernmental agency, WHO must rely on the annual World Health Assembly to set its aims, with the timing of policy statements determined by the director-general. But in the Essential Drugs group, at least, relying on Brundtland alone to decide when to speak out has meant missing opportunities to shape the wider global agenda of access to medicines.

When one reads the documents produced by WHO on essential medicines, many of MSF's messages appear again and again. WHO deems access to essential drugs a human right, and it argues that medicines are not simply another commodity to be traded. But it is MSF, not WHO, that has coordinated a strategy to implement the Doha Declaration. WHO was happy to follow quietly in its footsteps. Still, it would be wrong to suggest that departments within WHO are not trying to create a public dialogue to set high standards in WHO's work with the private sector. The director of the Essential Drugs and Medicines Policy group has raised important questions about public–private partnerships and commercial influences in research.[6] Moreover, a recent WHO effort to identify companies that produce the highest-quality medicines included generic manufacturers as well as multinational patent-holding pharmaceutical companies. The Indian generic producer Cipla has had nevirapine, zidovudine, and lamivudine all approved by WHO. This list of acceptable manufacturers is likely to encourage price competition and break the monopoly large companies have enjoyed over drug provision to the poorest countries.

There are also examples of quiet diplomatic pressure being brought to bear on the pharmaceutical sector. For instance, moves to create a new essential drugs list started in 2002. The Commission on Macroeconomics and Health argued that such a list should be the basis on which the pharmaceutical industry licenses its technologies to producers of high-quality generics for use in resource-poor countries. Industry has been nervous about the possibility that profitable patented drugs will be included on this WHO list. When the idea was first mooted, the US government, according to members of the Essential Drugs group, sent a long fax setting out its objections to such a maneuver. In many areas, therefore, WHO has to work behind the scenes to secure public health advances, and it must endure frustrating political pressures not faced by MSF. But its gentler approach to advocacy can be successful. The new essential medicines list, released at the end of April 2002, included ten new antiretroviral agents—all for the treatment of HIV in adults and children. WHO gave guidance on preferred combinations, and on starting and switching therapy. The agency also endorsed development of fixed-dose (single-pill) formulations—to improve adherence and efficacy, while delaying resistance—as a high priority for industry. These measures go a long way toward cutting through persistently applied industry and US government barriers to drug access.

This self-imposed reticence in the public arena has not characterized all areas of WHO policy. Tobacco control was one of Brundtland's crusading initiatives. She spoke publicly of the tobacco industry's "financial obligations for death and disease"; about an "industry which is massively focusing its marketing efforts on youth and women in developing countries"; and even of the "tobacco industry's manipulation of WHO's work." On tobacco, Brundtland was passionate, political, and unqualified in her criticism of business. It is unfortunate, therefore, that she did not speak out more forcefully about the pharmaceutical industry's global responsibilities. In this case, the demands of the private sector took precedence over public health principles.

The noncommunicable disease cluster, led by Derek Yach, also makes commerce a central issue in its policy work. In a recent address to the Washington International Business Council, Yach spoke about the damaging effects of not only tobacco but also alcohol, which kills about two million people every year. WHO, he said, is now turning its attention to "how best to curb marketing [of alcohol] to youth." For example, "restrictions" may be needed on "commercial speech" and higher taxes might be required on behaviors to be discouraged. Yach ended his lecture by reiterating that WHO's "overall goal of interaction [with business] is to make markets work for chronic disease control."

Yach has quickly come face-to-face with an industry that does not wish to listen to his message of public health responsibility. WHO launched its long-awaited report on diet, nutrition, and prevention of chronic diseases in April 2003. One of the report's targets was sugar, which it said should not, in added form, exceed 10 percent of a food's total energy content. But the Sugar Association in the US is asking Congress to cut American contributions to WHO because of its dislike for this expert advice. "We are very mad," said the president of the Sugar Association, Andrew Briscoe.

This uneven approach to the commercial sector worries some long-serving employees at WHO. Brundtland seemed willing to attack an easy target—tobacco—but receded from a full-blown challenge to the sector that is chiefly responsible for denying access to essential medicines. She made a great success of politicizing WHO's work to raise health higher on the global development agenda, but this politicization was a double-edged sword, and when it looked likely to incite donor disapproval, WHO's resolve collapsed.

Undoubtedly, Brundtland's greatest achievement was to make health a serious and credible political issue. The document that has done most to legitimize health in the political sphere has come from the Commission on Macroeconomics and Health. Its report is explicitly political, and claims to have produced evidence that will "reduce poverty, spur economic development, and promote global security." At a time when the Western world is examining its post–September 11 vulnerabilities to terrorism, this message is having an effect on political leaders. Former US President Bill Clinton was one of the first to link poverty reduction to counterterrorism: "We have to create more opportunity for those left behind by progress, thus reducing the pool of potential terrorists by increasing the number of potential partners. To make new partners, the wealthy world has to accept its obligation to promote more economic opportunity and help reduce poverty."[7]

Jeffrey Sachs, the Harvard economist and now UN adviser who chaired the commission, argued that unless his investment recommendations were heeded, the Millennium Development Goals laid down by world leaders would never be met. His case was mixed with moral and political urgency: "With globalization on trial as never before, the world must succeed in achieving its solemn commitments to reduce poverty and improve health." Brundtland called the commission "a turning point in the history of development." It was "a document to the governments of the world." Her former executive director, Julio Frenk, now minister of health in Mexico and a recent candidate to succeed her as director-general, underlined the political nature of the issue: "Directing greater political attention and financial resources to health is an overdue requirement for equity and sustainability."[8]

One of the key instruments for putting health at the forefront of development, and one strongly endorsed by the commission, is the Global Fund to Fight AIDS, Tuberculosis, and Malaria. Its purpose is to secure and distribute grant money to stem the effect of these diseases that together kill over five million people every year. Although questions have been raised about the likely effectiveness of the Global Fund,[9] a much more fundamental issue is how political forces will shape the work of the fund's governance, management, and decision-making. Behind the official claim that the Global Fund is independent of WHO, agency staff have had important parts to play in its administration and policy-making.

During a visit to Geneva in 2002, I attended a private board meeting of the Global Fund. The meeting, held at WHO's headquarters, was surprisingly chaotic; indeed, childishly point-scoring. The main items on the agenda were updates about the recruitment of an executive director and the appointment of a technical review panel to judge applications and make recommendations to the fund's board. Six hundred and twenty-one applications had been submitted for the post of executive director. Interviews were to take place in early April 2002 and three candidates would finally be presented to the board. France immediately lodged an objection. Despite previously agreed-upon procedures for interviews, its representative wanted a seat on the recruitment panel. The fund secretariat argued that the interview committee should be kept small. France remained insistent on being given a place. After much haggling, France was awarded observer status at the interviews. Ultimately Richard Feachem was appointed executive director of the fund in April 2002. He was not one of the shortlisted candidates, and it is not clear how he became the compromise choice.

Discussion about the technical review panel produced near gridlock. Seven hundred nominations had to be reduced to seventeen, taking account of specialist expertise, geographical balance, and gender. All delegates praised the "tremendous work" of the fund secretariat. But this polite veneer concealed a great deal of anger. Pakistan registered "deep disappointment" that none of its representatives had been chosen. A UNAIDS spokesman criticized the excessive time pressures on selection and the opacity of the process. The US representative raised concerns that many skilled individuals had been peremptorily "cut off" the final list. Excellence had been traded for international balance, he claimed. Most irritated of all was the private sector, whose representative pronounced herself "very unhappy" about the "flawed circumstances" and a "flawed result." The process had been "clouded by geography and gender balance." The UK delegate agreed. In return for its place on the board, the private sector has contributed only a tiny proportion of existing fund monies. So much for public–private partnerships.

The further opening of WHO's doors to the private sector has unsettled many inside and outside the agency.[10] The UN Millennium Declaration endorsed by heads of state and governments insisted on the development of "strong partnerships with the private sector." Brundtland recognized the risk of this new policy and the need for clear standards in dealing with industry. In a note to WHO's executive board dated December 5, 2001, she summarized her views on WHO's involvement with public–private interactions for health. She stressed that any interaction had to have a clear statement of purpose; conflicts of interest had to be avoided, or at least fully declared; and industry involvement had to be balanced by engagement with nongovernmental organizations. Brundtland acknowledged that WHO staff needed substantial further training for their dealings with commercial bodies. The aim remains independent "science-based setting of norms and standards," with decision-making "at a remove from the private sector." She was convinced that her policy is the right one to follow: "The alternative would have been less effective," she told me.

Although these words offered comfort to some critics, others will remain skeptical. Within the Essential Drugs group, for example, there is a strong belief that WHO has already given up too much independence. How can a senior member of the pharmaceutical industry be a credible adviser on generic drugs to the Commission on Macroeconomics and Health? And when such "an outrageous conflict of interest" was challenged, the concerns of WHO's own technical staff were ignored. The view of one senior WHO scientist was that, as a result, the commission "lacked authority."

The criticism that Brundtland failed to be an advocate for the world's poor is less just. Repeatedly, she promoted health as the key to poverty eradication. She did not understand the criticism leveled against her. "I don't measure what we achieve in changing the world by how many times I or other WHO staff members say certain things.... It is the impact of what they say, when they say it, and the follow up, and the way you are able to create movement."

She was also a fierce proponent of a gender-equal society. In a discussion devoted to International Women's Day in 2002, she reiterated that "poverty carries a woman's face," and that to improve women's health "means speaking out against all forms of violence." She was prepared to speak up for health in the most complex and sensitive of political settings. An escalation of violence in the Middle East, for example, led her in March 2002 to urge Israelis and Palestinians to accept the neutral role of doctors, nurses, and paramedical workers, and to allow them to continue their work in safety, especially in provision of services to children, pregnant women, and the disabled.

But although some criticisms can be rebutted, the strong feeling of administrative failure among Geneva staff was harder to explain away. In a survey of employees completed by the staff association in May 2001, over 80 percent rated WHO management's concern for employee well-being and satisfaction as bad or very bad. Coordination within WHO was rated as bad or very bad by three quarters of the 637 respondents. Forty percent rated morale bad or very bad. In a recent report to the executive board, WHO employees complained of nepotism and discrimination in appointments (there was Norwegian cronyism, said some), lack of training, poor staff security and safety, and inequalities in contracts, salaries, and benefits. Representatives of WHO claimed that Brundtland had "no direct contact with staff" despite her expressed wish to spend two thirds of her time in Geneva, and that she "disregarded" their views. Brundtland surrounded herself with two or three close advisers who controlled her access to other colleagues, even some of her most senior executive directors. She ran her office like a prime minister—she had "minders" and "handlers" who were quick to extinguish small rebellions, often brutally. I was told that staff were "reaching a point of confrontation on a big scale." An independent UN oversight unit recently confirmed some of these "shortcomings."[11] In polite understatement, its report concluded that "there is a need to reassert the value of the human capital of the Organization as a means of encouraging and motivating staff."

There is another view—namely, that some employees were resistant to change and that they disliked Brundtland's efforts to improve accountability throughout the agency. And to the charge that she tolerated no dissent, Brundtland, ever the politician, simply pointed to the Fresle letter: "This illustrates, I think, the freedom that people in this house have." But Fresle left partly because she felt that her views were ignored. Freedom to speak without any sign of being listened to is no freedom at all.

In a comprehensive analysis of WHO's history and impact, Jared Siddiqi[12] argued that politicization was the cause of WHO's "greatest dishonor." The origins of this corrosive force went back, Siddiqi claimed, to the politics of exclusion. Donor power and recipient weakness were the twin roots of "frustration and uncertainty" that threatened to starve WHO's future growth. Exactly the opposite has turned out to be true. The politicization of health by Brundtland injected fresh life into an agency suffering diminished influence. But Siddiqi was right in one important respect: the success of WHO will be judged not on the communiqués from lavish governmental conferences, but rather on the work of the organization at the country level.

Late in her tenure Brundtland started a program to strengthen WHO's performance in countries. This initiative comprised two parts. First, to define the core skills required of WHO's country representatives, including strengthening country teams according to need. Appointees as WHO representatives, commonly criticized outside the agency, will be held to new standards and trained in financial and staff management. Second, there will be better communications between countries, regions, and headquarters. Responsiveness to country needs will be a key aim. The product of these improved systems will be three-to-five-year country-cooperative strategies. Such strategies now exist for Uganda, Nicaragua, Indonesia, Cambodia, Bangladesh, Nepal, and several other Southeast Asian states.

The success of this upgrade in strategic thinking depends, of course, on results in the field. There are good reasons to be anxious about delivering on these promises. For example, countries asked for $1.2 billion in 2002 from the Global Fund to Fight AIDS, Tuberculosis, and

Malaria. The budget available was only $700 million. The gap between available funds and global needs widened in 2003. Demand clearly outstrips capacity, which will only be enhanced if the persistent brain drain of doctors and nurses from the developing world is stemmed.[13] That change will require better training programs and a commitment by donors and nongovernmental organizations not to poach local talent for their own ends. The disbursements from the Global Fund will fail without a stable human infrastructure in place. WHO has barely begun to articulate a strategy to address these problems.

The test case for WHO's new country focus is Afghanistan, where 90 percent of people live in villages, and six million of them have no access to medical care. WHO's Afghanistan representative, Mohammed Jama, reports that there is a desperate lack of health workers across the country in all sectors. His priorities are dauntingly large: controlling communicable disease, improving nutrition (250,000 Afghan children die every year from malnutrition), restoring reproductive health, and building health care institutions. Field workers are being trained and new WHO offices are being established. In March 2002, the agency issued a call for $60 million for 2002 alone to begin building an almost nonexistent health system. Fifty of the country's 220 districts have no medical facilities. But continued Western military activity in the country, together with extensive ethnic conflicts, an earthquake, and a refugee crisis, are turning a program for reconstruction and development into one of sheer survival. The challenge is not WHO's alone—its work must be coordinated with that of UNICEF and many nongovernmental organizations. Still, WHO is likely to be the most effective agency to organize such a complex process of repair.

In the immediate future, WHO plans to focus its annual reports on health systems (again) (2003) and health research (2004). Sustainable development has been Brundtland's most important next step to rehabilitate health as a political and economic issue. The World Summit on Sustainable Development, held in Johannesburg in August 2002, was a further opportunity to link health to development, this time in the context of the environment. But except for the work of a few, including Yasmin von Schirnding, WHO's key representative working on sustainable development, this issue has been a Cinderella area in WHO's repertoire of activities.

Although von Schirnding has argued that the WSSD is an "unprecedented opportunity for WHO," it has proved difficult for WHO to translate the concept of sustainable development into political programs, especially at the country level. Urbanization, climate change, extreme weather events, pollution, mismanagement of natural resources, tobacco use, poor access to clean water and sanitation, inadequate housing, violence, and the encroaching privatization of health systems all continue to threaten sustainability.[14] Strategies to meet the Millennium Development Goals remain obscure. Political will is fragmented and riven with self-interest. There is no consensus about how to translate the argument that health is the key to development into a feasible plan. WHO's aim is to continue to push the findings of the Commission on Macroeconomics and Health. There is a new initiative on children's health and the environment, incorporating food, sanitation, and household energy.

Nobody now calls for a debate about the future role of WHO. And yet Brundtland knew that her tenure would be judged on how well she implemented her vision. Sometimes, the prospects looked bleak. On gender, for instance, she only agreed on a policy within WHO—on staff recruitment, employment of gender specialists, creating a gender task force—almost four years after promising it as a priority. In one cabinet discussion I attended, executive directors debated at great length the words "gender" (unpopular), "gendered" (even more unpopular), "mainstreaming" (hackneyed), "concerns" (too negative), "approach" (better), and "perspective" (much more positive), together with their anxieties that WHO might be creating a "gender police." This trail through the thesaurus eventually returned to the issue at hand—namely, that only 29 percent of new WHO recruits are women, despite a Health Assembly resolution that WHO should have equal proportions of men and women.

Brundtland cited polio eradication as an example of WHO at its very best. Why? Because "the polio campaign," she said, "has reached out to places in the world and in remote parts of poor countries where no one has ever seen a health worker before." In 1988, the World Health Assembly passed a resolution mandating WHO to begin a campaign of polio eradication. The member states of the agency then faced over 350,000 cases in 125 polio-endemic countries. By the end of 2000, the number of confirmed cases had fallen to 2,979 across twenty nations. This dramatic success was achieved through synchronized national immunization days and "days of tranquility," on which vaccination could take place in conflict zones. In 2001, almost one tenth of the world's population—575 million children—received oral polio vaccine. By the end of that year, cases had fallen still further, to 483 in ten countries—India, Pakistan, Afghanistan, Niger, Nigeria, Ethiopia, Angola, Egypt, Sudan, and Somalia. In 2002, only India, Nigeria, and Pakistan had high levels of polio transmission (there was still low-intensity spread in Afghanistan, Egypt, Niger, and Somalia). But despite this geographical isolation, numbers of cases increased—to almost 1,500 by the end of the year. This upward blip is discouraging and has prompted renewed efforts to extend polio vaccine coverage. Still, the disease is expected to be certified as eradicated by 2005. That seems the sort of measurable effect that Brundtland might have meant when she spoke of making a difference. But can RBM, for example, really halve the burden of malarial disease? I was told by senior RBM staff that there will be "deep satisfaction" if they can "show reliably [that the] curve has started to turn down" for malaria by 2010. Here is the new equation for WHO to confront—the algebra of political expectation confounded by field reality.[15]

* * *

Jong Wook Lee—colleagues know him as J. W.—takes over Brundtland's position in July 2003. He is fifty-eight years old and has spent twenty years working for WHO, most recently leading programs on vaccines and tuberculosis. His election took many observers of the global health scene by surprise. After a former prime minister had held the position of director-general, there was an assumption that a person with similar high-level political skills would have been an advantage in the increasingly complex world of global health politics. But many Geneva headquarters staff wanted a public health specialist instead—and in J. W. Lee they certainly have someone with no shortage of technical health experience. What is more, as the only internal candidate to stand, his victory was seen as a vote of confidence in WHO's demoralized staff. Nevertheless, many senior global health leaders outside WHO are skeptical of Lee's ability to resist the sometimes bullying approach of the US government, WHO's largest donor, in the agency's affairs. They see him as a lightweight leader.

J. W. Lee has an engaging and open personal manner. He is quick to laugh. Over a drink he will pepper his conversation with many jokes at WHO's expense, and he is happy to be questioned about some of the most sensitive matters facing his tenure—usually preceded by an outrageous roar of feigned surprise that you would ever dare ask such a question. He is uncomfortable with the accoutrements of high UN office—as the newly elected director-general, a limousine follows him everywhere: he prefers to sit in the front seat for now. He says that he will not surround himself with minders, as did his predecessor, and that he will work hard to stay close to WHO's staff in Geneva—a major criticism of Brundtland, who rarely ate in the staff canteen and never wandered the corridors to meet colleagues. Lee is also keen to consult widely. Where Brundtland surrounded herself with a coterie of Norwegian advisers, Lee makes clear that he will appoint his team on merit—and that there may be a few unexpected appointments in the offing. But he admits that he feels enormous stress beneath a surface appearance of jovial calm. Immediately after his nomination in January 2003, he flew back to South Korea, intending to stay for a month of rest and contemplation of what was to come. After only one week of intense media scrutiny in his home country, he returned to the more orderly world of WHO's Geneva headquarters.

In his campaign manifesto, Lee stressed his loyalty to the poor: "to finally deliver on the promises to the poor that this world has so often failed to keep." For Lee, "health care is a right, not a commodity to be bought and sold by those who have the resources to do so." He has pledged to continue Brundtland's focus on Africa, but to broaden it to include Asia. His most radical plan—and most observers of WHO have not yet realized quite how radical this idea is—will be a massive internal reform and restructuring program at WHO. Presently 67 percent of the WHO's human and financial resources are in countries or regional offices, with the remaining third in Geneva. Lee has committed himself to decentralizing programs and people, with the goal of slimming headquarters to only 20 percent of the WHO's total budget by 2008. Such a rebalancing of its work will require courageous skills of persuasion within an institution already low on morale after years of dispute with the Brundtland regime over contracts, salaries, and conditions. Lee has promised a continuous program of internal audit to back up his reform plans.

Lee's manifesto and his answers to questions concerning the future priorities for WHO included no ideas on how he would like WHO to shape the global health agenda.[16] He is committed to achieving the Millennium Development Goals, and he wants his term of office to be judged according to progress made on these important measures. But that is no surprise since, as an intergovernmental organization, WHO can do nothing but be committed to those globally agreed-upon UN goals. The question still remains: What new programs will he launch to hasten progress in reaching not only these goals but also, if he still wishes to pursue this objective, health for all?

One possible program that has caught his early interest is child survival. The first official meeting that Lee attended after being nominated as director-general was held at the Rockefeller Foundation's Conference Center in Bellagio, Italy, in February 2003. This meeting was called to review progress in reducing the tremendous burden of child mortality in the world. Presently, 11 million children under the age of five die each year (20 percent of the global total annual number of deaths). Ninety-nine percent of these deaths occur in settings of acute poverty. This is a frustrating and shameful tragedy, so much so that one of the Millennium Development Goals is to reduce child mortality by two thirds by 2015.

The problem is concentrated in a limited number of countries. Fifty percent of annual under-five deaths occur in just fourteen nations: for example, 2.3 million deaths in India, 860,000 deaths in Nigeria, 735,000 deaths in China, 582,000 deaths in Pakistan, and 514,000 deaths in the Democratic Republic of Congo.[17] Almost two thirds owe their underlying cause to malnutrition. And deaths in the first month of life account for over 40 percent of the 11 million total because of serious infections, birth injuries, or prematurity.

What is so difficult to understand is why the pace of progress in improving child survival has slowed. Declines reached their peak in 1980. Since then, the rate of fall in child mortality has halved. This dramatic deceleration is partly because of the expanding HIV-AIDS epidemic, but not wholly. There have also been serious institutional failures during the past twenty years, and especially in the past decade. UNICEF and WHO have largely abandoned the world's children to die in poverty. For example, spending on immunization by UNICEF totaled $180 million in 1990. By 1998, that figure had fallen to around $50 million. And programs to manage childhood illnesses, while theoretically effective, have had only a weak impact in the field because of their poor coverage of those most in need. Matters had become so serious at WHO that in 2002 the agency's governing body, the World Health

Assembly, called on the director-general to devise a strategy for child and adolescent health. The barriers to improving child survival have been lack of money, insufficient advocacy and leadership, and a chronic failure to strengthen the health systems of the poorest nations. In a word, neglect.

There was great nervousness among WHO staff at the 2003 Bellagio meeting when rumors spread that Lee might come. Tomris Turmen, WHO's executive director responsible for child health, did not want the spotlight to fall on her failing WHO program so soon after his nomination. She argued strongly that he should not come, but when he signaled his interest she made sure that she accompanied him for the twenty-four hours that he was present. Although tired from his transcontinental travel schedule—his eyes closed momentarily during the presentations being made to him—he listened intently as the story of needless child mortality unfolded. Lee stood and spoke to the Bellagio group as he was about to leave. He recognized what he called the "beginning of a very, very important movement." "It's the time to take action," he said, and he promised that child survival will be "a very important agenda in the next five years for WHO." If he does make child survival a central plank of his administration, Lee will find that the task at hand is huge. But it is both morally and economically essential—for unless the lives of children are protected, the capacity of countries to work themselves out of poverty will be seriously harmed. And anyway, what kind of a world have we created where we allow so many millions of children to die unnecessarily before they have reached the age of five?

# HIGH HOPES

# 12

# HOW SICK IS MODERN MEDICINE?

AS MARCUS AURELIUS gathered his forces against German tribes in the second century AD, he summoned Claudius Galenus, an up-and-coming physician from Pergamum, to ride with him. Galen declined, politely and imaginatively, claiming a higher loyalty to "the contrary instructions of his personal patron god Asclepius."[1] This early instance of conscientious objection was accepted, it seems graciously. But in exchange for his indulgence, Marcus Aurelius ordered Galen to await his return and attend the health of his neophyte emperor son, the soon to be deranged Commodus.

Galen did his job rather too well, curing Commodus of an illness around 174 AD and unwittingly laying the ground for a murderous period of political instability some ten years or so later. Rome's long-term loss was medicine's great gain, for, as Galen later wrote,

> During this time I collected and brought into a coherent shape all that I had learned from my teachers or discovered for myself. I was still engaged in research on some topics, and I wrote a lot in connection with these researches, training myself in the solution of all sorts of medical and philosophical problems.

In addition to being a fine scholar and a wise court physician,

Galen was also the supreme polemicist of his day. The aggressive tendencies of his mother—"so bad-tempered that she would sometimes bite her maids"—provided a valuable store of endurance for Galen to draw on as he quarreled with his contemporaries. Indeed, his passion for conflict led him, at the age of twenty-eight, into the unusual role of physician to the gladiatorial school of Pergamum, a position, amid the flayed limbs, punctured chests, and eviscerated abdomens, that gave him a perfect vantage point for firsthand anatomical observation.

One of Galen's philosophical preoccupations was to understand how doctors came to know what they did about healing. He lived at a time when there was no consensus about how doctors should acquire knowledge. Empiricists relied entirely on experience, while Rationalists depended on reason from a prespecified theory of causation. A third group, the Methodists, rejected both experience and causal theory, putting all illnesses down to a tension between the flow of bodily discharges and their constipation. Galen was a deft eclectic. He scrutinized opposing arguments, identified their flaws, erased erroneous logic, and combined what remained into a practicable clinical method. He wished to assert the primacy of clinical observation and to bind an integrated (Hippocratic, Platonic, Alexandrian) theory of medical knowledge with its practice. But Galen wanted to achieve his unique synthesis neither as a remote theoretician nor as someone who had a reputation for being merely a "word doctor": "Rather, my practice of the art alone would suffice to indicate the level of my understanding."

In *The Rise and Fall of Modern Medicine*, James Le Fanu, a practicing London doctor, a prominent medical controversialist in the English press, and a person wholly dissatisfied with the huge power exerted by modern medical sects, has surveyed and systematized, processed and picked apart the past fifty years of medical discovery.[2] Like Galen, he is frustrated by what he sees as the misleading ideologies of today's widely accepted and lavishly praised medical epistemologists.

So just what has medicine achieved? If one believes the mainstream view of Western white male medical progress, it has been an astonishing success. The turn of the millennium saw many efforts to sum up what the editors of the *New England Journal of Medicine* have called "the astounding course of medical history over the past thousand years."[3] Medicine deserves such glorification, they said, because it "is one of the few spheres of human activity in which the purposes are unambiguously altruistic." Well, quite possibly, provided that academic tenure is speedily secured, research grants are generously awarded, salaries stay ahead of inflation, teaching loads are progressively lightened, managed care organizations try harder to be respectfully flexible, and patients keep their lawyers at a distance.

Is it also true to say, as the prolific British historian Roy Porter did, that Western medicine is "preoccupied with the self"? The narcissistic obsession with the body's personal cosmos has produced, Porter insists, a compulsion to celebrate historical winners. He defends this constant reverence for success:

> I do not think that "winners" should automatically be privileged by historians . . . but there is a good reason for bringing the winners to the foreground—not because they are "best" or "right" but because they are powerful.[4]

Other critics are less respectful of medicine's traditions. Richard Gordon, the British author of *Doctor in the House* and fourteen amusing sequels, is an agreeably arch cynic. He prefers the view that

> the history of medicine is not the testament of idealistic seekers after health and life. . . . The history of medicine is largely the substitution of ignorance by fallacies. . . . Medicine has persistently decked itself out in fashion's shamming achievements, while staying miserably bare on masterly discoveries.[5]

Despite his witty debunking, Gordon's personal résumé of premodern "masterly discoveries" largely conforms to the accepted medical canon. He includes William Harvey's discovery of the circulation of the blood (1628), Edward Jenner's exploitation of vaccination (1796), the discovery of anesthesia (in the 1840s), the elucidation of endocrine function by Claude Bernard (1850s), Charles Darwin's theory of evolution (1859), Lord Lister's invention of surgical antisepsis with carbolic acid (1865), the launch of bacteriology in the 1880s by Louis Pasteur and Robert Koch, the discovery of x rays by Wilhelm Roentgen (1895), and Freud's early forays into psychiatry. Great achievements, every one of them, even if we might quibble about Freud's staying power.

To which, after consulting antiquarian medical book dealers, physician-collectors of historical memorabilia, and doctors working at two well-established West Coast medical schools, the respected clinicians Meyer Friedman and Gerald Friedland added Andreas Vesalius's anatomic sketches (1543) and Antony Leeuwenhoek's visualization of bacteria (1676).[6] Friedman and Friedland also single out the work of William Harvey for special honor since it was he who "introduced the principle of *experimentation* for the first time in medicine."

In the twentieth century, medicine underwent something of a bifurcation. The physician Kerr L. White, a decisive figure in the study of American public health, has identified 1916 as the crucial point of separation between a medicine concerned with the health of individuals and one concerned with the health of populations.[7] It was in 1916 that the Rockefeller Foundation decided to create schools of public health independent of schools of medicine. The result was an abandonment of the social impulse within American medical education. This division contributed to the origination of two distinct histories of Western medicine, histories that had until then been indivisible.

By the end of the century, the separation of public health from clinical science was complete and officially recognized to be so. The "ten great public health achievements" of the twentieth century, according to the US Centers for Disease Control and Prevention, are vaccination, motor-vehicle safety, safer workplaces, control of infectious diseases, declines in deaths from coronary heart disease and stroke, safer and healthier foods, healthier mothers and babies, family planning, fluoridation of drinking water, and recognition of tobacco as a health hazard.[8] Compare these simple social milestones with those feats of technical discovery celebrated annually since 1901 in the Nobel Prize in Physiology or Medicine. All but a few distinguished laureates have come from the laboratory rather than the clinic, and few prizewinners reflect the tradition of public health.

This leaning of the Nobel committee to basic science has caused consternation among many in medicine. For some years, unsuccessfully, an annual letter-writing campaign has taken place to persuade the reluctant Swedes to give their prize to Richard Doll, the man who, among other achievements, codiscovered the link between smoking and lung cancer. He is ninety years old and time is ebbing away.

Le Fanu's thesis takes in this strange parallel evolution of laboratory science and public health, and he engagingly refuses to submit to convention about who should be applauded for their contributions to each. About Doll, for example, whom he agrees is "one of the world's most eminent cancer epidemiologists," Le Fanu is scathing. Doll's 1981 treatise, *The Causes of Cancer*, is found badly wanting: it "may look impressive, but appearances can be deceptive.... Intellectual rigor...is conspicuous only by its absence."

In the fifty years after World War II, Le Fanu argues, the Western world has undergone a "unique period of prodigious intellectual ferment." Drawing mainly on British and US experience, he goes on to select his personal ten definitive moments of discovery, arbitrarily he admits, from this half-century. But he also begins with a warning. Although there has been startling progress, medicine is now facing an era of perplexing stagnation. Doctors are disillusioned by their profession; they increasingly have to deal with "the worried well" rather than the genuinely sick; they have to contend with the puzzling and, for many physicians, irritating popularity of alternative medicine; and the costs of diagnosis and treatment are escalating at a rate that is not matched by advances in knowledge. From the 1970s on, there has been "a marked decline" in innovation. And, worst of all, doctors have experienced a "subversion, by authoritarian managers and litigious patients, of the authority and dignity of the profession."

The purpose of retelling standard histories of drug development (penicillin), physiology (cortisone), dramatic treatments (open-heart surgery), and identification of major causes of disease (the bacterium that causes peptic ulcers), as Le Fanu does in his "Lengthy Prologue," is to find common patterns in the social conditions that delivered these discoveries. Four characteristics appear time and time again, none of which supports the notion that medical progress is a rational enterprise. Le Fanu's reading of the postwar history of medicine marks him, in Galenic terms, as an extreme and unforgiving empiricist.

First, medicine must pay a great debt to chance. In cancer treatment, for example, "virtually all [drugs] owe their origins to chance observation or luck." They were mostly "stumbled upon," often by "accident." "The common theme," Le Fanu concludes, "running through the discovery of these cancer drugs was that there was no common theme." With respect to treatment of the childhood cancer acute lymphoblastic leukemia (ALL), "the most impressive achievement of the post-war years,"

> the cure of ALL is proof of the power of science to solve the apparently insoluble. But science can certainly not claim all the credit, for many aspects of the cure of ALL remain frankly inexplicable.

> The culprit is not technology itself, but the intellectual and emotional immaturity of the medical profession, which seemed unable to exert the necessary self-control over its new-found powers.

As doctors misunderstood and misused the tools available to them, they passed the responsibility for research to a new professional cadre of medical scientists. The "fall" was by now irreversible. Failures stacked up in all spheres of medicine, laboratory and clinical.

Basic science came to be dominated by molecular genetics. The discovery of DNA spawned new technologies that led to research into genetic engineering, genetic screening, and gene therapy. Naive investors, often ignorant about the wafer-thin credibility of the research they were paying for, poured millions into biotechnology companies. The result, according to Le Fanu, has been that "the impression of progress has not been vindicated by anything resembling the practical benefits originally anticipated."

Worse, gene therapy has largely turned out to be "not only expensive but useless." Why has the new genetics so far failed medicine? Le Fanu answers that "genetics is not a particularly significant factor in human disease." And, in any case, genes are "complex," "unpredictable," and "perverse." They are not amenable to easy understanding. Their involvement in disease is largely "incomprehensible."

And what of the clinic? Le Fanu believes the huge error that doctors made was to be "seduced" by "the Social Theory," an approach to the study of disease by which exposure to environmental hazards or to dangerous forms of human behavior are sought as the possible causes of diseases. These epidemiological inquiries suggested ways of preventing illness by altering the exposure or modifying a behavior.

Smoking is an obvious example. Le Fanu has no doubts about the link between smoking and lung cancer; but he believes the success of Richard Doll's early work has rendered doctors and the public prey to the foolish view that many diseases are caused by unhealthy lifestyles. Le Fanu's key exhibit for the prosecution is the dietary hypothesis of heart disease—namely, that what one eats will determine one's risk of a heart attack. This idea, according to Le Fanu, is "the great cholesterol deception." Accepting the mechanistic link between cholesterol and heart disease, he vehemently denies that diet can be counted on to cure it. He applies the same skepticism to similar claims about diet and cancer ("quackery"). Without any qualification, Le Fanu concludes that the Social Theory "is in error *in its entirety*" (his italics). He accuses epidemiologists of "deceit," "idealist utopianism," and "lack of insight." The consequence is that the epidemiological perspective

> has wasted hundreds of millions of pounds in futile research and health-education programmes while justifying the imposition of costly regulations to reduce yet further the minuscule levels of pollution in air and water. And to cap it all, it does not work. The promise of the prevention of thousands of deaths a year has not been fulfilled.

The fall of medicine was complete.

Le Fanu's criticism of wildly exaggerated claims and expectations for the new genetics is shared by many of those who are leaders in the field. David Weatherall, who ran the Institute of Molecular Medicine at the University of Oxford, once pointed out that

> the remarkable complexity of the genotype–phenotype relationship has undoubtedly been underestimated during the early period of the revolution in the biomedical sciences that followed the DNA era. It has led to many statements being made about the imminence of accurate predictive genetics that are simply not

> true. . . . It is far from certain that we will ever reach a stage in which we can accurately predict the occurrence of some of the common disorders of Western society at any particular stage in an individual's life.[9]

Research tends to support Le Fanu's view that genes are mostly a minor determinant of human disease. Studies of twins enable investigators to explore the genetic and environmental contributions to disease (although they tell us nothing about important interactions between the two). In one recent report, for example, evidence from twins showed "that the overwhelming contributor to the causation of cancer" was not genetic. If genes play an important part, then the risk of cancer should be substantially greater in identical twins than in nonidentical twins, and this was not the case.[10] For breast cancer, only 27 percent of all causes can be traced to genetic factors. Prostate cancer was the disease in which genes had the most important part to play (42 percent of risk was explained by genes).

Genetic fatalism about disease is a myth that needs to be exposed once and for all. It is very unlikely that a simple and directly causal link between genes and most common diseases will ever be found. This message is not one that many scientists want the public to hear; continued political support for funding genetic research depends on persistent public credulity.

The prevailing if rather private realism among some scientists about the contribution of genetics to our understanding of human disease makes the recent hoopla about a reported first draft of the human genome all the more difficult to accept. An editorial writer for *The Times* of London, under the nonsensical headline "Secrets of Creation," concluded with hundreds of other journalists that

> this is a breathtaking moment for genetic science, for human health, even for philosophy. . . . The greatest scientific journey of

> this century starts here, with this directory; as its alphabet is decoded, the prediction, treatment and understanding of disease should be revolutionised.... It could, in particular, revolutionise the treatment of cancer, which is caused by malfunctioning genes.[11]

Not so. The fact is that progress in exploiting the genome will be painfully slow. Its importance lies not in the existence of a working draft of the genome—by itself, this tells us very little—but rather in its opening up the possibility for sequencing multiple copies of the human genome to discover variations among individuals in health and in disease. Even knowing this variation—a precondition for practical application—is of limited value, since the chief task of research must now be to study how variations in gene sequences interact with different environmental exposures, and gradations of each exposure, so as to alter the conditions of risk. I doubt that we will get far along this path during my lifetime (I am forty-one).

Having emphasized the importance of humility in the face of unfettered journalistic hyperbole, I should also mention the isolated signs of small steps forward. Le Fanu mocks the lack of progress in gene therapy since the first report of successful treatment for a type of inherited severe combined immunodeficiency disorder (SCID) in 1990. The recipient of this intervention, Ashanti de Silva, is now sixteen years old. She received eleven infusions of gene-corrected cells thirteen years ago and she has, in the words of her doctor, "thrived" ever since.[12] Moreover, during the past decade, the techniques for giving new genes to patients with SCID have improved. In a recent report, the delivery of normal genes to two infants with SCID corrected their abnormal immune function. Ten months later, both children were living at home, growing and developing normally without any side effects. A third child has also been treated and was at home, fit and well, four months later.[13] While it is far too early to draw firm conclusions, technical improvements in gene delivery do seem to translate into clinical benefit. One should still be cautious here: SCID is a rare condition amenable to correction with a single gene. Most common diseases will not be so easy to deal with.

Le Fanu's opposition to the social theory of disease is, if anything, even greater than his skepticism of genetics. His vehement condemnation of the social theory is a regular subject in the columns he writes for the London *Sunday Telegraph*.[14] Epidemiological studies produce, he claims, "spurious statistical associations whose contribution to useful knowledge is zero." How has this "nonsense" come to be so ingrained in medicine? Le Fanu explains:

> First, this type of study is easy to do: it takes no special expertise to switch on a computer, trawl through the social habits of a large group of people and come up with a "new" finding. Second, they have the veneer of scientific objectivity, with lots of figures and statistics whose publication in a journal is visible evidence of the researcher's productivity.

Maybe. But it is Le Fanu's notions of causation that are more at fault here. Epidemiology aims to uncover associations. Sometimes these associations, as Le Fanu has to admit, turn out to be true causes—as with smoking and lung cancer. But at other times, associations hide more subtle relationships. Perhaps red wine, let's say, includes an as yet unidentified ingredient that explains why its consumption is linked to a particular outcome, such as a lower risk of heart disease. The idea that an association is equivalent to a cause is a fundamental error of epidemiological interpretation; but this does not mean it is futile to report associations. The conflicting reports of risk associations—for instance, that alcohol is or is not good for you—reflect the to and fro of scientific debate, not some essential flaw in the methods being used. What human science produces the entirely unequivocal and unchallengeable results that Le Fanu so yearns for?

He also expresses heartfelt discontent that the medical research industry, despite vast government and private investment, has so few certainties to show for its endeavors. But I think his conception of the research process is seriously mistaken. Clinical research never produces definitive conclusions for the simple reason that it depends on human beings, maddeningly variable and contrary subjects. Although medical science is reported as a series of discontinuous events—a new gene for this, a fresh cure for that—in truth it is nothing more than a continuous many-sided conversation whose progress is marked not by the discovery of a single correct answer but by the refinement of precision around a tendency, a trend, or a probability.

Advances in diagnosis and treatment depend on averaging the results from many thousands of people who take part in clinical trials. The paradoxical difficulty is that these averages, although valid statistically, tell us very little about what is likely to take place in a single person. Reading the findings of medical research and combining their deceptively exact numbers with the complexities of a patient's circumstances is more of an interpretative than an evidence-based process. The aim is to shave off sharp corners of uncertainty, not to search for a perfect sphere of indisputable truth that does not and never could exist. In this way the process of research is often more important than the end result. It does not have the drama and heroism that Le Fanu dwells on in his ten definitive moments. But these moments are not typical of what most medical researchers do.

What should be clear is that Le Fanu is on shaky ground in rejecting the argument that changes in lifestyle have contributed to the rise and fall of heart disease in the US and Canada since the 1950s. He cites inconsistent findings that seem to prove a widespread confusion surrounding this orthodoxy. Superficially, his case is fair because risk factors related to lifestyles have usually been studied one at a time, providing a chaotic and conflicting picture overall. One recent study done at Harvard, however, has attempted to circumvent this problem by looking at the interplay of risk factors in a single large group of middle-aged women. The results will not please Le Fanu.

The small group who collectively did not smoke, remained reasonably thin, drank alcohol moderately, exercised regularly, and ate a diet rich in fiber and low in saturated fat reduced their risk of heart disease during a fourteen-year period by over 80 percent. Whichever way you interpret these data, how you live influences how you die. The Harvard epidemiologists conclude that their findings "support the hypothesis that adopting a more healthful lifestyle could prevent a substantial majority of coronary disease events in women."[15] The social theory of disease may not explain everything about life and death, but it would be wrong to cast epidemiology into oblivion just yet.

Le Fanu ends his review of medicine's demise in typically unflinching style: "By the 1970s much of what was 'do-able' had been done." His interpretation of the past fifty years is that medical science has reached its natural limit:

> The main burden of disease had been squeezed towards the extremes of life. Infant mortality was heading towards its irreducible minimum, while the vast majority of the population was now living out its natural lifespan to become vulnerable to diseases strongly determined by ageing.

Any solution to the diseases that now affect human longevity

> means discarding the intellectual falsehoods of The Social Theory and the intellectual pretensions of The New Genetics.... The simple expedient of closing down most university departments of epidemiology could both extinguish this endlessly fertile source of anxiety-mongering while simultaneously releasing funds for serious research.

Le Fanu misreads the ills of present-day medicine. But his approach to the discoveries of the past does bring into clear relief important social changes in the way medical research is done today, changes that should influence professional, public, and political attitudes toward contemporary medicine.

Clinical research had become highly specialized, often eliminating the ordinary doctor from the process of day-to-day investigation. This upheaval in the way research was done accelerated during the 1970s, at the time Le Fanu identifies as being the start of medicine's precipitous fall. There was a hiatus in dramatic discoveries, it is true, but that now seems to be coming to an end. As research moved from the bedside to the laboratory, doctors in clinics were left empty-handed, with little to contribute to the production of medical knowledge. But a far more important instrument was being given to them —the randomized controlled clinical trial.

The clinical trial is a human experiment, enabling physicians to study the safety and effectiveness of interventions, whether in the form of drugs, devices, or prescribed changes in behavior. According to the Declaration of Helsinki, in principle a trial must be sanctioned by an ethics committee and the patients involved must give informed consent to taking part in it. These conditions are not always met, particularly in the developing world. But still, the randomized trial has become the foundation of current clinical knowledge. Clinicians are increasingly being drawn into trial networks. Far from being divorced from medical research, doctors are now back at the center of its most powerful new means of discovery.

The centrality of clinical trials to twenty-first-century medicine means that further definitive moments, unlike those in earlier times, may not always be instances of positively beneficial discovery. "Negative" results—proving that a drug either does not work or causes more harm than good—can be equally if not more important in shaping medical knowledge. Trials allow scientific concepts to be tested experimentally and these theories can sometimes be proven embarrassingly mistaken.

For example, stroke is a leading cause of death and disability in the Western world. In the early 1990s animal experiments suggested that brain damage after a stroke occurred when chemicals released during an episode of oxygen starvation overstimulated surrounding neurons. A theory was developed and tested in the laboratory in which blocking the effects of these chemicals protected the brain from further harm. Recently reported trials have shown this carefully worked out theory to be either wrong or, at best, seriously oversimplified.[16]

The new genetics is likely to expand, not contract, the potential for drug discovery. Genes code for proteins. Now that most of the human genome sequence is available to us, the total protein complement of the human cell (the proteome) is within reach. Since proteins control most cell processes, they are important natural targets for drugs. Not only will the genome and proteome yield new sites for drug action, but finding the pattern for the ways genes and proteins are expressed in each disease state will enable much more precise classification of diseases. Subtle differences in diseases, notably cancers, which were previously thought to be homogenous pathological entities, are now being found, with significant implications for prognosis and treatment. Currently accepted disease classifications will soon be torn up. For example, one type of blood cancer that previously had an unpredictable outcome after treatment has recently been shown to consist of two separate categories of disease, categories that were distinguished from one another by their different molecular fingerprints. These two types of cancer had clearly distinct clinical outcomes. The confusion caused by lumping together two diseases as one was finally resolved.[17]

As these developments change the semantics of human disease, so they will reveal ever more clearly the vast inequalities in health between North and South. These differences have been with us for many years, but they have been all too openly emphasized by the excruciating brutality of the HIV/AIDS epidemic. The introduction of highly active antiretroviral treatment has cut the rate of illness by over 90 percent for the two million people living with AIDS in the developed world. But for the 32 million HIV-infected people living in poorer countries, access to these drugs is denied because of their high cost. According to a recent report from Médecins Sans Frontières, "In most poor countries the prices of HIV drugs condemn people with AIDS to premature death."[18] Contrary to Le Fanu, then, the major issue in medicine is not maintaining the past pace of discovery but making sure there is equitable access, throughout the world, to the discoveries we have already made.

There is another aspect of medicine, hardly touched on by Le Fanu, which has probably caused deeper and more impassioned disagreement among today's medical sects than any other issue during the past two decades. Screening for disease should bring about the successful convergence of epidemiology and clinical medicine. A group of people apparently free from disease is screened for a disorder that, once found, is treated. Since the condition is identified early, the chances of cure are high. Mammography, the Pap test, colonoscopy, prostate specific antigen—all of these investigations should throw up early warning signs of potentially fatal illnesses. Controversy is bound to arise over what to do when a result is positive. But these skirmishes are nothing compared with the terrifying choices that will be presented when genetic tests become more widely available.

Women with the gene mutations BRCA1 or BRCA2, which were first reported in 1994 and 1995, respectively, have a lifetime risk of breast cancer ranging up to 85 percent. If such a mutation is discovered in a woman, what should she do? She might have no identifiable disease at the time the mutation is found. Should she choose what may, for her, lead to peace of mind (prophylactic mastectomy) or should she choose regular surveillance? The little research that has been done suggests that about half of women with a risk mutation will choose prophylactic surgery, and that those who do so tend to be parents and of younger age.[19] Genetic testing poses immensely difficult life choices for women at moments when the conflict between fear and apparent good health is unresolvable. Fear seems to drive the decision for surgery. As a leading team in genetic research on breast cancer recently wrote:

> Prophylactic mastectomy is a mutilating and irreversible intervention, affecting body image and sexual relations. There is much concern about the potential psychological harm of DNA testing for BRCA1 and BRCA2 and prophylactic surgery, in particular mastectomy. However, in our experience and that of others, women who had mastectomy after adequate counselling rarely express regret, instead they are relieved from fear of cancer.

Finally, the separation of clinical medicine from public health seems as intractable as ever. And yet, oddly, it may be here that Le Fanu's twin evils of genetics and social theory might find a useful meeting point. If one knows that a gene is in some way related to a disease, the study of those genes in populations can help one to plan the health services that will be needed to take care of those affected.

That is exactly what Shanthimala de Silva and her colleagues have done in Sri Lanka.[20] They used chemical fingerprints for thalassemia, a genetically determined blood disorder causing severe anemia, to calculate that the island had over two thousand persons requiring treatment. To take appropriate care of these people would require about 5 percent of the country's total health budget—$5 million, a large sum of money for a small nation. Yet it would be better to know what costs will be involved and to try to raise the money domestically and internationally than to ignore the disease. These findings have implications throughout the entire Indian subcontinent and Southeast Asia, where the gene frequencies for thalassemia are even higher than they are in Sri Lanka.

By improving the clarity of questions that medical practice poses and by diminishing the uncertainty of our answers to those questions, geneticists and social theorists have not damaged the "intellectual integrity" of medicine, as Le Fanu claims. They have simply blurred old and reassuring certainties. Le Fanu longs for the past authority enjoyed by doctors and for the deference that such authority demanded from patients. He berates these researchers for their erosion of medicine's moral base. But just as scientists do not have ultimate control, despite their intense efforts to the contrary, over the interpretations others place on their work, so it seems ludicrous to impose a moral imperative on their motivations. Medical science is just as self-serving as any other branch of human inquiry. To claim a special moral purpose for medicine or even a beneficent altruism is simply delusional.

Many doctors do feel under pressure from the bureaucracy of managed care, the opportunism of zealous litigants, and the overwhelming weight of new knowledge that they are expected to assimilate. With all of these extraneous forces, is Le Fanu correct when he concludes that today "medicine is duller"? I doubt it. Medicine is as unpredictable, baffling, ambiguous, fallible, and absurd as it ever was.

And medicine is vulnerable too. We take its successes for granted. If one consults a book about a particular disease, one aimed at patients rather than doctors, the likelihood is that clinical trials will not figure prominently. The natural history of the condition in question will be given, together with characteristic symptoms and signs for self-diagnosis. And when it comes to treatment recommendations, clear directions are common. Patients naturally seek certainty. Careful critiques of contrary evidence from one trial or another would confuse rather than enlighten. The contribution of clinical trials to medicine is mostly hidden from the public eye. And yet we have now reached a time when the accumulated benefits of a half-century of clinical trial research are being seriously eroded. Just as the positive value of trials is hidden, so the current visibility of the problems of trials has created a perverse imbalance in public perception that now threatens them—and medicine itself.

In February 2000, *The Lancet* published the results of a randomized trial examining the efficacy of interferon in Behçet's disease.[21] Shortly afterward, a letter arrived from one of the alleged co-authors. It read:

> Sir—I do not regularly read *The Lancet* but I happened to see my name on an article supposedly by Haluk Demiroglu and colleagues.... I am totally unaware of the patients who were enrolled in that study and I have done nothing in the running of the study. I have signed no copyright agreement and, therefore, do not share any kind of scientific or legal responsibility that may arise in the future concerning that paper.

The corresponding author could not explain the basis of this letter, or two similar letters from other "co-authors." I wrote to the dean of Hacettepe University Medical School in Turkey, who formed an "investigational committee." His inquiry revealed that authors' signatures on the paper had been forged, that no ethics committee approval had been secured (the paper said otherwise), that no written informed consent was sought (the paper said otherwise), and that "some fabrication and falsification might have taken place." I retracted the paper eight months after its original publication. Similar recent cases of outright fraud have gained wide publicity. A 1995 paper from Werner Bezwoda, a South African oncologist, was retracted after an extensive investigation.[22] Patient records and diagnoses were unverifiable, and what records were verifiable were insufficient. Most patients were, in any case, improperly entered into the study.

Research misconduct is not confined, however, to the thoroughly disreputable. The INSIGHT study was a well-conducted randomized trial. But even so, the trial included 254 patients who were "withdrawn for misconduct," and "monitoring led to withdrawal of nine centres, in which existence of some patients could not be proved, or other serious violations of good clinical practice had occurred."[23]

Critics of those, such as myself, who raise the issue of scientific misconduct argue that the fire of publicity surrounding rare cases deserves to be dampened down rather than fanned. Certainly a proportionate response is necessary. But there is strong evidence that the community of medicine should not ignore these high-profile examples of fraud, for they may be an indicator of something far worse. A survey of 442 medical statisticians found that half of all respondents knew of at least one fraudulent project done in the previous ten years. Forty-three (26 percent) statisticians reported fabrication and falsification, thirty-two (20 percent) described deceptive reporting of data, thirty-one (19 percent) knew of data suppression, and sixteen (10 percent) were aware of instances of deceptive design and analysis. Worse still, a third of this sample had themselves engaged in a fraudulent project.

In Europe, committees to investigate allegations of fraud have sprung up in many countries. In the United States, the Office of Research Integrity (ORI) remains preeminent in this effort. And it is now flexing its muscles. In a 2000 report focusing on editors, ORI invited us to take this issue more seriously: "Requiring that the data supporting all submitted manuscripts be deposited may not be feasible. However, authors could be explicitly informed that their data may be requested during the review process or if questions arise following publication."[24] In desperation, editors are being asked to become the science police.

In March 2001, the *New England Journal of Medicine* published the results of efforts to transplant human embryonic dopamine neurons into the brains of patients with Parkinson's disease.[25] The investigators conducted a randomized trial in forty patients. Half received cultured tissue from four embryos, while half underwent sham surgery with holes drilled into the skull only. The one-year endpoint (a score measuring improvement or deterioration in symptoms) was no different between the groups. Of great concern, however, was the finding that in five transplant patients there were late-onset and debilitating side effects. The authors were cautious in their conclusions: "The surgical technique may need further refinement," they wrote. But this study was reported in the media as a severe setback in Parkinson's research. In one typical example, the headline of a press report was "Trial and Error." The opening paragraph read: "Medical research needs human guinea pigs. But the news this week of patients irreversibly damaged by a new treatment for Parkinson's disease has highlighted the risks. When is it worth it?"[26] Throughout the piece, the writer's emphasis was on concepts such as risk, guinea pigs, experiments, chance, and error. Although the value of clinical trials was discussed, the overwhelming impression left by this report was that "clinical trials remain highly risky, and public concern is understandable."

Organized research, such as that exemplified by the clinical trial, is easily open to skepticism and scare. The results of a trial are likely to have a high degree of validity, and they can be trusted by journalists. When a trial reveals harm from a potential new treatment, that result is more reliable and compelling than, say, a problem identified in an individual case report. The journalist will feel on safe ground reporting the harmful effects of a treatment studied in a trial. Yet success stories reported in the press tend to focus on the anecdotal. This bias is also understandable. Journalists need human stories that connect with their readers. The story of a single person's victory over a terminal disease (for example, on receipt of a new mechanical heart pump[27]) is far easier to convey than the complexities, methodological as well as interpretive, of a clinical trial. This challenge of understanding is damaging the public's perception of the trial process. The peer review system is sacrosanct in medicine. Yet if we summarize all we know about peer review we can hardly avoid the conclusion that the present system for verifying scientific information is the worst best system we could possibly have. Only in the past few years have readers of clinical trials been reassured that what they are reading is a complete and accurate report of what took place, but there is further room for improvement.

There is another reason why users of clinical trial data might have reason to pause. The influence of industry in trial research is not new. But the debate about potential and real malign influences of the sponsor has now reached such a pitch that the fragile foundation of integrity supporting the research enterprise could easily crack. Thomas Bodenheimer recently summed up the difficulties of this "uneasy alliance."[28] He drew attention to the way in which commercial networks were taking over clinical trial research. The academic medical center was now adopting a secondary role in the research process. Investigators seemed willing to promulgate opinions based on who was paying for their hospitality. Sponsored studies and industry-supported symposia appeared to be more favorable to the company than nonsponsored trials or events. Bodenheimer highlighted the influence of industry in trial design, data analysis, and publication. He concluded that there were serious and substantial conflicts in academic–industry partnerships, which produced "potential public and physician skepticism about the results of clinical drug trials." Marcia Angell, a former editor of the *New England Journal of Medicine*, urged that "academic institutions and their clinical faculty members must take care not to be open to the charge that they are for sale."[29]

Assuming that we can trust what a clinical trial report says, what do its results actually mean? This question was tackled by Michael Clarke and Iain Chalmers in a survey of twenty-six randomized trial reports published in leading medical journals.[30] They found that only two articles included a review of earlier research work. Clarke and Chalmers concluded:

> The public is often confused by the conflicting messages it receives as a result of piecemeal reporting of research. To deserve the public's continued support and trust, researchers and journals need to ensure that reports of research end with scientifically defensible answers to [the] question, "What does it mean, anyway?"

There is a further issue, one based on the interpretive boundaries placed on readers by the text or by the readers themselves. Unless we investigate these processes in medicine, we will misunderstand how and why doctors interpret clinical trial data in the way they do. We need to know the how and why of interpretation if we are to get some sense of the impact of trials on medicine. I call this "interpretive medicine."

The premise of this approach is that the research paper is, first and foremost, a document produced by a group of authors presenting an argument to the reader.[31] The task for the reader is to judge the validity of that argument. In medicine, and for clinical trials in particular, editors, clinical trialists, and biostatisticians have set rules for controlling the interpretion of a text.[32] The research paper has a formal structure (introduction, methods, results, and discussion). A structured abstract directs the reader to the key facts about the research report. Adherence to guidelines relieves the risk of biased reporting. The insistence on framing a result in several ways prevents the reader from taking an overly optimistic (or pessimistic) view of the treatment being tested. Hierarchies of evidence tell readers to pay more attention to particular study types. And the notion of structured discussions may assist more accurate appraisal of research data.[33]

An additional way to set boundaries on interpretations is to invoke rules of reading.[34] These rules can be divided into two categories—those relating to the text and those relating to the reader. Textual rules derive from the idea that meaning rests in words and numbers, tables and figures. The capacity to understand research papers can be acquired through training in clinical epidemiology and biostatistics. The assumption here is that the text has an objectively attainable meaning, available to readers if they have the right skills. An alternative view is that readers make meaning, not texts. To understand how the reader ascribes meaning to a clinical trial result, we need to know something about the subjectivity of interpretation. For example, what is the role of respected opinion leaders, celebrity authors, famous institutions, a journal's historical reputation, and the largesse of the sponsor in shaping the response to a clinical trial result? Presently, we have intuitions but no answers to these questions. If we are interested in putting the results of clinical trials to good use, this seems to warrant further study.

In November 2000, David J. Rothman, a respected medical ethicist, wrote an article in *The New York Review of Books* entitled "The Shame of Medical Research."[35] In this polemical essay, he drew on evidence of clinical trials conducted in resource-poor countries to charge that trialists were exploiting the vulnerable; seeking participation by coercion, not consent; failing in their obligations to offer the highest standard of care to individuals not receiving the experimental treatment; failing to offer decent post-trial care; and taking advantage of weak institutional review boards. He argued that research "practice has overwhelmed ethics."

Rothman's claims have resonance in the North as well as the South. September 17, 1999, was a turning point for medical research in the United States. On that day, Jesse Gelsinger died. He was an eighteen-year-old volunteer in a gene therapy trial at the University of Pennsylvania in Philadelphia. Further trials were quickly suspended. Subsequent scientific soul-searching was matched only by the intrusive zeal of federal officials. In direct response to the death of Gelsinger, Donna Shalala, then US secretary of health and human services, wrote about four "disturbing" trends in clinical research.[36] First, "researchers may not be doing enough to ensure that subjects fully understand all the potential risks and benefits of a clinical trial." Second, "too many researchers are not adhering to standards of good clinical practice." Third, institutional review boards "are under increasing strain" and oversight is often "inadequate." Finally, the integrity of clinical trials is now being compromised by the force of commerce. These trends had "seriously shaken" public confidence, she argued. This was an "appalling state of affairs." Shalala offered six prescriptions: improved education and training for investigators, clearer guidance on informed consent, a requirement for more detailed monitoring of clinical trials, stricter regulations about conflicts of interests, financial penalties for violations of these codes, and an expanded role for the Office of Human Research Protections. She also asked the Institute of Medicine to review the structure and function of human research participant protection programs.

The subsequent report, *Preserving Public Trust*, was published in 2001.[37] The Institute of Medicine proposed the creation of Human Research Participant Protection Programs, together with a new independent accreditation body that would set standards for these programs. Research participants and representatives of other organizations would be included in these standard-setting exercises. Here are the beginnings of regulatory hypertrophy. Indeed, the tone of this response is persecutory rather than merely proscriptive. The summary of the report circulated to news organizations began by referring to "crimes committed by Nazi scientists during World War II." On the same page, the fate of Jesse Gelsinger was reported as the principal motivation for the inquiry: "As the circumstances and events leading up to his death emerged, it became apparent that the system intended to protect him from unacceptable research risks instead failed him." The reader cannot fail to see the report's wish to equate a war crime with a present-day "science crime." We live in a time of enormous regulatory activity predicated on a few tragic errors and a great deal of misunderstanding. But a backlash is coming. William J. Burman and his colleagues have discussed how a culture of obsessive oversight—"rigid enforcement of outmoded regulations that do not contribute to patient safety" —is causing a crisis in clinical trials.[38] It seems that in the rush to add layers of administrative checks and balances, the whole purpose of the clinical trial—to benefit patients by providing reliable information for their care—has been forgotten.

The evidence supporting these propositions indicates that the clinical trial process is approaching a critical moment. Indeed, public skepticism is already producing problems in patient recruitment. A March 2001 article on BBC *Online* entitled "Medical Advances 'In Jeopardy'" began, "A desperate lack of patients for clinical trials of new drugs for cancer may be costing lives, say experts." Part of the reason is because "patients in general do not want to become 'guinea pigs' for medicines." Are there ways forward? All those who take part in clinical trials must become far more powerful advocates for those trials. The hidden benefits of clinical trials must be hidden no longer. Iain Chalmers has written, "We should make a more concerted effort to help the public understand how biases and the play of chance can lead to dangerously incorrect conclusions about the effects of healthcare interventions."[39]

Such public outreach needs to involve governments, science policy agencies (such as the National Institutes of Health), schools, and patient organizations. The media might be another avenue to pursue. However, as any self-respecting journalist will admit, the reporter is there to report the news and not to be an instrument of public education. Nevertheless, trialists could do more to help journalists report trials more accurately. They must also show deeper concern for the threatened integrity of the clinical trial process. A part of this anxiety naturally centers on the issue of research misconduct. Limited oversight of research is valuable and reporting instances of proven misconduct as soon as they come to light is part of the scientist's responsibility to patients.

Researchers also need to think more critically about the practical aspects of the studies they undertake. While the large, simple, randomized trial has huge and obvious merits, there are clearly problems. In a qualitative study of cancer trials, for example, Carole Langley and her colleagues found that clinicians felt they were being asked to enroll patients "at a very vulnerable stage" in their care.[40] The notion of randomization (deciding treatment "out of an envelope") was anathema. In addition, patients were often surprised by the degree of uncertainty displayed by their doctors. Langley concluded, "Action is needed to promote awareness of randomized trials under way, to ensure that trials address issues of importance, are acceptable to patients and clinicians, and that practical support is provided for participating centres." Perhaps an emphasis on the better care a patient receives in a clinical trial would be one way ahead. Research into written trial information for patients is also an urgent need.

One of the most challenging problems facing trialists remains informed consent. In a study of attitudes toward trials, Italian investigators invited family physicians to ask patients to complete a questionnaire about their views of the trial process.[41] Knowledge about informed consent was poor and depended on the educational level of the patient. Over 80 percent of patients were not interested in taking part in "a controlled scientific study involving the administration of a new drug potentially useful to you but not yet evaluated in human beings for its usefulness and its adverse effects." More attention to these practical issues is rarely mentioned by advocates of trials. Yet unless these rather mundane matters are taken up, and they are only very rarely, the problems of clinical trials will not be addressed and public skepticism will only increase further.

# 13

## DNA: THE LIFE OF A DEAD MOLECULE

JAMES WATSON AND Francis Crick ended their April 25, 1953 paper in *Nature* describing the structure of DNA with the now notoriously casual line, "It has not escaped our notice that the specific pairing we have postulated immediately suggests a possible copying mechanism for the genetic material."[1] Disarming insight or false modesty—who can tell? For Watson and Crick were certainly aware of the power their simple model held for explaining the molecular basis of biological reproduction. In self-conscious homage to this work, the International Human Genome Sequencing Consortium ended its 2001 *Nature* report describing its initial analysis of human DNA in respectfully parallel fashion: "Finally, it has not escaped our notice that the more we learn about the human genome, the more there is to explore."[2] The words interlock with one another and seem to twist into their own historical double helix. Is the sequence of DNA indeed the code of codes, or is DNA, as the biologist Richard Lewontin once called it, "a dead molecule"?

On February 12, 2001, the Consortium published its complex and nearly complete map of human DNA. (The final draft was ready two years later.) Dr. Michael Dexter, then director of the Wellcome Trust, used a simple metaphor to underline the importance of this new piece of biological cartography:

> Maps are a timeless resource—you don't have to visit every part of them at once for them to be of value. It's worth knowing that Oxford is south of Birmingham and west of London, even if you don't plan to visit any of the places tomorrow. The same is true of the Human Genome Project—it will guide researchers for centuries, even if every inch isn't explored or used tomorrow.

Dexter had good reason to be proud of this collaborative achievement involving more than twenty laboratories. The Wellcome Trust committed £210 million to the Human Genome Project. Its sequencing hub was the Sanger Centre in Hinxton, Cambridgeshire, England, where a third of the draft genome was decoded. But all was not so peacefully collegial among the scientists who had worked on the gene hunt. As Jeremy Black made clear in his *Maps and Politics*,[3] an atlas does not provide a neutral depiction of objective fact. From the headline title to its shadings of color, a map is a plan, a "product and recorder of human agency." Black wrote that such plans "reflect a society that both seeks to understand and that can create, construct and control." In sum, maps are "instruments of power."

Nothing could be more true of the conflict surrounding the human genome. Its story was less about the detail of what the genome had revealed and more about the stand-off between the publicly funded Consortium and a private-sector company, Celera Genomics, led by Dr. J. Craig Venter. Celera, too, has published a report on its own genome sequence, in *Nature*'s chief competitor, *Science*.[4] Yet Venter has become something of a hate figure among many of his peers. Whereas the publicly funded sequence is fully accessible and usable by any third party, Celera put severe restrictions on who could obtain and use its sequence. At the end of the *Science* paper, Venter stated that "for commercial scientists wishing to verify the results presented here, the genome data are available upon signing a Material Transfer Agreement."

I wanted to compare the Celera genome with its Consortium rival.

I went to www.celera.com and read the long series of terms and conditions of use: the definition of an acceptable academic user; how one must cite the Celera sequence; the laws governing warranty, liability, and indemnity; and warnings about intellectual property rights, registration information, and confidentiality. I was refused access. My e-mail address did "not appear to represent an academic, governmental or non-profit institution." I e-mailed Celera to appeal their decision. They did not reply. The Consortium, meanwhile, is furious that Venter has hidden his sequence behind a commercial veil. John Sulston, former director of the Sanger Centre, said: "Others want to charge the rest of the human race a fortune to read our own genetic code, but we're here to tell them that the human genome is not for sale." He declared Celera's policy to be "criminal." The upshot of Celera's secrecy came two years later when, in 2003, the US National Academy of Sciences launched UPSIDE—the Universal Principle of Sharing Integral Data Expeditiously. The goal of the Academy was to ensure that all DNA sequences were quickly released and freely accessible on public databases. The genome belongs to all of us, they were saying, not merely to those trying to exploit its commercial opportunities. Yet these complaints belie the fact that Celera achieved something quite remarkable. The Human Genome Project was launched in 1990, and the Consortium's sequence was reported the same week as Celera's. But Venter only began his sequencing program in September 1999. He finished nine months later. And instead of relying on multiple contributions from laboratories worldwide, his team completed its work in a single facility in Maryland.

The row between these research groups, often a principal focus of attention in the media, also included sniping attacks by the Consortium on Celera's methods of determining the genome sequence. Celera was charged with insufficiently acknowledging its appropriation of—stealing, some might call it—data from the Consortium Web site, which was freely available and updated daily. Sulston argued that the methods Celera used had "failed by their own standards," although he conceded that Venter's sequence was more complete than his own. A press release issued by the Wellcome Trust claimed that Celera's approach "had been found wanting."

By the time these acrimonious exchanges had subsided, the only substantive news left to be reported was that the number of human genes seemed to be fewer than expected—"a major surprise," according to Venter. Early estimates had put the number of human genes at around 100,000. The highest guess was over 140,000. A few years ago, biologists such as E. O. Wilson and Steve Jones revised this figure downward, putting the minimum complement of human genes at 50,000. We now know that the number is closer to 30,000 to 40,000. Yet beyond the personalities, their fallings-out, and an unexpectedly small number of genes, what does the human genome actually reveal?

The human hereditary mechanism was first conceived as a "code-script" not by a biologist but by the physicist Erwin Schrödinger. It was this code-script that, according to Schrödinger in his 1944 book *What Is Life?*, determined whether a fertilized egg "would develop, under suitable conditions, into a black cock or into a speckled hen, into a fly or a maize plant, a rhododendron, a beetle, a mouse or a woman." He imagined that the gene was "the hypothetical material carrier of a definite hereditary feature." There is nothing hypothetical about the 3.2 gigabases of DNA reported in *Nature*. This is the size of the whole human sequence.

But the first question one might ask is, whose genome is it that we are reading? For the Human Genome Project, blood samples were taken from twelve anonymous human donors who replied to advertisements near the two laboratories responsible for building DNA libraries. These laboratories were in California. Donors came from "diverse backgrounds"—not specified—and were included on a first-come, first-DNA-taken basis. Written informed consent was given, but from that moment on, all connections between donor and DNA were broken. Identities were erased, labels destroyed, and samples for sequencing pulled out randomly. The identity of those persons whose genomes we are now reading will forever remain a mystery.

Celera's approach was very different. They wanted to avoid random sampling of the human DNA pool. Instead, they selected five donors to give their sequencing effort proven diversity: two men and three women; one African-American, one Asian Chinese, one Hispanic Mexican, and two Caucasians. And although privacy was initially maintained, their identities are known. The very notion, therefore, of a single human genome is mistaken. The DNA so far described is a composite of many genomes.

The care with which genes are examined and cataloged is not unlike the fidelity of observation shown by museum curators. Venter even writes about "human curators" of genes. Human DNA, tightly packed, resides in forty-six chromosomes: twenty-two matching pairs and the sex chromosomes X and Y. The published Consortium genome map begins by showing pictures of these chromosomes as seen under a high-powered microscope. Beneath these pictures are linear representations of the chromosomal content arranged in twelve horizontal tracks, each mapping selected aspects of genetic information. The first track is a scale dividing the length of DNA into equal-sized segments, each one megabase long. Chromosome 1, for example, is the longest human chromosome, running to 263 megabases. It has two arms, one (the p arm) slightly shorter than the other (the q arm). A second track couples the positions of dark bands seen on stained chromosomes under a microscope with DNA itself. The map plots what can be seen with the human eye with what cannot. The third track is a mix of red, yellow, and orange blocks, reflecting the degree of completeness of the sequence. Only red areas indicate finished genome, and these seem oddly few in number.

Now the genome map becomes more labyrinthine. It exposes strange configurations of content and bizarre architectures of component bases. The fourth mapping track focuses on GC content. DNA is composed of four nucleotide bases: adenine (A) pairs with thymine (T), and guanine (G) with cytosine (C). Variations in GC content are thought to reflect subtle differences in biological function, such as gene density. A fifth track measures the frequency of repeated DNA sequences. Only 5 percent of human DNA codes for protein production. Half of the genome is made up of repeats; this "junk DNA" seems peculiarly useless padding. But all human trash, if one only looks hard enough, leaves a telling footprint. And so it is with junk DNA. These ubiquitous ancient duplications point to important schisms in human heredity. The Consortium calls them "an extraordinary trove of information about biological processes...a rich palaeontological record, holding crucial clues about evolutionary events and forces."

The human genome's practical value is thought to lie not in the sequence itself but rather in the genetic variation that exists between individuals. This variation is indicated by the presence of single nucleotide polymorphisms, referred to as SNPs (pronounced "snips"). SNPs are points of substantial variation in the DNA sequence, and their frequency is shown in the sixth horizontal track on the human genome map. There are an incredible 2.1 million SNPs in human DNA, according to Celera's calculations. They are important because identifying genetic variation should open the way to finding genes linked to diseases, both for diagnosis and treatment. At least that is the standard accepted theory. But a persistent critic of the human genome endeavor, Richard Lewontin—a distinguished geneticist himself—resists the idea that human variation is straightforwardly determined. In his book *The Triple Helix*, Lewontin argues that "the organism does not compute itself from its genes" and so "random processes must underlie a great deal of the variation observed between individuals."[5] The dominant theme running through the Consortium's report is that genes rule. By contrast, Venter counsels against the fallacy of easy determinism.

A once-inflexible law of information flow in biological systems—its so-called central dogma, formulated by James Watson—was that DNA makes RNA makes protein. We have known for many years that this simple precept is wrong. DNA alone does not make protein. Indeed, RNA can "make" DNA, an inversion of the usual process that requires a special enzyme called reverse transcriptase. This important discovery was made by David Baltimore, who received a Nobel Prize in 1975. RNA is an essential molecule in regulating cell function, notably in building proteins from their constituent amino acids. The human genome contains tracts of DNA coding for RNA that does not eventually go on to make protein. Information transfer from the genome stops at RNA. This "non-coding RNA" is shown as brown and light orange bands on the genome map. An even more elusive finding in human DNA is the strange CpG island. CpG is a molecule of two bases, C and G, bound together. The density of CpG islands seems to correlate with the beginning of a gene, but the precise relation between the two is obscure. Regions of human DNA with higher than expected CpG levels are shown as green bars on the eighth track of the genome map. The ninth, tenth, and eleventh tracks describe, respectively, regions of similarity with another organism (the one chosen is the puffer fish, *Tetraodon nigroviridis*), further molecular clues to the presence of genes (called expressed sequence tags), and ticks to signal predicted starts of new genes.

This long mapping prologue culminates in the final track—the genes themselves. On the Consortium atlas, the genes are divided into two categories. One is labeled red, indicating disease genes. The other is blue, representing the rest. I counted 777 red genes, although the Consortium makes clear that they are aware of several omissions and misplacements. They find the distribution of genes to be extraordinarily uneven. Some chromosomes seem packed with genes, while others are comparatively empty. And on any one chromosome, gene distribution varies enormously. As much as one fifth of the human genome is gene desert.

But this multilinear map of human DNA is only one of many

selective representations of the human genome. The sequence map shows a string of As, Ts, Cs, and Gs. The SNPS map reveals variations in that sequence. A telomere map uncovers DNA sequences at the tips of chromosomes, which seem to be important in human aging. A radiation hybrid map gives a physical picture of the major landmarks along the DNA sequence. The cytogenetic map gives a wide-angle view of the human genome by looking at all the chromosomes together. And a transcriptome map draws patterns of gene expression, which should help to fit diseases to specific genes—or so geneticists hope. Each of these maps gives a very different perspective—every one a distortion, perhaps—of human DNA's topography.

What does publication of the human genetic sequence signal for writers who have speculated long and hard on the biological meaning, cultural importance, and medical implications of the genome? Surely there can now be some reckoning in the harassed debate that first took seed in 1953. The truth is that publication of the human genome has not lessened our anxiety about issues such as genetic screening of embryos, selective abortion, the ethics of embryo storage, genetic diagnosis, cloning, and the use of genetic information by employers or insurers. As Steve Jones wrote after the first release of genome data in 2000, "Biology has told us little about human affairs that we did not know before." The problem is that—in Jones's words again—"the public is obsessed with genes." Partly, one wants to add, because of the likes of Jones himself. In fact, his message is confusingly ambiguous. When he writes, for example, that "the completion of the DNA map marks the triumph of genetics as a science.... At last we understand what sex really means, why we age and die, and how nature and nurture combine to make us what we are,"[6] scientists know that he is enjoying a riff of wild, if entertaining, exaggeration. Most definitely, we do not understand what sex means. If we did, at anything beyond the molecular structure of X and Y, it would be possible to understand why some people adopt behaviors that put them at high risk of acquiring HIV. Aging is still a riddle. And we have only a back-of-the-envelope idea about how we develop into what we are. The extent of our lack of understanding makes release of the human genome a crushing anticlimax.

Since the draft genome was published, the personal controversies have continued. A research team led by Bo Yuan at Ohio State University reported in 2001 that when it ran all the available human DNA sequences through a powerful computer, the number of genes came out to twice as many as Celera and the Human Genome Project estimated—about 66,000. British genome scientists repudiated this finding. But we still do not know for sure how many genes it takes to build a human being.

Meanwhile, Venter stepped down from Celera in 2002, as the company sought to exploit its discoveries in the pharmaceutical sector. He disclosed that some of the DNA used to create the Celera sequence was actually his own. He has turned his attention to providing a sequencing service for the public, costing about $700,000 for a personalized genome to be burned onto a CD. He predicted that by 2010, parents of newborn children would be taking their child's genome sequence home with them from hospital. Venter saw this technology as the ultimate expression of preventive medicine. If a particular gene known to increase the risk of colon cancer is found, for example, that disease can be rooted out more quickly. Does knowing your own DNA give you greater control over your own destiny? I must disclose a personal bias. My birth father, whom I never met, although we did exchange several letters toward the end of his life (he lived in Johannesburg, South Africa), died, so I believe, from the complications of breast cancer. I have not met my birth mother. My genetic heritage is, therefore, rather obscure. What I do know is the contribution my adoptive parents made to my life experience—an aversion to smoking, exercise, milk, and vegetables. These are risks that readily make sense to me, and to my destiny.

The debate about genetics has moved well beyond genes. The pressing field of inquiry now is ontogeny—how our biological form, shape, structure, mind, and capabilities develop from the instant an egg is fertilized until the moment we die. The ontogenetic challenge is formidable. How do nerve cells end up in the brain and cardiac muscle cells in the heart? How is this process controlled and integrated into an overall strategy for interpreting the genetic message? Ontogenetic questions expose the weaknesses of present genome maps. Understanding gene expression cannot be achieved in two dimensions. DNA is a duplex wrapped up into chromosomes and bound to proteins in discrete packets. Already we need a new map of the spatial and temporal organization and orchestration of genes in human development. Structure is meaningless without function. Lewontin would go further. He doubts our ability to secure any complete explanation of a biological system. In his view, genes do "not specify a unique outcome of development." Questions about shape will not find answers in our genome. The confounding problem facing developmental biology, according to Lewontin, will always be an incalculable random noise of events buffeting a gene acting within its environment.

And what of larger matters, such as human culture? In his book *Consilience*,[7] E. O. Wilson makes the case that our "world is orderly and can be explained by a small number of natural laws." One of these laws is that genes and culture are "inseparably linked." Although human culture evolves rapidly, its bond with the genome will always remain intact. Just as the gene is the basic unit of human heredity, Wilson tries to find its sibling in culture. He opts for Richard Dawkins's concept of "meme" but defines the meme more precisely than Dawkins as a "node of semantic memory"—conferring meaning by connecting one object or idea with another—which somehow correlates with brain activity. Genes and memes intersect and coevolve because genes help to create an environment—a culture—in which the meme will thrive. Wilson, an unapologetic reductionist whose special interest is behavioral genetics, sees the genome as only one means to study the gene–culture interaction. While always emphasizing the limitations of a genetic theory of human behavior, he insists that genes do set more or less prescribed boundaries on our perceptual capacities.

The point of his argument lies in the predictions it forces. Knowledge of the genome should usher in a new phase of volitional evolution. Old Darwinian laws will be put to one side, and "hereditary change will soon depend less on natural selection than on social choice." The overriding cultural question will become: How much should people be allowed to mutate themselves and their descendants? A human genome map does not help to answer this question, except that it confirms there is no direct causal link between a gene and a common behavior. Such a connection remains, for my liking at least, reassuringly cloudy. A few gaps in the clouds are appearing. And with these gaps are coming new perspectives on how genes influence human life. Matt Ridley has summarized these shifts in thinking in the title of his book *Nature Via Nurture*. He argues that we should invert our present understanding of the gene–environment balance: it is nurture that is less amenable to change than nature. This is "one of the least recognized and most significant discoveries in recent years," he claims. It is our environment that governs which genes are switched on and when, and so "genes are at the mercy of our behavior." They exist simply to extract information from our surroundings. There is nothing inevitable about the effect genes have on our lives. By the time I had finished reading Ridley's plea for this new thesis, I was actually beginning to feel sorry for the poor little creatures we call genes, which he describes as sadly "vulnerable."

The imprecise consequences of these permanent genetic endowments mean that any therapeutic advances are likely to be incremental rather than revolutionary. An expectation that medical applications of the human genome would be its most powerful benefit was the single most important justification for funding the project. A payback is sorely needed. But without a functional understanding of what genes do, it is hard to know what the genome will add to our understanding of disease. It remains only a promissory note. For example, we know that excision of DNA from the p arm of chromosome 1 is commonly associated with cancer. But how? And what can we do about it? We have already learned that a simplistic conception of gene replacement is one of the great conceits of modern genetics. Still, a quick trawl through the Consortium map has already thrown up new gene candidates that could be responsible for drug addiction. Future physicians are likely to think of diseases more as delicate perturbations in cell function than as gross organ pathologies. Since the publication of the draft genome, gaps have been filled and tears repaired. Each chromosome is now being reported separately and in detail, displaying the precise links between genes and very rare genetic diseases.[8]

April 25, 2003, marked the fiftieth anniversary of Watson and Crick's description of the double helix. That occasion provided ample opportunity for reflection about DNA's likely contribution to medicine. A truly important discovery, which depends entirely on a close understanding of how the genome works—or rather fails to work—in disease has been the drug imatinib mesylate (better know by its trade name, Gleevec). In chronic myeloid leukemia, this chemical binds to and blocks the actions of a protein that is the product of a gene created by a mixup of genetic material (technically called a translocation) between two chromosomes, 9 and 22. Once this protein is neutralized, the driving force behind the cell proliferation that makes chronic myeloid leukemia what it is—a life-threatening disease—is diminished.

The Regius Professor of Medicine at the University of Oxford, John Bell, who is William Osler's successor by a generation or two, shares the optimism that such discoveries have fostered. Writing in a special issue of *Nature* to mark DNA's fiftieth anniversary, he concluded that "while public health and antibiotics produced important healthcare outcomes in the past 50 years, the next 50 are likely to belong to genetics and molecular medicine." But he also admitted that "progress has been slow." And he cautioned optimists to bear in mind that DNA "will not, however, answer all of the questions about human health, nor will it provide all the answers for optimizing clinical practice."

Beyond the genome, in the world of post-genomics, the goal is to catalog a new library, this time of human proteins—the proteome. It is proteins that offer the most possibilities as new targets for drugs and as means for more accurate diagnosis. Just as there is a Human Genome Organization to lobby governments and the public for research money, so there is a Human Proteome Organization to do the same for "proteomics." Its first meeting took place in Virginia in April 2001. The aim will be to do for biology in the twenty-first century what the Manhattan Project did for physics in the twentieth. There is also optimism about the way genetic information will come to be used in health care. Once doctors understand how genes contribute to disease, they will be able to label every child with a risk profile for heart disease, cancer, dementia, or anything else one cares to worry about. Some geneticists see this prospect as a reason for joy, somehow vindicating their claims about the power of genes. Except for those conditions where the risk is great, such as breast cancer, I am not so sure.

Put to one side for a moment the technical issue of how genes interact with external environmental influences and random events to produce disease. There is still some value, it seems to me, in preserving a freedom to live life without the perpetually pressing knowledge that genes can be fractioned and totaled into a finite risk of, say, a heart attack. I already know that fact, since heart disease is the commonest cause of death in the Western world. It is here, especially, that Lewontin's critique becomes important. When he argues, as he does in *The Triple Helix*, that "the organism is determined neither by its genes nor by its environment nor even by the interaction between them, but bears a significant mark of random processes," geneticists—and doctors—should pause. Random events are neither programmed nor predictable, which makes the assertion that a disease is associated with a gene not only practically unhelpful but also dangerously misleading. And, in any case, when one looks at the causes of illness worldwide, genes are largely irrelevant. The Human Genome Project is a scientific self-indulgence when set beside the challenges of malnutrition, poor water systems, unsafe sex, and unbridled tobacco use.

Despite my skepticism about the projected role of the genome in medicine, one cannot deny the tremendous technical progress in gene manipulation. In January 2001, an Oregonian research team described the birth of the world's first transgenic primate. These scientists had engineered a gene for a fluorescent green protein from jellyfish into a rhesus monkey. In one instance, a male embryo survived. The fluorescent dye glowed in the toenails of a stillborn relation, proving that the gene had been successfully transferred. Researchers called their live baby monkey ANDi, for "inserted DNA" (read backward). But the significance of this experiment, which has no benefit whatsoever for either monkey or man other than to prove a principle, is not yet obvious. And human cloning, reproductive rather than therapeutic, is first and foremost a technical challenge rather than a human imperative.

What does the human genome tell us about who we are? Is it true that, as Steve Jones concludes, "DNA grinds [mankind's] face into the biological mud"? The notion that a modest number of genes somehow puts *Homo sapiens* in its place—"a blow to the idea of human uniqueness," as anthropologist Svante Paabo has called it—seems ludicrous to me. To be sure, we have many genes in common with the fly, worm, and mustard weed. And there is even evidence that a whole raft of bacterial genes took up residence in our genome at some point in the past (one of which is linked to depression). But Venter shows that human beings have substantially expanded gene repertoires for immunity, brain function, tissue development, and blood clotting. These essential control networks are, at the most obvious level, what distinguish us genetically from other organisms. We should all feel a little humbled by our genome but not, I think, too much. Perhaps the male has most to fear. The Y chromosome contains many dead genes riddled with mutations. And it has been savagely cut down to a deformed stub. A lesson, here, not to anthropomorphize the genome.

The geneticist J. B. S. Haldane, in his essay "On Being the Right Size," explored why a human could never be sixty feet tall and why an insect is in acute danger whenever it goes for a drink. Haldane's purpose was to explain how each animal has a convenient size. He argued that animals are not larger because they are more complicated. Rather, the reverse. We are more complicated because we are larger. One important meaning of the genome lies within this Haldanian transposition. Our biological and cognitive complexity has its origins not in our genes, our environment, the interaction between the two over time, or even in random events. We are what we are, in genetic terms, because of what has gone before us. Despite the work of Celera and of the Consortium, the contours of our own gene past remain in shadow. To find our way around them, we need a compass, not a map.

The most controversial area that has been explored from the standpoint of genes is human behavior. Historians of homosexuality will judge much twentieth-century "science" harshly when they come to reflect on the prejudice, myth, and downright dishonesty that litter modern academic research on sexuality. Take, for example, the lugubrious statements of once-respected investigators. Here is Sandor Feldman, a well-known psychotherapist, in 1956:

> It is the consensus of many contemporary psychoanalytic workers that permanent homosexuals, like all perverts, are neurotics.[9]

Or consider the remarks of the criminologist Herbert Hendin:

> Homosexuality, crime, and drug and alcohol abuse appear to be barometers of social stress.... Criminals help produce other criminals, drug abusers other drug abusers, and homosexuals other homosexuals.[10]

The notion of the homosexual as a deeply disturbed deviant in need of treatment was the orthodoxy until only recently. Bernard J. Oliver Jr., a psychiatrist specializing in sexual medicine, wrote in 1967:

> Dr. Edmond Bergler feels that the homosexual's real enemy is not so much his perversion but [*sic*] ignorance of the possibility that he can be helped, plus his psychic masochism which leads him to shun treatment....
>
> There is good reason to believe now, more than ever before, that many homosexuals can be successfully treated by psychotherapy, and we should encourage homosexuals to seek this help.[11]

Such views about the origin of homosexual preferences have become part of American political culture as well. When, in 1992, Vice President Dan Quayle offered the view that homosexuality "is more of a choice than a biological situation.... It is a wrong choice,"[12] he merely reasserted the belief that homosexuality reflected psychological conditioning with little biological basis, and certainly without being influenced by a person's biological inheritance.

And more recently we have had the much-publicized spectacle—*Time* magazine took up the story in a dramatic feature entitled "Search for a Gay Gene"[13]—of homosexuality's origins being revealed in the lowly fruit fly, *Drosophila*.[14] Males and females of this, one has to admit, rather distant relation adopt courtship behavior that led two researchers at the US National Institutes of Health to draw extravagant parallels with human beings.

Shang-Ding Zhang and Ward F. Odenwald found that what they

took to be homosexual behavior among male fruit flies—touching male partners with forelegs, licking their genitalia, and curling their bodies to allow genital contact—could be induced by techniques that abnormally activated a gene called *w* (for "white," so called because of its effect on eye color). Widespread activation (or "expression") of the white gene in *Drosophila* produced male-to-male rituals that took place in chains or circles of five or more flies. If female fruit flies lurked nearby, male flies would only rarely be tempted away from their male companions. These findings, which have apparently been reproduced by others, led the investigators to conclude that "*w* misexpression has a profound effect on male sexual behavior."

Zhang and Odenwald speculated that the expression of *w* could lead to severe shortages of serotonin, an important chemical signal that enables nerve cells to communicate with one another. The authors conjecture that mass activation of *w* diminishes brain serotonin by promoting its use elsewhere in the body. Indeed, cats, rabbits, and rats all show some elements of "gay" behavior when their brain serotonin concentrations fall. Intriguing and, you might think, convincing evidence.

Yet, although *w* is found in modified form in human beings, it is a huge (and, it seems to me, an obviously dangerous) leap to extrapolate observations from fruit flies to humans. In truth, when the recent data are interpreted literally we find that (a) the *w* gene induces male group sex behavior in highly ritualized linear or circular configurations, and (b) while these tend more toward homosexual than straight preferences, they are truly bisexual (as pointed out by Larry Thompson in *Time*). Zhang and Odenwald force their experimental results with fruit flies to fit their preconceived notions of homosexuality. How simplistic it seems to equate genital licking in *Drosophila* with complex individual and social behavior patterns in humans. Can notions of homosexuality apply uniformly across the biological gulf that divides human beings and insects? Such arguments by analogy seem hopelessly inadequate.

By contrast, the work of Simon LeVay, Dean Hamer, and a small group of researchers concerned to distinguish biological and genetic influences on sexual behavior has discredited much of the loose rhetoric that has been used about homosexuality. In August 1991, LeVay, a neuroscientist who went on to direct the Institute of Gay and Lesbian Education in southern California, published in the magazine *Science* findings from autopsies of men and women of known sexual preference. He found that a tiny region in the center of the brain—the interstitial nucleus of the anterior hypothalamus (INAH 3)—was, on average, substantially smaller in nineteen gay men who died from AIDS than among sixteen heterosexual men.[15]

The observation that the male brain could take two different forms, depending on one's sexual preference, was a stunning discovery. The hypothalamus—a small, intricate mass of cells lying at the base of the brain—was long believed to have a role in sexual behavior, but direct evidence that it did so was weak. Yet LeVay expressed caution. Although his data showed that human sexual preference "is amenable to study at the biological level," he noted that it was impossible to be certain whether the anatomical differences between the brains of gay and straight men were a cause or a consequence of their preference.[16]

In the thirteen persuasive essays that make up *The Sexual Brain*, LeVay takes account of the current biobehavioral controversy over the science of sex.[17] From the union of wiry sperm and bloated ovum to the child-rearing practices of mammals and humans, for which mothers are largely responsible, he writes (metaphorically), that the "male is little more than a parasite who takes advantage of [the female's] dedication to reproduction." He goes on to draw from a wide range of sources to support his contentious assertion that "there are separate centers within the hypothalamus for the generation of male-typical and female-typical sexual behavior and feelings." He argues that a connection—the details of which remain mysterious—between brain and behavior exists through hormones such as testosterone.

The most convincing evidence he puts forward to support his view comes from women with congenital adrenal hyperplasia. This condition, in which masculine characteristics, such as androgenized genitalia, including clitoral enlargement and partially fused labia, become pronounced in women, is caused by excessive testosterone production and leads, in adulthood, to an increased frequency of lesbianism affecting up to half of all the women who have the condition. The theory, still unproven, that is proposed to explain these behavioral effects of hormones is that one or more chemical signals act during a brief early critical period in the development of most males to alter permanently both the brain and the pattern of their later adult behavior. Unless this hormonal influence is switched on, a female pattern of development will follow automatically.

What might be the origin of biological differences underlying male sexual preference? In 1993 Dean H. Hamer and his colleagues at the National Cancer Institute discovered a preliminary but nevertheless tantalizing clue.[18] Hamer began his painstaking search for a genetic contribution to sexual behavior by studying the rates of homosexuality among male relatives of seventy-six known gay men. He found that the incidence of homosexual preference in these family members was strikingly higher (13.5 percent) than the rate of homosexuality among the whole sample (2 percent). When he looked at the patterns of sexual orientation among these families, he discovered more gay relatives on the maternal side. Homosexuality seemed, at least, to be passed from generation to generation through women.

Maternal inheritance could be explained if there was a gene influencing sexual orientation on the X chromosome, one of the two human sex chromosomes that bear genes determining the sex of offspring.[19] Men have both X and Y chromosomes, while women have two X chromosomes. A male sex-determining gene, called SRY, is found on the Y chromosome. Indeed, the Y chromosome is the most obvious site for defining male sexuality since it is the only one of the forty-six human chromosomes to be found in men alone. The SRY gene is the most likely candidate both to turn on a gene that prevents female development and to trigger testosterone production. Since the female has no Y chromosome, she lacks this masculinizing gene. In forty pairs of homosexual brothers, Hamer and his team looked for associations between the DNA on the X chromosome and the homosexual trait. They found that thirty-three pairs of brothers shared the same five X chromosomal DNA "markers," or genetic signatures, at a region near the end of the long arm of the X chromosome designated Xq28.[20] The possibility that this observation could have occurred by chance was only 1 in 10,000.

LeVay takes a broad philosophical perspective in his discussion of human sexuality by placing his research in the context of animal evolution. Hamer, on the other hand, has written, with the assistance of the journalist Peter Copeland, a more focused popular account of his research, *The Science of Desire and the Search for the Gay Gene and the Biology of Behavior.*[21] He conceived his project after reflecting on a decade of laborious research on yeast genes. Although the project was approved by the National Institutes of Health after navigating a labyrinthine course through government agencies, it remained rather meagerly funded.

Taken together, the scientific papers of both LeVay and Hamer and the books that their first reports spawned[22] make a forceful but by no means definitive case for the view that biological and genetic influences have an important—perhaps even decisive—part in determining sexual preference among males. LeVay writes, for example, that "the scientific evidence presently available points to a strong influence of nature, and only a modest influence of nurture." But there is no broad scientific agreement on these findings. They have become mired in a quasi-scientific debate. What happened?

To begin with, we must ask what LeVay and Hamer have not shown. LeVay has found no proof of any direct link between the size of INAH 3 and sexual behavior. Size differences alone prove nothing. He was also unable to exclude the possibility that AIDS has an influence on brain structure, although this seemed unlikely, since six of the heterosexual men he studied also had AIDS. Moreover, Hamer did not find a gene for homosexuality; what he discovered was data suggesting some influence of one or more genes on one particular type of sexual preference in one group of people. Seven pairs of brothers did not have the Xq28 genetic marker, yet these brothers were all gay. Xq28 is clearly not a sine qua non for homosexuality; it is neither a necessary nor a sufficient cause by itself.

And what about women? Although the genitalia of women as well as men are clearly biologically determined, no data exist to prove a genetic link, or a link based on brain structure, with female sexual preferences, whether heterosexual or homosexual. Finally, neither study has been replicated by other researchers, the necessary standard of scientific proof. Indeed, there is every reason to suppose that the INAH 3 data will be extremely difficult to confirm. Only a few years ago INAH 1 (located close to INAH 3) was also thought to be larger in men than in women. Two groups, including LeVay's, have failed to reproduce this result.

Most of these limitations are clearly acknowledged by both LeVay and Hamer in their original scientific papers and are reinforced at length in their books. But reactions to their findings have nevertheless been harshly critical. For instance, after pointing out several potential weaknesses in Hamer's study and criticizing his decision to publish in *Science* at a time when gay "lives are at stake," two biologists, Anne Fausto-Sterling and Evan Balaban, asked "whether it might not have been prudent for the authors and the editors of *Science* to have waited until more of the holes in the study had been plugged...."[23] Their somewhat hysterical reaction has been followed by more careful comment by other scientists.[24]

Lack of prudence also characterized the response in the press. In

London, the conservative *Daily Telegraph* ran the clumsy headline, "Claim that homosexuality is inherited prompts fears that science could be used to eradicate it." Another story began, "A lot of mothers are going to feel guilty," while another was entitled "Genetic tyranny."

These headlines are part of the popular rhetoric about DNA, which supposes that a gene represents an irreducible and immutable unit of the human self. The correlation between a potentially active gene and a behavior pattern is assumed to indicate cause and effect. Was Hamer himself guilty of overinterpretation? In his original paper, he went to extraordinary lengths to qualify his findings. He and his co-authors offer no fewer than ten statements advising a cautious reading of their data, and they note that "replication and confirmation of our results are essential." Neither the hyperbolic press response with its relentless message of genetic determinism nor the ill-judged scientific criticism was appropriate.

Nevertheless, there are three conceptual issues raised by these reports—namely, heritability, sexual categorization, and the meaning of the phrase "biological basis of behavior"—which have been largely ignored in the scramble to publish instant analyses of the findings of LeVay and Hamer, among others.

Heritability is a measure of the resemblance between relatives; it is expressed as the proportion of variability in an observable characteristic that can be attributed to genetic factors. Eye color, for example, is 100 percent heritable, whereas we know that most behavioral traits have genetic contributions of well below 50 percent. Heritability is a quarrelsome issue among geneticists, and its proportional value is often quoted without the necessary qualifications. Variation in any trait is accounted for by the influence of genes (including, importantly, the interaction among genes), environment (the family and one's wider life experience), and the interaction between one or more genes and one or more environmental variables. The standard measure of heritability is the sum of all genetic influences, and it ignores potentially complex interactions—for example, the influence of the family milieu on the behavioral expression of a gene influencing sexual preference. The most common error made by those who discuss genetic contributions to behavior is to forget that heritability is a property only of the population under study at one particular time. It cannot be generalized to characterize the behavior itself.

When we apply these considerations to Hamer's data, we make a surprising discovery. If we accept his own hypothesis of the relation between the xq28 marker and the behavioral trait, the maximum heritability of homosexuality in the group he studied is 67 percent, which may seem a remarkably high figure. Yet this group was a particularly selected one: the seventy-six study participants openly acknowledged being gay, and had volunteered for the study. What Hamer's results do not tell us is what the influence of the xq28 marker in the general population might be. He infers from various mathematical calculations "that xq28 plays some role in about 5 to 30 percent of gay men." But he admits that this is merely a preliminary estimate and that accurate measuring of xq28 heritability in the general population remains to be done. In fact, a frequent criticism of Hamer's *Science* paper was that he did not measure the incidence of xq28 markers among heterosexual brothers of gay sibling pairs. Without this information, it is impossible to guess the influence of any genes that might be located at xq28. Their effects will be unpredictable at best, and any interaction with the environment will assume critical importance.

At this point, science inches uneasily toward dogma and diatribe. Hamer cites Richard Lewontin's *Not in Our Genes*[25] as one of his early inspirations to change the direction of his research. Hamer writes that he

> knew that [Lewontin] had criticized the idea that behavior is genetic, arguing instead that it is a product of class-based social

> structures.... Why was Lewontin, a formidable geneticist, so determined not to believe that behavior could be inherited? He couldn't disprove the genetics of behavior in a lab, so he wrote a political polemic against it.

Indeed, Lewontin has frequently provided cogent arguments against the view that heritability can help delineate the effects of genes on human behavior.[26] He has described the separation of behavioral variation into genetic and environmental contributions and the interaction between the two as "illusory."[27] For him and his co-writers, such a model "cannot produce information about causes of phenotypic difference," that is, differences in observable physical and mental traits. The precise meaning of heritability forces the inevitable conclusion, Lewontin has written, that whatever proportion is quoted, it "is nearly equivalent to no information at all for any serious problem in human genetics."

Imagine Dean Hamer's astonishment, therefore, when he received a letter from Richard Lewontin in 1992. A Harvard professor teaching genetics and behavior had invited Hamer to submit a pamphlet describing his research as an example of "conceptual advances" in "modern behavior genetic studies." He had willingly complied, but only later discovered that it had been ruled "scientifically unacceptable" by Ruth Hubbard, an emeritus professor at the Harvard Biological Laboratories who was deeply skeptical about determinism. In his letter, Hamer writes, Lewontin

> went on to theorize that human behaviors must be "very, very far from the genes" because "there are some at least that we know for sure are not influenced by genes as, for example, the particular language one speaks." That made about as much sense as saying that since some people eat tacos and some eat hamburgers, there is no biological drive to eat.

Hamer, tongue firmly in cheek, offered to give Lewontin's students a lecture on how good research into behavior genetics is done. Lewontin accepted. On the day of his scheduled talk, Hamer faced not only Lewontin but also Ruth Hubbard and Evan Balaban (a co-author, with Anne Fausto-Sterling, of the hostile letter later published in *Science*). Hamer described his methods carefully and stressed that his research could identify only potential genetic influences and not isolate specific genetic causes of behavior. At the end of the lecture, Lewontin indicated that he had no dispute with Hamer after all, and left the classroom without further comment.

Although it is true that heritability is only a crude measure of genetic influence, it remains a valuable research tool if, as one scientist has said, the researchers realize that

> genetic influence on behavior appears to involve multiple genes rather than one or two major genes, and nongenetic sources of variance are at least as important as genetic factors.... This should not be interpreted to mean that genes do not affect human behavior; it only demonstrates that genetic influence on behavior is not due to major-gene effects.[28]

More important, one can move beyond the "lump sum" theory of genetic influences to study the way in which genes affect behavior over time, or to discover how a gene influences different but possibly related behaviors, for instance both sexual preference and aggression.

Lewontin also cited the "terrible mischief" that could result from a research program based on heritability as his reason to suggest stopping "the endless search for better methods of estimating useless quantities."[29] Hamer agrees that precise genetic determinacy is an impossible goal; his 1993 article for *Science* on DNA markers also ended with an unusual admonition:

> We believe that it would be fundamentally unethical to use [this] information to try to assess or alter a person's current or future sexual orientation, either heterosexual or homosexual, or other normal attributes of human behavior. Rather, scientists, educators, policy-makers, and the public should work together to ensure that such research is used to benefit all members of society.

If scientists who have opposed research on heritability would accept that it can have, when it is carried out in this spirit, an important place in the study of behavior, that would add much-needed weight to calls to expand, and improve, research on human sexuality.

Although Hamer and LeVay have both expressed cautious confidence in their results, they are evidently uneasy about their own categorizations of men as *either* gay *or* straight. Hamer writes:

> In truth, I don't think that there is such a thing as "the" rate of homosexuality in the population at large. It all depends on the definition, how it's measured, and who is measured.

Classifying sexuality into homosexual and heterosexual categories may have benefits of simplicity for researchers, but how closely does this division fit the real world? Poorly is the answer. Sexual behavior and styles of life among men and women vary from day to day and year to year, and a conclusion about whether or not sexual experience is characterized as homosexual frequently depends on the definition one uses.[30] The slippery nature of our crude categories should alert us to beware of conclusions about groups labeled as "homosexual" or "heterosexual."

Moreover, the concept of sexuality itself cannot easily be analyzed. It exists at several levels—chromosomal, genital, brain, preference, gender self-image, gender role, and a range of subtle influences on behavior (hair color, eye color, and many more). Each of these can be grouped together with the others to produce a single measurable component on a scale, devised by Alfred Kinsey in the 1940s, that allegedly shows a person's degree of homosexual preference. Hamer used this scale somewhat uncritically to categorize his volunteers. Stephen B. Levine, a medical expert on sexual behavior, has noted that the conflated and crude Kinsey scale "does not do justice to the diversity among homosexual women and men."[31]

One of Hamer's severest critics, Anne Fausto-Sterling, a developmental geneticist at Brown University, has tried to extend sexual categories beyond the binary divisions of male and female.[32] She suggests adding three more groups based on "intersex" humans: herms (true hermaphrodites who possess one testis and one ovary), merms (individuals who have testes, no ovaries, but some female genitalia), and ferms (who have ovaries, no testes, but some male characteristics). This attempt to create multiple categories is, however, futile. It tries to systematize the unsystematizable by proposing a neatly divided-up continuum of sexuality, while, in fact, very different and mutually exclusive factors may be at work in particular cases. It is an impossible and intellectually misguided task.

Two major studies examining the historical origins of modern sexual categories show how social groupings that evolve over time can mislead one into supposing that inherent biological classes exist in some unchangeable sense. Michel Foucault chronicled the history of sexual norms by concentrating on the fluid notion of "homosexuality."[33] He denounced what he called "Freud's conformism" in taking heterosexuality to be the normal standard in psychoanalysis. He concluded:

> We must not forget that the psychological, psychiatric, medical category of homosexuality was constituted from the moment it was characterized—Westphal's famous article of 1870 on "contrary sexual sensations" can stand as its date of birth[34]—less by

> a type of sexual relations than by a certain quality of sexual sensibility.... The sodomite had been a temporary aberration; the homosexual was now a species.

This analysis, it seems to me, points to a critical error in the research of both Hamer and LeVay. Both, in spite of their qualifications, adopt the idea of the homosexual as a physical "species" different from the heterosexual. But there are no convincing historical grounds for this view. As Foucault points out, at the time of Plato,

> People did not have the notion of two distinct appetites allotted to different individuals or at odds with each other in the same soul; rather, they saw two ways of enjoying one's pleasure....

The cultural historian Jonathan Katz has recently attacked the naive partitioning of sexual orientation by tracing the dominance of the norm—heterosexuality—throughout history.[35] He provides a convincing argument that the "just-is hypothesis" of heterosexuality—that is, that the word corresponds to a true behavioral norm—is an "invented tradition." He shows that the categories of gay and straight are gradually dissolving as notions of the family become more various. Basing his view more on intuition than on sociological evidence, he predicts "the declining significance of sexual orientation."

The final issue that has confused the interpretation of research into sexuality is the meaning of "biological influence." Unfortunately, both LeVay and Hamer, in their effort to popularize their findings, ignore the subtlety of this question. As has been noted, LeVay is unambiguous about his own position on biological determinism:

> The most promising area for exploration is the identification of genes that influence sexual behavior and the study of when, where, and how these genes exert their effects.

Both researchers ignore the central issue in the debate over nature and nurture: How do genes get you from a biochemical program that instructs cells to make proteins to an unpredictable interplay of behavioral impulses—fantasy, courtship, arousal, sexual selection—that constitutes "sexuality"? The question remains unresolved. The classic fall-back position is to claim that genes merely provide a basis, at most a predisposition, to a particular behavior. But such statements lack a precise or testable meaning.

Perhaps we are asking the wrong question when we set out to find whether there is a gene for sexual orientation. We know that genes are responsible for the development of our lungs, larynx, mouth, and the speech areas of our brain. And we understand that this complexity cannot be collapsed into the notion of a gene for "talking." Similarly, what possible basis can there be for concluding that there is a single gene for sexuality, even though we accept that there are genes that direct the development of our penises, vaginas, and brains? This analogy is not to deny the importance of genes, but merely to recast their role in a different conceptual setting, one devoid of dualist prejudice.

The search for a single dominant gene—the O-GOD (one gene, one disorder) hypothesis—that would influence a behavioral variant is likely to be fruitless. Many different genes, together with many different environmental factors, will interact in unpredictable ways to guide behavioral preferences. Each component will contribute small quanta of influence. One result of such a quantum theory of behavior is that it makes irrelevant the overstretched speculations of both Hamer and LeVay about *why* a gene for homosexuality still exists when it apparently has little apparent survival value in evolutionary terms. The quest for a teleological explanation to identify a reason for the existence of a "gay gene" becomes pointless when one understands that there is not now, and never was, a single and final reason for being gay or straight, or having any other identity along the continuum of sexual preference.

* * *

Does this complexity, together with an adverse and polarized social milieu, preclude successful research efforts concerning human sexuality? In 1974, Lewontin wrote that reconstruction of man's genetic past is "an activity of leisure rather than of necessity."[36] Perhaps so. But, as Robert Plomin argues, the value of studying inheritance in behavior lies in its importance

> per se rather than in its usefulness for revealing how genes work. Some of society's most pressing problems, such as drug abuse, mental illness, and mental retardation, are behavioral problems. Behavior is also a key in health as well as illness, in abilities as well as disabilities, and in the personal pluses of life, such as sense of well-being and the ability to love and work.[37]

What research into human sexuality, then, lies ahead? Dean Hamer has repeated his initial work among male homosexuals in an entirely new group of families and has included a much-needed analysis of women. He has also compared the frequency of the Xq28 marker among pairs of gay siblings and their heterosexual brothers, important control data that he did not acquire the first time around. In work published in 1995, Hamer and his colleagues found linkage between Xq28 and sexual preference for gay male families, but not for lesbians.[38] Subsequent research has failed to corroborate these findings, although George Rice and his Canadian co-workers emphasized that their "results do not preclude the possibility of detectable gene effects [on sexual preference] elsewhere in the genome."[39]

To track down and sequence the DNA from one or more relevant genes, wherever they might lie, seems an almost insuperable task. To read the molecular script of DNA involves deciphering millions of constituent elements. Moreover, each gene will have to be studied individually and many more pairs of gay brothers will be needed to achieve this goal. The work will be extremely difficult for a single laboratory to undertake on its own. Hamer's request for a federally funded center for research into sexuality—a National Institute of Sexual Health—is therefore timely, for the study of differences between the sexes has reached a critical, though admittedly fragmented, stage and a coordinated research program would be valuable.

Inevitably, the idea of biological determinism carries with it the threat of manipulating the genes or the brain in order to adapt to the prevailing norm. As I have noted, Hamer was acutely aware of this possibility when he wrote his paper. But the prospects for pinpointing genetic risk have moved rapidly and worryingly forward with the recent availability of genetic screening techniques for, among other diseases, several cancers, including a small proportion of cancers of the breast, colon, and thyroid. Most such techniques are used without any current prospect for gene therapy or for any other effective treatment of the conditions identified. Geneticists such as Francis Collins, director of the Human Genome Project, have opposed unrestricted and unregulated screening techniques, describing their recent uses as "alarming"[40] because we are "treading into a territory which the genetics community has felt rather strongly is still [in the stage of] research." Hamer's words opposing genetic manipulation are likely to mean little in the marketplace if his work eventually leads to the isolation of a gene that has an effect on sexual preference, even if it has only a small effect that is present in only a limited number of people. US state legislatures are slowly responding to these issues. In the mid-1990s Colorado became the eleventh state to enact a law preventing information derived from genetic testing to be used in a discriminatory fashion.

But sex-based research has already run into political trouble. The Council for Citizens Against Government Waste has charged that some NIH research is a misuse of taxpayer's money. Tom Schatz, CCAGW's president, has criticized twenty such studies, including one involving research into sex offenders. Rex Cowdry, acting director of the National Institute of Mental Health, argued that "for these grants, I think first you have to believe that the factors that motivate and control sexual behavior are worth knowing about... you have to believe that knowing more about how men and women are both similar and different is important."[41]

With such partisan pressures dominating the future of the research agenda, the circulation of uninformed opinions couched in scholarly prose is a cause for anxiety. In an otherwise superb and iconoclastic critique of the history of heterosexuality, Jonathan Katz ends with a sweeping and badly informed declaration:

> Biological determinism is misconceived intellectually, as well as politically loathsome.... Contrary to today's bio-belief, the heterosexual/homosexual binary is not in nature, but is socially constructed, therefore deconstructable.

LeVay and Hamer on the one hand, and Katz on the other, evidently have taken completely antithetical positions. But Katz's extreme intellectual reductionism makes him as guilty as the more simplistic biologists and journalists who inflate claims about every new genetic discovery. After convincingly undermining the distinction between gay and straight, he then accepts the naive dualism of nature versus nurture. It is such attempts as Katz's to put into opposition forces that are not in opposition which argue so strongly for a serious research program free from the ideological temptations that he succumbs to. Biological research into sexuality will indeed be misconceived if we assume that we already understand the differences between the sexes. In part the results of that research often contradict any such assumption. Katz demands that "we need to look less to oracles [presumably biological], and trust more in our desires, visions, and political organizing." But to take this path risks perpetuating a debate based on ignorance rather than one based on evidence.

The research of Hamer and LeVay represented a genuine epistemological break away from the past's rigid and withered conceptions of sexual preference. The pursuit of understanding about the origins of human sexuality—the quest to find an answer to the question, What does it mean to be gay and/or straight?—offers the possibility of eliminating what can be the most oppressive of cultural forces, the prejudiced social norm.[42]

Still, medicine is nothing if not a practical discipline. We may seek meaning from the genome, whether in the origins of disease or human behavior, but the true test of its value will come in its therapeutic application at the bedside. And it is here that there are genuine tremors of excitement about the future. The cause of this clinical brouhaha is called RNA interference (RNAi), a phenomenon that "shows several features that border on the mystical."[43] The idea is a simple one. Strands of small interfering RNA (siRNA) are able to block gene expression. This ability was initially used to study gene function in worms. The effect is strong and highly specific. It has been confirmed in fruit flies, plants, and, of most relevance for humans, the vertebrate zebrafish and the mouse.[44]

Clinical applications of siRNA are beginning to emerge, at least in laboratory animals. For example, injecting thousands of siRNA into the bloodstream of mice protects them from hepatitis.[45] This description, in 2003, of switching off a disease process was the first proof of RNAi's therapeutic power. It could turn out to be a landmark in post-genomic medicine. But if it is, we will have the worm, *Caenorhabditis elegans*, to thank, and not the human genome. There is irony in the language of the genome after all.

# 14

# PROTECTING THE BREAST

THERE IS LITTLE that annoys professional medical historians more than the plodding feet of doctors past their prime who see it as their retirement right to stomp across fields they are wholly ill-prepared for. An eminent physician will blindly wade into a complex historical debate, ignoring reams of fine documentary analysis, only to deploy his (naturally superior) intellectual skills in identifying a single medical fact that solves the puzzle at hand. It is all the more enjoyable, therefore, to see a respected nonmedical historian engage in the same game. In *Bathsheba's Breast: Women, Cancer, and History*, James S. Olson has, for the first time I think, surveyed the interplay between the science of breast cancer and the wider culture of which it is a part.[1] His approach compels him to take on big issues.

Although not the first person to make the connection, Olson's boldest speculation is that "while Hitler contemplated the liquidation of millions of Jews... perhaps, in a warped inner vision, he remembered a Jew tormenting his mother." Klara Hitler died in her forties of breast cancer in December 1907, at a time when the young Adolf was preparing to leave his home in the provincial Austrian city of Linz for Vienna. It was a formative moment. He was close to his mother. As Ian Kershaw puts it in the first volume of his biography of Hitler, the future dictator was the recipient of her "smothering protectiveness."

Klara told Dr. Eduard Bloch, the Hitler family doctor, of the lump growing in her breast in January 1907. He arranged a mastectomy; she rallied, but quickly declined as the year progressed. After her death, Bloch wrote that "I have never seen anyone so prostrate with grief as Adolf Hitler."

The notion that Hitler's anti-Semitism solidified into a violent hatred because of a single Jewish doctor's failure to save his mother from breast cancer certainly has its attractions, and these bare facts became grist to the psychoanalytic mill. In 1947, Gertrud Kurth wrote an article in *The Psychoanalytic Quarterly* entitled "The Jew and Adolf Hitler." She asked, "Why did Adolf Hitler kill six million Jews?" and went on to claim that she had "discovered a valuable and hitherto unknown addition" to the evidence—namely, the existence of Dr. Bloch. True, Hitler was outwardly thankful to Bloch. He sent expressions of gratitude to the doctor on self-painted postcards from Vienna. He helped Bloch escape from Austria to the US after the *Anschluss* in 1938 by providing him with a visa and travel permits. The relationship appeared to be reciprocated: Bloch wrote, "Your Excellency: Before passing the border I want to express my thanks for the protection which I have received." But Kurth argued that Hitler's unconscious thoughts—she believed that he "experienced a father-transference to the doctor"—somehow explained why he attributed "all positive traits to the doctor and... negative ones to the Jew." Bloch was responsible, she wrote, for brutally assaulting and mutilating his dear mother. Logically enough, the Jew became Hitler's subsequent object of loathing.

Rudolf Binion, an opportunistic American historian, stumbled across Kurth's paper in the 1970s and built a case around Bloch as the one Jew who triggered Hitler's later genocidal policies. He discovered Bloch's 1907 medical casebook and believed he could prove that Bloch had overdosed Klara on iodoform. This treatment was applied directly to her suppurating breast wound, which had become studded with recurrent cancer, over forty-six consecutive days in the last weeks of her life. The iodoform caused Klara immense and intractable pain. According to Binion, here lay the subconscious origin of Hitler's hatred of the "Jewish cancer" and the "Jewish poison."

James Olson, although he cites neither Kurth nor Binion, stretches his attempt to weave breast cancer into the world's wider history by reiterating and endorsing the arguments of both writers. This causal chain seems a little too simple to me. Still, Olson's broad view of the important historical role of breast cancer is amply justified by the many examples of celebrities (Shirley Temple Black, Betty Ford, Nancy Reagan) whose breast cancer shaped the way doctors, scientists, and the public viewed this disease. The publicity surrounding the revelations that these women suffered from the disease not only did much to remove its stigma but also helped change its usual consequences—surgically removing or disfiguring a breast.

Olson has an unusual qualification to write about what is, of course, a disease which mostly affects women. He has struggled for over two decades with cancer himself, a sarcoma in his left arm. Like many women, he confronted a choice between full-blown amputation or lumpectomy, the local removal of the cancerous mass. At first, he opted to keep his arm by selecting only a restricted excision of his cancer. The tumor quickly recurred and again he chose the least deforming therapy. But a second recurrence by 1987 was too much of a threat. A hand and part of his arm were removed. Olson writes: "Although I know nothing of what it is like to lose a breast, I do understand the confusion of Hobson's choices, the anxiety of confronting one's own mortality, and the trauma of saying goodbye to a body part."

The history of breast cancer is the history of a waxing and waning concept. Until the 1970s, the prevailing view among breast cancer specialists was that the disease remained, at least at first, confined to the breast. If the tumor was caught late, it was likely to have spread, but metastasis was not thought to occur at an early stage. The logic of this view was best summed up by the Philadelphia physician Benjamin Rush, who concluded in the early nineteenth century that the "remedy is the knife." Cutting came of age with the radical mastectomy, pioneered by a brilliant but increasingly cocaine-addicted surgeon at Johns Hopkins Hospital, William Halstead. In a scientific paper published in 1894, Halstead reported the results of his operation on fifty women "for the cure of cancer of the breast." Beating the disease, he concluded, demanded unflinching aggression.[3]

Looking afresh at the drawings and photographs in that same paper today, there is both a beauty and a horror to what he was advocating. In one plate, a woman is lying on her back, her chest exposed and her right arm extended horizontally on the bed. An incision is shown near her armpit, curving around the medial part of her breast, and finally encircling the entire breast to meet the sweep of the first cut. A triangular flap of skin over the chest wall has been gently and evenly pulled back from the collarbone downward. The operation appears clean and straightforward, almost languorous. Another plate, a photograph, strips away this illusory precision and displays the real carnage of the procedure. It shows a deep bloody wound opened across a woman's chest. The breast is almost completely severed and hangs loosely from her side. The underlying dissected tissues are exposed for examination. Subsequent photographs show examples of freshly amputated breasts—skin, tissue, muscle, glands, blood vessels, and, in one case, part of a sawed-off collarbone. Halstead's efforts to remove as much of the woman's chest as possible were helped by advances in cleanliness (for example, rubber gloves), anesthesia, and blood transfusion.

Yet unbelievable as it may seem, Halstead was ultra-conservative next to some of his more adventurous colleagues. By the 1950s, the super-radical mastectomy (which eliminated a further string of lymph nodes from the chest) was in vogue, and then came the additional removal of ovaries, adrenal glands, and the pituitary gland, an organ that lies deep within the skull. Olson interprets these "extraordinary" procedures as the product of a new cultural phenomenon. Technological change in medicine implied progress, and with that progress came a greater trust in doctors. Women submitted themselves to these alarmingly elaborate operations because they believed that they were the only path to a cure.

But even while Halstead was publishing his early and apparently encouraging results, others were voicing contrary opinions, albeit cautiously. One American surgeon described as "fallacious" the belief that improved results could be explained by the increasing extent of the operation. A British doctor, Geoffrey Keynes (the brother of John Maynard), believed that the operation was just too debilitating for most women to bear. And in the 1920s, editorials in medical journals warned that success in treating breast cancer would not come from ever-greater agility with the knife, which, according to one commentator, had been "pushed to its practical limits." But women had to wait until the 1960s to see the radical mastectomy recede, and this revision at first took place only in Europe. In America, surgeons were more powerful and resisted important developments in radiotherapy and chemotherapy, notably because, according to Olson, "there was more money for surgeons in radical mastectomies than in more conservative procedures."

What finally made American surgeons stop butchering women? Certainly not science. Fifty years of skepticism did little to change surgical attitudes. Olson presents two possible explanations. He favors a cultural force—the "unprecedented fetish of the female breast." The birth of Hugh Hefner's *Playboy* in 1953 opened a broader market for pornography, one that led to breasts becoming "the physical icons of American popular culture, the sina [*sic*] qua non of eroticism and beauty." Thus was born the "mystique of the breast," and with it a woman's desire to hold onto them at all costs, even in the face of breast cancer.

Olson ties this emerging fetish to feminism. He argues that Shirley Temple Black helped drive the change in approach. When she discovered her breast cancer in 1972 she opted for less radical surgery, proclaiming that it was her "right to do with my body exactly what I wish to do." This statement might seem tame today, but it was said at a time when medical attitudes toward women were characterized by astonishing condescension. A leading American advocate of hormone replacement therapy (HRT) argued that estrogen would make "women adorable, even-tempered, and generally easy to live with." Against this culture of contempt for women's health, cancer survivors, together with a few like-minded doctors such as Susan Love, created the National Breast Cancer Coalition in 1991 "to be the voice, the obnoxious voice" on behalf of women. The coalition quickly became a strong political force, bringing about the release of millions of government dollars for research and changes in the law to enable uninsured women to have access to free treatment.

Another view is that doctors with an interest in proving the efficacy or harm of a particular treatment eventually created a body of evidence that was impossible to ignore, even by surgeons desperately trying to defend the income they received from performing mastectomies. One man did more than any other to transform the way women and their doctors thought about breast cancer—the tough, irascible Pittsburgh surgeon Bernard Fisher. In the 1960s, Fisher challenged the dominant consensus that breast cancer was a local disease. He argued that from the very start of a tumor's growth, cancerous cells were thrown off into the bloodstream to relocate elsewhere in the body. By 1970, he had concluded that "nobody really knows what the best treatment for breast cancer is." And by the end of the 1980s, he had shown that lumpectomy plus radiation treatment was better than Halstead's brutal radical mastectomy; that chemotherapy prolonged life; and that women taking the drug tamoxifen, which stops estrogen from driving cancerous growth, had lower rates of recurrent disease. The impact of these findings was dramatic, and their quick adoption into practice produced a remarkable result: a drop in breast cancer deaths by a quarter between 1987 and 1997—after almost no progress for centuries.

Strangely, Olson seems ambivalent about the benefits of research in medicine. He argues that the "university setting depersonalized medicine," and that the early triumph of radical surgery "rested on the twin pillars of male dominance and scientific objectivity." Yet when Fisher refused simply to run with the herd and instead asked difficult questions about the evidence of benefit from mutilating surgery—in other words, was ruthlessly scientific about breast cancer treatment—it led to tremendous advances in care. A cultural force of strong advocacy was important, but it had to be applied to a mass of credible evidence. It was Fisher's clinical trials, not *Playboy*, that provided this evidence.

But science does not always fall into line with the activist agenda. Sometimes new research findings leave women with hard decisions about how to reduce their chances of developing cancer. One such decision concerns breast-feeding. When all the best data in the world on the relation between breast cancer and breast-feeding are combined, the clear result is that the more children women give birth to and the longer they breast-feed, the more they will be protected against breast cancer. The incidence of breast cancer could be reduced by half if we changed our attitudes toward childbirth and breast-feeding. As Olson succinctly puts it, "Breasts without function can be dangerous." Even more pointedly, he quotes one activist who asked, "Do I have to be a skinny homemaker with a house full of kids to protect myself?"

The truth is that lifestyle changes might be more modest than many Western women fear—if each woman had two children and breast-fed each child for six months longer than is currently the norm, 25,000 breast cancer occurrences could be prevented across the world. The decision to have children is not usually made with prevention of breast cancer in mind. I doubt that exploiting female fertility will catch on as a technique to reduce the chances of breast cancer, even though it is, unquestionably, natural. There is, of course, the possibility of mimicking the hormonal changes of pregnancy and breast-feeding. The question is not only for women to answer, but also for all of us to ask of our governments: Do we want to create a society that supports women and families sufficiently to make these reductions in breast cancer risk possible? Incredibly, this is not a serious political issue in most Western countries today. It should be.

There remain unresolved and academically vicious disputes about technologies and treatments already in widespread use. Take two examples: screening mammography and hormone replacement therapy. The cumulative evidence of benefit from screening women for breast cancer just does not exist. When the results of clinical trials are combined and graded according to their quality, screening turns out to have no impact whatsoever on the likelihood of a woman dying of breast cancer. This fact seems impossible to comprehend given that screening services are such an entrenched part of health care in most Western countries, and it is fiercely contested by most screening advocates. Screening has become a sign of society's commitment to women's health. Olson gives the example of how women's health advocates successfully lobbied US state legislators to force insurance companies to pay for mammograms. To reverse such a long and bitterly won fight for screening is politically inconceivable. But the reality is that there is an urgent need for new research into the benefits and harm of modern screening methods. For example, does screening lead to unnecessary surgery by identifying changes in the breast that are not life-threatening?

Meanwhile, in 2002 a large US trial of hormone replacement therapy was stopped early because the rates of invasive breast cancer exceeded an acceptable limit—there was a 26 percent increase in numbers of new breast cancers. This risk sounds large, but it is actually quite small in terms of the *total* number of women. If ten thousand women took hormone replacement for one year, there would only be eight additional cases of invasive breast cancer. That might seem a reasonable trade-off if the benefits of hormone replacement were more substantial. But over many years, and among millions of women taking this type of therapy, these risks add up. A treatment that had been widely advocated to prevent chronic diseases, such as heart disease and osteoporosis, sadly causes more harm than we are willing to accept.

Women are also harmed by the excessive intrusion of politics into health and, according to Olson, the recklessness of journalists who hype new research in order to sell copy. The most dramatic political intervention in cancer was President Nixon's call for a "War on Cancer" in 1971. After a generation of massive investment, has this war been won? Although the incidence of breast cancer is falling in some countries, most common cancers continue to cause enormous suffering. Costly new drugs are developed, new surgical techniques are tried, and new schemes for irradiating tumors are devised—but no major breakthrough has taken place to cut substantially the overall toll of cancer on society. There are a few exceptions—for example, cancer of the testis and some childhood malignancies. A great deal of optimism erupted after the human genome was sequenced, but for every "breakthrough" you read about in the newspapers, ask yourself whether any lives will be saved by what has been reported. The answer will usually be: not one. Indeed, the pressure is so great to find something that causes a significant change in treatment that some doctors are tempted to deceive. One of Bernard Fisher's collaborators falsified his research results in the desperate belief that somehow he was helping women.

Olson portrays modern medicine's assault on breast cancer as a success story. In part, he is right to do so. But taken in context—the vast suffering that continues for thousands of women and the limited progress for most other cancers—the unavoidable conclusion must be that medicine is, at best, only holding the line against a pressing threat, one that will surely advance as our aging populations become more susceptible to malignant diseases. A report from the US National Cancer Institute in 2002 predicted that the number of cancer cases will double by 2050 as more people pass the age (seventy) at which cancer is typically diagnosed.

The question Olson does not address seems the one most obviously in need of an answer: Why has breast cancer become the defining illness of the women's health movement? Partly because breast cancer is a survivable disease, and so women go on to live life afresh. And partly because breasts are symbols of sex, in Swinburne's words "more soft than a dove's, that tremble with tenderer breath." Breast cancer is the central health issue for feminist advocacy. Yet it is not the most troubling cancer that faces women today. A far greater concern must surely be lung cancer, which is now becoming the leading cause of malignancy among women. Smoking—about nine out of ten cases of lung cancer are due to smoking—is still perceived to be largely a male problem. But tobacco use among women is a quietly growing burden. There are already over 200 million women smokers in the world today. That global figure is expected to triple by 2025, thanks to marketing, especially in films, that links smoking with images of health, liberation, independence, self-confidence, and slimness. Tobacco manufacturers see women worldwide as a lucrative new market. The past decade has seen a feminization of the cigarette, with milder, "lighter" brands that appear more safe. But they kill just as successfully as other cigarettes.

Two further questions follow. First, since smoking also contributes to breast cancer, why have breast cancer advocacy groups not raised their "obnoxious voice" against the tobacco industry? In recent years, the National Breast Cancer Coalition has issued statements about medical privacy, genetic discrimination, and treatment for low-income women, but nothing about smoking. Second, why do activists claim that we are enduring an epidemic of breast cancer, which is manifestly not true, when the real epidemic is tobacco use? This perversity shows all too clearly how cultural forces adversely influence public debates about breast cancer. Prevention is deemed less important than treatment, and tobacco is a less incendiary political issue than impossible technologies, such as human reproductive cloning. The lesson seems to be that we are unable to change the way we live today to reduce the risks we are storing up for tomorrow.

# 15

# THE FINAL CUT

SURGEONS HAVE A reputation for being cold, unprofessional, and indifferent to their patients' concerns. They overwhelm, psychologically as well as physically, those they incise. These are not my own prejudices. I know surgeons who can be kind when they try. But when Nalini Ambady studied surgeons' tones of voice, she found that these descriptions not only defined how surgeons behaved but also seemed to be linked to the likelihood of subsequent litigation for malpractice.[1] Not surprisingly, fast, loud, and harsh words in the clinic or at the bedside conveyed a lack of empathy and understanding. And when surgery went wrong, as it inevitably did from time to time, the patient had ample verbal grounds on which to feel bitter and angry.

Not every critic takes such a skeptical view of the surgical persona. According to Roy Porter, who until his unexpected death was one of Britain's most influential medical historians, medicine (as opposed to surgery) is passing through a period of profound uncertainty, even pessimism.[2] The "public climate is one not of optimism but of new-millennial anxiety." There has been an "erosion of confidence about doctors." The contribution of medicine "to the broader health of humankind remains... questionable"; medicine has simply become "another line of business." The hospital has been transformed into "a soulless, anonymous, wasteful and inefficient medical factory." It is little more than "the headquarters and power-base for the medical elite." Fewer miracle drugs are being bought to market, and doctors have forsaken Hippocratic principles for a damaging mix of technology and bureaucracy.

Amid all this gloom, Porter takes a quite different view of the present state of surgery. He begins with an obligatory Hippocratic aphorism: "He who wishes to be a surgeon should go to war." Indeed, the battlefield was the school of surgery for several centuries, and wound management its staple lesson. Gunpowder added helpfully to surgical skills by expanding the kinds of wounds and sources of infection that the surgeon had to contend with. Eventually, the discipline of surgery broadened and thrived with traveling tooth pullers, lithotomists, and "hernia-masters" who specialized in fitting trusses. In these early days, surgery was not for the fainthearted. As one commentator put it, cutting required "an eagle's eye, a lion's courage, and a woman's hand." Slowly, surgery became systematized. Anesthesia, antibiotics, and radiography dramatically altered surgical practice, and surgery rose steadily in professional standing. Surgeons even turned to experimentation, changing their work from an apprenticed craft to a physiological science. It is true that surgery has spawned the occasional cavalier madman—Sir William Arbuthnot, a British surgeon, excised great loops of gut as a means of preventing constipation—but Porter spares surgery much of the criticism he hurls at medicine. The removal of organs has now given way to their repair, restoration, and replacement. He concludes that surgery "knows no frontiers," that its practitioners have become the superstars of modern medicine.

Porter was a spectator of surgery, not a surgeon himself. A wholly different perspective has been eloquently and often movingly described by Atul Gawande, a surgical resident working in Boston who is not a triumphalist advocate of what the scalpel can achieve. Instead, he divides the essays in *Complications*,[3] his treatise on surgical practice, into three unusual groups: Fallibility, Mystery, and Uncertainty—the new trinity of the knife-god. Gawande writes brilliant extended case studies, showing the reader what he has learned as a surgeon—and, more important, how he has learned. Contrary to conventional histories, perhaps even to present-day public beliefs, he portrays surgery as a messy affair, an imperfect science, one that is "mostly hidden and often misunderstood." He describes how he became addicted and exhilarated by the "calculated violence" of the art. He made mistakes and learned through experience, now admitting that "it is people we practice upon." He also confesses that this truth is kept from patients. Honesty is not part of the language of surgery. Gawande's analysis is a long disputation about the origins of this duplicity.

The learning curve, for example, hides and dignifies the errors that are always made whenever any new procedure is developed or learned. The fate for the first few patients in either circumstance is often worse than it would have been with an older procedure or a more experienced doctor. In Gawande's stark words, "surgeons trying something new got worse before they got better." My reading of his argument is that he wants nothing less than to reinvent the covenant between surgeon and patient. It is not simply a matter of the tone of the surgeon's voice. The erosion of trust that medicine has suffered, so well chronicled by Porter, from malpractice suits to hopelessly contradictory scientific evidence about everyday risks (is a vaccine unsafe, or is it one of the greatest benefits to humankind), is based on the doctor's failure to explain to the public what medicine is truly about. Doctors have created expectations of perfection that they are unable to fulfill. Complete disclosure of surgery's failures and limitations needs to accompany the confidence surgeons have in their own commitment and ability. This is Gawande's call to arms. But he underplays the genuine crisis that surgery is now facing.

How satisfied are surgeons? For American surgeons, the answer is, not very. A survey of over twelve thousand US doctors in the late

1990s revealed that general surgery was a far less attractive career than family practice (the least attractive specialties were obstetrics and gynecology). A fifth of surgeons reported being dissatisfied with what they were doing. There was no single explanation for this pervading misery. Rising and unreasonable expectations of perfection, loss of income, loss of freedom to practice surgery in the way that they wished, long hours, and worsening conditions in which to provide high-quality care were all cited as reasons for discontent. These findings, together with Gawande's arguments about the essential dishonesty of surgery, raise the alarming hypothesis that, to put it mildly, not all is well in the state of surgery. To find out if this is so, one has to look deeper at subspecialties within the surgical corpus.

Cardiothoracic surgery is the dean of surgical subdisciplines. Physically demanding, highly technical, and the subject of extraordinary research effort, cardiothoracic specialization was the only surgical field to surpass family practice in career satisfaction.[4] But Timothy J. Gardner, the president of the American Association for Thoracic Surgery, has prophesied apocalypse for his own specialty.[5] In his 2002 presidential address, he spoke of "a loss of societal respect and esteem for the medical profession on the basis of a barely concealed suspicion that high-tech medical and surgical care are, in some way, being driven by a crass profit motive." Surgical trainees "often struggle just to find employment." They are "frustrated and angry." Government support for cardiothoracic specialists had ebbed and there had been "declining support for surgeon-researchers by the National Institutes of Health." This weakening of the research base had led to a "leakage of surgery activity from academic centers." There was "palpable demoralization and generalized ennui" among his colleagues. He questioned whether there were even grounds for encouraging enthusiastic students and surgical trainees to enter the cardiothoracic field. Was his an isolated opinion? No.

Thomas J. Krizek, a vice-president of the American College of

Surgeons, tried to examine the nature of this threat in more detail.[6] He asked a question that seemed incredible given the accumulated progress of surgical science and practice: Was there something now inherent in surgery that impaired its practitioners? He took as his starting point the unexpected suicides of four surgical colleagues, who were also longstanding personal friends and respected fellows of the American College of Surgeons. He wrote, almost in bemusement:

> All were involved in academic medicine and were considered successful; two were about to assume presidency or chairmanship of national organizations. Some observers ascribed the pressures of academic medicine as contributing factors. None of their acts has a rational explanation. But neither have their deaths been criticized; none was condemned.

He suggested that surgeons were suffering from "moral dyslexia." "It is hard for us to read the handwriting on the wall when our backs are against it," he wrote. Fewer medical students were entering surgery. Positions in practice were being left unfilled. Surgeons often felt a lack of support from colleagues. The specialty "is not as collegial as we like to think." Working environments were becoming increasingly hostile, and some surgeons were driven to "outbursts of anger" and "control through fear and intimidation." Krizek concluded, "Surgery is not as happy a career as it was in the past." The incidence of "impairment is high and is having a direct or indirect negative impact on our entire profession."

How has this perilous state of affairs come about? There seems to be no one all-encompassing answer. Training is too long, work hours destroy family life, the emotional burden of operating is draining, high standards are harder to maintain, and surgery has become fragmented to the point where the discipline has lost some of its binding values and common identity. Finally, the way mistakes are handled too often sets patient against surgeon. As Krizek wrote: "It is a profoundly human desire when we have made a mistake or an error to seek forgiveness. There is all too often no place in our profession . . . in which we can ask for forgiveness."

This erosion of confidence in a discipline that must surely rank as one of medicine's technically most successful has forced a good deal of philosophical soul-searching. Miles Little, director of the Centre for Values, Ethics, and the Law in Medicine at the University of Sydney, Australia, has tried to define the aspects of surgery that are unique to the discipline and so to pinpoint the surgeon's special relationship with his or her patient.[7] The person undergoing an operative procedure experiences an unusually intense sense of *rescue* thanks to the power that the surgeon wields. The physical proximity between the two also brings with it extreme *intimacy*. The *ordeal* of the surgical experience and its *aftermath* leave mental as well as bodily scars. In sum, Little argues, this dramatic psychological trauma shows how important it is for the surgeon to be *present* with the patient during the entire diagnostic, operative, and recovery process. These features make up "the moral domain of the surgical relationship." It is this moral domain that seems to have been fractured in recent years, and which is now driving the likes of Gawande, Gardner, and Krizek to reassess how surgery can recover the trust of the public and profession alike. Little puts it this way, and I think that Gawande would agree:

> Undergoing major surgery is an extreme experience, which changes people's lives. Surgeons are therefore repeatedly involved in the extreme experiences of others. This in itself is also a form of extreme experience, which changes their own lives. The grounds of understanding between patient and surgeon are therefore created by the nature and the acts of surgical practice. Surgeons . . . have only to open themselves to the stories of their

patients and to their own stories in order to develop a relevant ethics of surgical care.

* * *

What lies at the root of this professional despair among surgeons? An important and largely unrecognized element of this malaise is the profound way in which the acquisition of surgical knowledge is changing and is likely to change further over coming years. In other words, the problems facing surgery are epistemological as well as existential and ethical.

NB

The traditional course of surgical progress is the introduction of a bold new operation matched, perhaps, by a technological innovation. Take robotic surgery, the latest ingenious gadgetry to have captured the imagination of surgeons. The early reports of robotic revascularization of blocked arteries in the heart do cause one to pause with awe.[8] Without the need to crack open the chest, patients with heart disease can now undergo coronary artery bypass grafting by means of a system relying completely on a fiber optic endoscope to manipulate micro-instruments. The left lung is simply deflated and three holes are bored into the chest wall to introduce the necessary tools for arterial repair. These tiny surgical instruments are designed to work in a way that mimics the human wrist. A three-dimensional image of the surgical field is transmitted to a video screen for the surgeon to follow what he cannot see with his own eyes. A new vessel for the heart can be harvested from the chest wall and sutured into place remotely. The operation is not an easy one to learn or to perform. Some of the first patients to undergo this procedure lived in Germany, and in a quarter of cases surgeons had to open the chest in the old-fashioned way to resolve episodes of uncontrollable bleeding or vessel injury. But as these same surgeons slowly learned the technique, the risks seemed to diminish. And the benefits were great—the chest cavity remained intact, the cosmetic result was infinitely better than before, and the risks of infection were reduced (since there was no longer a large wound to get infected).

But describing what happened to a small series of patients who have enthusiastically consented to a heroic new procedure is no way—actually, it is the worst way—to evaluate an original surgical technique. In 1923, a medical statistician named Major Greenwood wrote, "I should like to shame [surgeons] out of the comic opera performances which they suppose are statistics of operations." His point was that surgeons took too little time to study properly what they were doing. Surgical knowledge was acquired through a mix of bravery and anecdote, with little or no science intervening between the scalpel blade and the patient. As a result, surgery was exciting and courageous. But nobody had any real idea what worked and what didn't. Unbelievably, this approach to surgery remains largely the same today. The now standard means for evaluating any new discovery in medicine—the randomized controlled trial—is a rare event in the surgical arts.[9] This is a scandalous situation since patients cannot be assured that the techniques being used by their surgeons have been subjected to careful and rigorous testing. Their surgeons might well be skilled, but skilled at doing the wrong operation. Surgeons dislike being challenged about their lack of interest in studying what they do. They often resort to the argument that surgery is a craft, not a science, and that the test of a good surgeon lies in his or her (usually his) learning a procedure carefully, not studying it in some abstract, highly controlled way. As one respected British surgeon once wrote: "The problem is that surgery is not like a pill which is refined and guaranteed to be similar; each procedure introduces a variable that is uncontrolled... frankly, these randomised trials do not advance knowledge."[10]

It would be a caricature to claim that all of surgery is a science-free zone. The formal evaluation of surgical procedures has taken place for several diseases and in a few notably committed countries. These examples are often forgotten by surgeons, such as the one just quoted, who get defensive about what they do and how they have come to do it. For example, advances in the surgical management of breast cancer and cancer of the colon have relied greatly on evidence from clinical trials. The Netherlands, unlike the UK and much of continental Europe, has a particularly strong tradition of conducting clinical trials: operations to cure peptic ulcers, repair hernias, ameliorate stomach cancer, and resect rectal cancer have all been refined through a remarkable series of trials performed in the Netherlands during the past decade.[11] For some reason that not even their own surgeons can explain (and I have asked them), the Dutch do, and think about, surgery differently from the rest of the world.

There are also signs that surgeons now recognize that when there is a choice between a surgical and a medical approach to a clinical problem, that dilemma can best be resolved by an experiment: the controlled trial. For the patient living with severe heart disease, for instance, the choice facing the doctor (and patient) presently is either a full-blown operation (opening the chest with a saw and bypassing the diseased vessels; gentle robotic manipulations are still a rare option) or a procedure called percutaneous transluminal coronary angioplasty. During an angioplasty, a collapsed balloon is introduced into the diseased vessel of the heart via a thin tube usually inserted through the groin. This balloon is then inflated, forcing the vessel to open once again. The vessel wall is often severely damaged by this traumatic solution, and the damage can cause the vessel to close again rapidly in the months following the angioplasty. Vessels can now be kept open by placing a metal tube—called a stent—into the artery. It has taken many years of performing large clinical trials, involving thousands of patients, to work out the benefits and dangers of one technique over another.[12] For patients with heart disease today, the trial has been a triumph in defining the best way to approach their condition. Indeed, in one review of all surgical research published during the 1980s and 1990s, the numbers of randomized trials almost doubled. But these encouraging signs should not be overinterpreted. In this survey, the increase in numbers of trials was pitifully small—from 2 percent to only 4 percent of the total published quantity of surgical research.[13] This unwillingness to take evaluation seriously is compounded by the fact that many of the trials done are of very poor quality.[14]

Is it fair to argue, in defense of surgeons, that surgery somehow differs from other parts of medicine? And if so, do these differences justify an alternative approach to acquiring sound surgical knowledge? In an important essay on the problems of surgical knowledge, Peter McCulloch and his colleagues from Britain and Japan argued that the dogma of clinical trials—that they are the *only* valid way to test new ideas—ignores some very real practical difficulties specific to surgery.[15] For a start, surgery has been around for several thousand years, whereas clinical trials only became embedded within medicine during the 1940s and 1950s—exactly the time when the pharmaceutical industry was born. It was relatively easy to integrate the testing of drugs into a new culture of clinical trials—but less so for the ancient traditions of surgery. Surgery, unlike the rest of medicine, has also depended on its personalities to invent, develop, and proselytize advances. Today the era of great physician figures, such as William Osler, has long passed. It is now great institutions, not individuals, that dominate the landscape of medicine. It is the industry of research that draws prestige, not the personal wisdom of physicians. But surgery is unlike any other medical discipline, as Little has pointed out, in its extraordinary intimacy. The consent of patients to allow surgeons to commit calculated acts of violence in their name reflects Alexanderian trust taken to its absolute extreme. And it invests the surgeon with not only power but also, or so some surgeons seem to believe, proprietary rights over the patient and the products of their surgical sculpting.

This power naturally reinforces a strong self-belief in the value of what the surgeon does. This is partly a good thing. If you are going to be put under the care of a person wielding a knife, better that person is confident of his skills than timid. As a patient I may prefer my surgeon to offer me certainty, not the toss of a coin that comes with a randomized trial. Surgeons also face strong commercial pressures to introduce new techniques quickly. Being at the leading edge of surgical technology draws prestige and money—attractive rewards for a surgeon whose career will have likely taken decades to build. And these incentives can induce a state of torpor when it comes to rigorous scientific investigation, especially if such studies are not, unlike for new drugs, required by law. So surgery is, to some degree at least, different. A research culture is slowly encroaching on the tried and not so tested practices of surgeons. But what do these shifts mean for the future of surgery?

Surgery is all about action, not reflection. But information is sometimes critical, even in the operating room. In 2002, surgeons in Australia were working frantically to save the life of a critically injured man. One of the surgeons recalled that he had read an article in a medical journal that he was sure would help his team right there and then. The problem was that he could not remember which article. What could he do? A call was put out to the British Library archives. Although it was received at 3 AM British time, library staff were able to track down the 1996 paper in the *European Journal of Emergency Medicine* within twenty minutes and send it to the desperate Australian surgeons.

Not all surgical situations demand such instant information. But the architecture of evidence that surgeons are building to work out the safety and efficacy of new techniques shows that the range of questions they must answer poses particular challenges. For example, in 2001 a quarter (350,000) of all coronary artery bypass grafts in the US were performed on a beating heart—that is, without the need to stop the heart, as is the usual practice, and divert the body's blood through a mechanical pump. There are many different ways to evaluate this relatively new but now widely used technique. One large randomized trial cannot provide the single answer the surgeon needs because there is no one single straightforward answer to be had[16]—only many answers to many different questions. The surgeon obviously needs to know if patients survive "off-pump," as it is called, as well as if they had been hooked up to an artificial pump. But surgeons also need to know which patients will do best with this new technique—and who will do worse. They need some measure of whether the new vessels grafted onto the heart remain open, how much blood is lost, whether the kidneys hold up during the stress of the operation, what adverse events might affect the brain, and how long the patient needs to stay in the hospital. Surgical procedures often raise more complex questions than those that surround the introduction of a new drug—and which can be resolved by a single large clinical trial. This complexity is reflected in the most controversial concept in surgery today—the learning curve.

Many surgeons I have met do not find it easy discussing the learning curve—that is, the increased morbidity and mortality among patients that may occur when a surgeon is learning a new procedure or technique. But the learning curve is a fact of surgical life. For example, in a rare investigation of the learning curve, a group of Australian surgeons found that their early results with an endoscopic method to remove the spleen were far worse than what they were able to achieve after this "practice phase." Operations failed in 40 percent of cases in the early period (only 6 percent thereafter), the operating time was almost an hour longer, the time spent in hospital was eleven days instead of four, bleeding was worse early on, and a third of patients had complications (and one person died) compared with neither complication nor death in the later phase.[17] The Australian team admitted that "there is a learning curve during which complications do occur." This experience has important implications in today's new culture of surgical transparency.

Surgery is passing through a difficult and disillusioning period of transition. Professional, political, and social forces are making surgical practice more difficult. Atul Gawande is not alone in calling for efforts to bring honesty about the fallibility and uncertainty of surgery out into the open. Surgeons are having to learn to be accountable and willing to defend their work in front of a questioning, occasionally hostile, public.

An example of this cultural change is to be found in Britain. The deaths of thirty-five children in Bristol, England, during the 1990s while they were under the care of heart specialists sent a seismic shock through the previously complacent British medical establishment. An inquiry found that the standard of care given to these children in and out of the operating room was appalling. There were professional and system failures on such a scale that the government was forced to make heart surgeons disclose their surgical results. The goal is to begin publishing these figures by individual surgeon in 2004. But surgeons are finding this new accountability difficult to adjust to. Professor Tom Treasure, an experienced heart surgeon working in London, wrote in 2002:

> The identity and reputation of the surgeon is on the line.... The rules under which we must now live and work are being made "to stop Bristol happening again." ...As we use surgeon specific outcome data to try to improve things for the patients we actually make things worse. There is no doubt...that it is much harder to persuade a surgeon to take on the more risky...cases. These are the rules that were intended to protect patients from their imagined coterie of unskilled surgeons who are as arrogant as they are reckless. It is in the higher risk cases that we make the biggest impact on survival and yet the new rules may deprive those patients of care.[18]

NB

The problems of transparency not only concern the learning curve and the rising levels of fear that will stop surgeons from operating on high-risk patients. These difficulties will also affect the pace of innovation itself. The introduction of a new technique is fraught with risk for the patient. Sometimes these risks pay off, sometimes not. On balance, there is probably benefit, although without formal testing in clinical trials it is hard to know. Here is a recent example of what can happen not only when the risks prove too great but also when they are not properly disclosed to patients.

In 1996, surgeons at one of the most prestigious specialist heart centers in the world—the Cleveland Clinic in Ohio—embarked on a project that would bring their institution to public attention for exposing patients to a procedure that had not been properly tested. A Cleveland Clinic team traveled to Brazil to investigate a new operation to treat heart failure, a condition in which the heart is unable to pump blood around the body effectively. Five million Americans are estimated to suffer from this condition. An unknown surgeon, Dr. Randas Batista, had developed a completely original way to strengthen the heart's own muscle. Counterintuitively, the procedure involved removing a wedge-shaped piece of tissue from the left ventricle, the main chamber of the heart. Batista claimed huge success for the four hundred patients under his care. The Cleveland Clinic team were sufficiently encouraged by what they saw to try out Batista's procedure for themselves. Sixty-two patients underwent this stunningly innovative operation back at the clinic. They all gave their consent after, in the words of the surgeons, "verbal and written discussion of risks, alternatives, and perceived benefits."[19] But the technique proved to be a failure. Fewer than two thirds of the patients were alive after three years, and only a quarter were free from heart failure.

Instead of hailing a careful investigation of a promising new procedure, surgical colleagues criticized the Cleveland Clinic team for their lax standards. Martin F. McKneally, a heart surgeon and ethicist from

Toronto, asked whether patients had been sufficiently informed about the study (he argued not) and whether the study had been formally reviewed by the clinic's Institutional Review Board (he said not).[20] McKneally was troubled by the lack of information concerning the Batista procedure at the time it was being offered to patients:

> The Batista operation is a *non-validated procedure*. Cardiologists and surgeons did not know the answers to such questions as these: Does the operation really work? Which patients will benefit?

The US Office of Human Research Protections later found that the clinic's procedures had broken federal rules for safeguarding research volunteers. Surgeons were performing a research study on these sixty-two patients, but they had not disclosed this fact at the time of the patients' consent. The clinic's surgical team took a different view. They did not conduct a randomized trial to fully test the procedure, they argued, because "comparing the earliest 'learning curve' results of this complex operation to established therapies without some preliminary experience with patient selection, operative technique, and perioperative care seemed premature." In other words, their early efforts to understand this technique were, they claimed, simply part of a learning curve. But it was a learning curve with an untested technique that eventually harmed patients. McKneally argued that what surgery now needed was a consent form "emphasizing novelty [and] the learning curve."

Yet not all risks of this sort turn out so badly. In regulating surgical practice and protecting patients from harm, failure must not extinguish genuine and carefully won hope, as the example of liver transplantation shows. After undergoing coronary artery bypass grafting in 1990, Thomas E. Starzl, who pioneered liver replacement, decided that "what I had experienced might help someone else who feared along the way that their best efforts were leading nowhere." He went on to write, somewhat reluctantly, his memoir, *The Puzzle People.*[21] Starzl began his early work in transplantation in 1958. He practiced removing a liver and sewing it back into place in about two hundred dogs. He and his colleagues confronted what then seemed like insuperable challenges, such as stopping and then restoring blood flow to the organ graft. Most of the animals he worked on died within a few days of the procedure. Yet he built up his confidence and skill sufficiently to believe that liver transplantation was possible in a human being.

On March 1, 1963, Starzl conducted his first attempt to replace a human liver—in a terminally ill three-year-old boy. The procedure was much more difficult than he had anticipated and his patient bled to death on the operating table. He tried four more liver transplants in 1963, but all ended in failure caused by a combination of infection, hemorrhages, and blood clots. The program was going nowhere, and parallel initiatives in Boston and France also collapsed. Starzl wrote that "our primary mission of liver transplantation had failed." He suspended all work on human beings for three years.

But he had not given up his hopes entirely. He continued to work on perfecting his technique in dogs. By March 1964, one dog had survived longer than most, and it continued to live for another twelve years. Drugs to treat organ rejection were finally becoming available. Why was the procedure working now, when it had been such a spectacular failure only a few months before? "Successes came steadily. These were not attributable to any single factor, but were due to accretion of small details in surgical skills and postoperative management."

The pressure on surgeons trying to reintroduce liver transplantation into humans was intense—and occasionally fatal. Lawrence Brettschneider was a gifted surgeon who worked with Starzl in the 1960s. He devised a successful method for preserving the donor liver. But he damaged his finger in a baseball injury, so badly that he found it hard to operate safely or successfully. His frustration was simply too great.

"He put a gun in his mouth," Starzl wrote, "and with the defective finger, pulled the trigger."

In 1967, facing strong opposition from many surgical colleagues, Starzl resumed liver transplantation in humans. The first seven children he operated on proved to be technical successes, but four died several months after the procedure. By 1969, he had treated twenty-six patients, reaching the "grim conclusion [that] liver transplantation was a feasible but impractical way to treat end-stage liver disease." Despite this feeling of enormous failure, he pressed on, transplanting livers in 170 patients by 1979—only twenty-nine of whom were alive by 1992. The event that ushered in a new era for liver transplantation was the discovery of cyclosporin in 1971—a drug that was soon found to prevent organ rejection.

But now science hit surgery head-on. Despite the clear benefits of cyclosporin for Starzl's transplant patients, he came under immense pressure to subject this new drug to formal testing in a randomized controlled trial. Starzl resisted, arguing that a trial which would deny some patients the most effective drug available to treat episodes of organ rejection—since half of all patients in the study would, by random allocation, not receive cyclosporin—was far more unethical than not conducting a trial at all. But he had no choice. A trial was launched and, as Starzl had predicted, it failed when it proved impossible to persuade patients to enter a life-or-death lottery for a drug they knew was essential for the operation's success. This experience left Starzl furious. As a scientist who had spent thirty years perfecting liver transplantation in the laboratory, he concluded that "the randomized trial had not been an instrument of discovery, but a validation of a conclusion already reached in previous patients."

In 1980, Starzl moved to Pittsburgh to set up the world's first liver transplant program. Although he was treating over twenty patients each year, liver transplantation was still classified as an experimental procedure. Only in June 1983, twenty-five years after the first experiments in dogs, and after several dramatic reversals of fortune, did the National Institutes of Health eventually agree that liver transplantation was a successful service worth offering to patients and not a hit-or-miss experiment. A lifetime's work had finally been vindicated.

The experience of liver transplantation shows that had there been heavy regulation of surgical research in human beings and harsh media scrutiny of the early years of liver transplant failure, what eventually turned out to be a tremendously successful procedure could easily have been killed off. Many of the patients who first took part in the embryonic liver replacement programs were undoubtedly taking part in high-risk research—research that not only had a predictably uncertain learning curve but also offered little likelihood of success without, in retrospect, the drugs necessary to treat organ rejection. Informed consent by today's standards would have almost certainly stalled the program from the start. Full disclosure of the prospects for failure would have revealed the futility of the procedure, and the savage truth that patients who were being operated on were little more than laboratory animals. But these were absolutely necessary experiments if surgical progress was to be made. An institutional review board in the modern era would surely have blocked Starzl's early work in human beings—and successful liver transplantation would have been needlessly delayed.

In a recent survey of American surgeons, most believed that the government should not impose further regulations on innovative surgery.[22] Some surgeons argued that existing regulations were sufficient. Others preferred to rely on "honest discussion between patient and investigator." There was genuine anxiety that progress in surgery would be stifled by continued government intrusion into the research process. And yet this is the likely outcome of a culture that requires complete transparency, punishment of error, and certainty of success. Gawande's call for a new covenant of honesty between patient and surgeon is surely correct. But its unintended and seemingly inescapable consequence will be a choking off of innovation when the reality of research and its early human toll becomes clear. I might be wrong, of course. Altruism may overcome suspicion and cynicism, but the recent history of medicine's relations with our wider culture suggest that transparency, shone through the lens of an aggressive media, breeds mistrust, not confidence. And with mistrust comes profound anxiety. The dangers of litigation and professional humiliation for the surgeon who takes risks will become simply too great. And so we will arrive at a moment that could truly be called the end of surgery.

NB

# 16

## IN THE DANGER ZONE

TO ENTER A hospital is to pass into a zone of occasional and unusual danger. Many illnesses invite well-tried treatments with normally uncomplicated outcomes. But unintended catastrophe is always at hand. In *Intensive Care: A Doctor's Journal*,[1] John F. Murray's unsettling account of life on the intensive care unit at San Francisco General Hospital, one story exemplifies the intrusion of unexpected disaster.

Day twenty-six of Murray's month on service. Julius Upshaw, who drinks too much, injects himself with heroin, and earns a lean living as a panhandler, has been admitted three weeks before with an infected human bite. The story is that he has been caught in a brawl, the outcome of which has left his hand trapped between the clenched jaws of his opponent. The human mouth is a paradise for bacteria, and Mr. Upshaw's swollen hand is now oozing thick pus. Crimson threads—infected lymph vessels—track toward his armpit.

Treatment is straightforward: intravenous antibiotics. But without a ready supply of alcohol, Mr. Upshaw quickly begins to shake uncontrollably from acute withdrawal. He is sedated, and immediately aspirates vomit into his lungs. A nasty pneumonia ensues that, in the presence of a serious blood infection, tips his kidneys into failure. He develops a syndrome in which his entire body swells with fluid, turning him into a ball of human flesh. The retained fluid begins to spill into Mr. Upshaw's lungs. Quite reasonably, it is decided to remove some of this fluid with a needle to prevent him from drowning. The lung, less reasonably, collapses and surgeons are summoned to place a tube into his now hollow chest cavity. By this time, there is only one safe place for this unlucky patient to go: the intensive care unit.

Murray's diary of daily patient admissions—sixty in all—puts the reader at the center of the tense decision-making that frequently takes place in a crisis setting. San Francisco General is a tough frontline city hospital for the disadvantaged, founded in 1850 during a bitter cholera epidemic. It faces the raw edge of urban living.

Despite these pressures, Murray's clinical approach is methodical. Each day's account opens with a brief introduction to a large issue—misdiagnoses, the language of medicine, the threat of infection—which is then illustrated by a case or two from the day's admissions. Murray ties his narrative together by interweaving the stories of patients already in the ICU with the experiences of his new patients.[2] This device enables him to select and discuss aspects of their clinical course that throw light on both the inexact arts of intensive care and intensely personal issues, such as how one dies.

His "chief purpose" is "to inform people about what really goes on in ICUs.... Few have this information, but it concerns everyone." By writing in depth about this one specialty of medicine, and for a broad general audience rather than for other physicians alone, Murray follows a long twentieth-century tradition of clinical narratives. This genre was inaugurated by William Carlos Williams in *The Doctor Stories*.[3] In essays such as "The Use of Force," medicine was shown to be a messy affair, with many predicaments that seem far away from the orderly clinic or antiseptic operating room.

The approach that Williams used so well has been further and finely developed by Richard Selzer, a surgeon, who, in books such as *Letters to a Young Doctor* and *Mortal Lessons*,[4] used the confessional and interpretative essay to describe some of the most unexplored trenches of medicine. An example of a recent new voice in this tradition is Frank Huyler's *The Blood of Strangers*.[5] This narrative vein of medical writing has become gorged to such a degree that its study has become an academic discipline in its own right.[6]

But Murray has a larger purpose than simply to develop the heritage of doctor as writer or to open a window for those curious enough to look through. He is disturbed that the view of ICU medicine presented to the public seriously distorts the truth. For instance, the success rate for resuscitations acted out in television series such as *ER* is 75 percent. The true figure is 15 percent. Murray's observations—he has worked in intensive care for much of his career—lead him to two conclusions. First, "that death is an ever-present part of the ICU story." And second, "that death is not a correctable biological condition—it is everyone's ultimate destiny."

We might think that ICUs work miracles. They do not. They fail more often than they succeed. That reality is not a comfortable one to admit, but it matters because it forces us to confront issues such as physician-assisted suicide with an honest understanding of what medicine can fairly be expected to achieve. The evidence that Murray accumulates from his sixty patients allows him to construct a persuasive argument. In sum, it is "that the current decision-making process [in ICUs] can and should be improved."

This critical look at intensive care is a surprising and important departure for Murray. His academic reputation rests largely on his co-editorship of a comprehensive review of respiratory medicine,[7] which was first published in 1988. A third edition came out in 2000. In the preface to the first edition, Murray and Jay A. Nadel emphasized their belief in the logical scientific basis of respiratory medicine: "A strong foundation in these basic sciences will make possible a rational and scientific approach to the more specialized clinical material." In the past twenty years, his research and other writings have concentrated on tuberculosis, HIV, and the interplay between these two lethal infections. In other words, Murray has been a sober academic commentator on a highly technical discipline. Something striking seems to have taken place to lead him to write for a new audience.

Murray's sardonic description of the tribal nature of hospital life makes his case that much more convincing. He creates a telling picture of the ICU. At the apex of the tribal hierarchy is the attending physician who has overall responsibility for patient care and who gives out "orders" each day. A cadre of young doctors—from confident first-year residents to wiser third-year residents—carry out these instructions, do the scut work, and cover nights while their bosses sleep or, as Murray once admits, sneak off during the day to play the occasional game of tennis. Residents throughout the world have a highly variable sense of respect for their attending physicians. Murray is self-consciously aware that his ways are seen as old-fogeyish by some of his younger colleagues.

Nurses, not doctors, hold the ICU together. They know more about their patients than any doctor and they are frequently more experienced than residents at the technical aspects of ICU care. There are competing specialists too. Surgeons are impatient aggressors, holding their scalpels poised to slice through the procrastinations of dithering colleagues. Murray is sensitive to their highly charged presence:

> Surgeons routinely perform technical feats no internist would ever conceive of undertaking, and they bring those brilliant skills with them when they consult on a patient. But they often bring their giant egos and short fuses as well. A surgeon friend of mine has characterized his confreres as "Often wrong, but never in doubt." By contrast, the call to arms for internists is "Don't just do something, stand there." It is undoubtedly good for the profession that it includes men and women of instant

> action as well as those of prolonged reflection; but when these polar temperaments meet at the bedside of a sick person, things can heat up.

Somehow these tribes do work together, in a balance of often ferocious suspicion.

Doctors also take part in rituals that strengthen their traditional tribal loyalties. At San Francisco General Hospital, as elsewhere, these rituals have included daily ward rounds, morning report, weekly grand rounds with a retinue of residents, and even "liver rounds," at which a drink or three was taken to celebrate the end of the week. Murray is nostalgic about these rituals because he sees the ethos that they embody—and so the spirit that binds the medical team together—now being irrevocably eroded. Bedside ward rounds are being diminished by the false notion that to discuss a patient's care next to the patient is somehow demeaning; grand rounds by academic arrogance and the perfidious intrusions of the pharmaceutical industry; and "liver rounds" by the replacement of beer and pretzels with more socially correct ice cream and cookies.

It is in the daily detail of an ICU at work that Murray wonderfully depicts a place of function and dysfunction. His account is based on the stories of his sixty admissions, all with various combinations of failing hearts, lungs, brains, kidneys, livers, and intestines. Causes of death range from bizarre accidents (a carrot lodged in a bronchus) to repeated episodes of self-harm (alcohol, heroin, cocaine, and other undiscovered substances) to the familiar ravages of old age (cancer, stroke, and heart attack).

Murray shows that the ICU is a place of small successes rather than triumphant victories. He does not hide the rougher side of intensive care: the need for strong prisonlike restraints to tie down agitated patients; the lethal presence of hospital-acquired infections; the crude indignities that a lack of privacy forces on ICU patients and their families; the psychic terrors that afflict some of those under his care; the threats of litigation from worried relatives ("We'll be watching you.... Don't pull the plug on him, Doc. Don't you dare"); and the frustrations of a system stretched beyond the point at which it can operate safely (for example, missing radiographs: "I have complained to the chief of radiology, screamed at file clerks, and thrown fits in the reading room. Nothing has ever worked; now I just shrug—beaten by the system—and do what I can without the film").

He also opens the usually closed issue of iatrogenesis—that is, illnesses caused by medical examination or treatment—and describes several instances of such illness during his month on ICU. One man was given intravenous penicillin, to which he was allergic. Astonishingly, he was given the same antibiotic again during the same admission, which gave him a ticket that took him immediately to the ICU. In another case, a woman with pneumonia was pushed into pulmonary edema—a condition in which the lungs fill with water—by overzealous infusions of intravenous fluids. Murray reports twelve cases of iatrogenic pulmonary edema during his month, and he rails at the "careless physicians" who paid too little attention to preventing this serious complication.

Part of the difficulty, Murray argues, is that doctors have come to rely too heavily on laboratory tests and radiographs to make diagnoses and to monitor treatments. The skills of history-taking and careful physical examination are not endowed with the mystique of a new and expensive technical investigation. And so they are neglected. Murray's belief in the centrality of these old-fashioned values is confirmed by reading his textbook. In this multiauthored treatise, the chapter on history and physical examination was written by Murray alone. There he affirms the importance of a doctor's communication skills, which form "the foundation for the physician–patient relationship." But he also argues that "communication is not just words but is an interaction with sequences and quality." These subtle transitions between doctor and patient are vital influences "on subsequent trust, understanding, concern, and compliance."

> It follows, therefore, that the medical interview, which is nearly always the first event in the continuum of physician–patient communication and which is the most frequently used tool in clinical medicine, has considerable effect on the outcome of the patient's illness.

A reliance on technology can make doctors overconfident or, worse, plain lazy. Murray gives an example of how the discovery, by computed tomography, of "free air" in a patient's abdomen almost led to a major operation to locate a presumed rupture of an internal organ. And yet a thorough clinical examination revealed the "free air" finding to be a red herring. The radiologist, confronted with the negative clinical examination but clinging to his x-ray proof, began to lose touch with reality. "It doesn't matter what your examination shows," he exclaimed. "That's free air, take my word for it." It was not, and Murray sums up his views about this incident. He is scathing:

> A CT [scan] of his abdomen, which was probably not indicated in the first place, revealed a "finding" that I decided not to act on, but that could have sent him to the operating room. In addition, the turmoil of going to the x-ray department for the CT study in the early morning, when he would have been better off sleeping, and the multiple examinations to resolve the debate, have only served to make poor Mr. McVicker much more terrified and confused than he already was.

These unusually frank reflections raise the issue of why Murray has written this critical account of ICU medicine. His experiences have led him to ask two large questions. First, is there any point in having an ICU when patients' outcomes seem so poor? And second, given that the ICU is a place where people frequently die, have we paid enough attention to how they die? His answers to both questions are not wholly reassuring.

A plainly distressed first-year resident challenged Murray directly. "This is my second month at 'The General' and almost all my patients have been losers. In the ICU alone, of my five patients, three were drunks and two were junkies.... They're all trying to kill themselves. What's the point? Why are we doing this?"

Her observations will ring true for many doctors. And Murray, although he tries to quell her skepticism with a passionate speech about "commitment," "victims of social bad luck," and the occasional "brilliant success," shares some of her doubts. Drug users are, he concludes, "notoriously bad at complying with therapy." After one patient suffered a huge stroke as a complication of injecting drugs, Murray cannot refrain from remarking: "It is incomprehensible to me how this young man—or anyone—could wreak such destruction on his own body. Yet it happens over and over again." Add to drug abuse the effects of alcohol and smoking and one has the holy trinity of self-harm. ICU does nothing to tackle these root causes of acute illness.

Murray's verdict on his month's work—the real answer to his resident's question—can be inferred from his stark summary of the outcomes among his sixty admissions: twenty-seven alcoholics and drug users patched up, in all likelihood, only to return again soon, but in ever worsening shape; eighteen episodes of iatrogenic disease; fifteen deaths; nine "notable failures"; and two patients who survived but who now have irreversible brain damage. There were only seven "gratifying rescues," at a total monthly ICU cost of $1.15 million. Murray asks bluntly whether such "huge expenditures" can be justified.

Physicians use what they call the f-word to describe these situations—futility. Clinical judgment about how to manage the ruinously ill is reduced to estimating a probability: What is the chance of a given intervention achieving a particular goal? Below a certain threshold that intervention is pronounced futile and is thus deemed pointless. Such brutal rationalism may seem fair. But it is almost impossible to put into practice.

Who defines, for example, the threshold of probability? Must the chance of success be better than one in two, one in four, or one in ten? Who decides? How does one calculate a probability reliably and accurately? Murray points out how difficult it is to pinpoint the moment when an illness crosses "the invisible threshold from potentially curable . . . to hopeless." And what should the final goal of treatment be? The purpose of the ICU is to preserve life, to restore the patient to near-normal functional capacity, and to limit morbidity. But the aims of intervening may be more modest and yet equally reasonable. Murray describes an instance in which he kept a comatose patient peacefully alive to allow the family to come to terms with an approaching death. The purpose of intervention shifted, humanely, from patient to family. These value judgments force decisions about what is futile to be made jointly among the patient, family, and medical team. There is no precise calculus that can be appealed to, and decisions can rarely be extrapolated from one setting to another.

There is an additional problem. The concept of futility is often confused with rationing, and Murray sometimes seems to conflate the two. The cost of ICU medicine is high. To husband limited resources more effectively, one might ask how much we are willing to spend on intensive treatments. But the issue of equitable resource allocation between critical and noncritical care is not equivalent to guessing when a chance of treatment is worth taking or not. These are entirely separate issues. To mix cash flow so intimately with clinical decision-making risks a dangerous ethical shortcut.

In any case, such theorizing may ignore the reality at the bedside. If it was your son, daughter, mother, or father lying in an ICU bed, could you make a rational judgment about the probable outcome? My guess is no. You are more likely to want everything done that reasonably could be done in the absence of undue suffering, even if, when one examined the evidence and weighed the probabilities, the outlook was poor. A probability is, after all, only a probability. Your case could be the one that beats the odds.

Is there a way out of this apparent impasse between a desire to do all one can and making a decision based on probable outcomes? The impediment to answering this question is that, even today, the ICU is an obscure "black box" within the hospital. Cory M. Franklin, the respected Chicago expert on intensive care, wrote in 1998 that the ICU is

> an intricate assemblage of high-tech equipment where patients enter as "input variables" at one end and emerge sometime later from the other end as "outcomes." Tellingly, unless they have specific business there, outsiders tend to avoid venturing into the ICU. Medical students, residents, and consultants from other disciplines often speak of doing training rotations or visiting the ICU simply to find out exactly what goes on there.[8]

Murray succeeds in demystifying the ICU by telling its story. But one can also turn to research for answers. In an effort to devise ways of predicting a patient's outcome, several models for calculating risk have been tested. The best studied is the Acute Physiology and Chronic Health Evaluation (APACHE), first introduced in 1981 and now in its third revision. Risk is calculated according to the patient's physiological status, age, and preexisting health. To these variables are added predictive equations reflecting the diagnosis and a large database of additional clinical information. Although these models have identified important aspects of a patient's physiological state that confer poor prognosis, they are used mainly for research and their place in everyday patient care remains undecided. APACHE III is not a reliable way to differentiate survivors from nonsurvivors.

Yet there is an urgent need for some means of evaluating intensive care. Murray himself deplores "the impossibility of ever knowing whether each of the many decisions I make is right or wrong." The hope is that explicit approaches to the calculation of risk will enable the work of ICU physicians to be assessed fairly and outcomes to be defined as accurately as possible. This transparency in setting goals might reduce the desire of all parties to embark on a course of futile treatment.

The motive for seeking intervention in dire circumstances can be fostered by mistrust, confusion, and ignorance. Laying out for discussion the factors that are likely to govern an individual's outlook should lessen all three of these threats to compassionate and appropriate care. But the truth is that all such decisions are going to be imprecise judgments. After twenty years of trying to use the methods of science to answer these impenetrably human questions, I get the sense that many doctors now accept that the best we can do is to do our best. The prop of spurious statistics is at last being discarded.[9]

In 1821, William Hazlitt reflected on the very issue that Murray draws our attention to at the end of his diary, an issue that causes more angry struggle today than any other in the swamps of modern medical ethics:

> It has been thought by some that life is like the exploring of a passage that grows narrower and darker the farther we advance, without a possibility of ever turning back, and where we are stifled for want of breath at last. For myself, I do not complain of the greater thickness of the atmosphere as I approach the narrow house.... I should like to have some friendly hand to consign me

> to the grave. On these conditions I am ready, if not willing, to depart. I could then write on my tomb—grateful and contented.[10]

Whose friendly hand should do the consigning remains disputed, and it is a question that certainly perplexes Murray. Of one patient whose life was lost, he notes that "what distressed me was that there was no room in our system for me to leave her alone and let her die peacefully. I was obliged by the rules to intervene." He writes that these efforts sometimes seem like inducing "a long period of torture" and that "dying in increments with a tube in your windpipe and another in your chest is infinitely miserable."

A friendly hand can be gripped more tightly or less. The lightest touch is the DNR—do not resuscitate—order that prevents futile clinical intervention if a patient has a potentially fatal crisis, such as a respiratory arrest. England is now in the throes of a critical reexamination of the DNR notice. For years doctors have written DNR orders on patients' case notes without their consent or knowledge. When a woman with cancer recently survived her ordeal and examined her hospital notes she discovered with horror her medical team's decision to deny her resuscitation should she require it. She had not been consulted about her intended fate and her case reignited issues of patient autonomy, medical paternalism, and clinical futility, which the British still seem to have great difficulty confronting.

A physician can take a slightly firmer hold if there is an advance directive to turn to. Murray and his wife both have "living wills," and those who possess such documents can prevent a hopeless endeavor to repair the irreparable. While advance directives deserve to be encouraged—the 1991 American Patient Self-Determination Act obliges US health care providers to offer patients written information about living wills—they do not, as yet, provide a solution to the puzzle of when to accept the inevitability of death and withhold or withdraw treatment. Too few patients (Murray cites a figure of around 15 percent) have created advance directives; their doctors may be unaware that such an instruction exists; and there is some evidence that, in any case, advance directives may have only a limited impact on decision-making in the end-of-life setting.

All of which leads to Murray's final argument, which he lays out briefly in an epilogue. His long working experience of the ICU has led him to believe that a proportion of his present patients should have been offered one of "the many infinitely more humane alternatives to ICU care." He raises, but never tries to answer, questions of physician-assisted suicide and euthanasia. His tone suggests that he is out of sympathy with advocates of either solution to fatal illness. "Doctors are," he writes, "invariably less enthusiastic than the general public about their would-be role as executioners."

Still, he acknowledges that this professional mood may be starting to shift. Surveys indicate that more doctors now seem willing to contemplate assisted suicide.[11] And he agrees that the evidence from Oregon, where a 1997 Death with Dignity Act legalized physician-assisted suicide within narrowly proscribed rules, seems to suggest that such a law can be implemented without ushering in mass medical slaughter. Importantly,

> Contrary to the fears of some, there was no indication that physician-assisted suicide was disproportionately chosen by or forced on terminally ill patients who were poor, uneducated, uninsured, or worried about financial loss.

Further experience of Oregon's statute shows that only one in six requests for physician-assisted suicide was being granted.[12] Crucially, although a fifth of patients requesting assistance committing suicide were clinically depressed, none with treatable symptoms received a lethal prescription. Findings such as these strengthen the argument that assisted suicide can be practiced free from abuse.

The momentum of support for euthanasia is increasing. Practices in the Netherlands have now been enshrined in law—since 2001, it has been legal for a doctor to help a patient to die. An individual seeking an end to life must have an incurable disease, be experiencing "unbearable suffering," be of sound mind, and have given consent. If a person makes a request to die in his will, the doctor must consider that request seriously. The Netherlands was the first country to legalize euthanasia. A psychological barrier had been breached. Christian groups protested by reading from the Bible on the steps of The Hague's senate building. Others predicted death tourism. The Polish bishop Tadeusz Pieronek compared Dutch practices with those of Nazi Germany. By contrast, doctors in the Netherlands largely welcomed legal clarification of a position that had left them open to criminal challenge.

Belgium went on to legalize euthanasia in 2002. France's health minister, Bernard Kouchner, admitted that he had practiced mercy killing while serving in wars in Vietnam and the Lebanon. (But French courts jailed Christine Malevre, the so-called "Madonna of euthanasia," for ten years in 2003 after she had been found guilty of murdering six terminally ill patients.) South Korean doctors have backed "passive" euthanasia, and a British woman traveled to Switzerland in 2003 to enable her husband to end his life in a clinic run by the assisted suicide group Dignitas. In Australia, a doctor has produced an "exit bag" to fit over the head. It is designed to starve a sleeping person of oxygen and so, according to Dr. Philip Nitschke, the director of Exit Australia, bring about a "peaceful death."

But I sense that Murray remains reluctant to allow the physician to cross a line from a position of withdrawing treatment and providing only symptomatic relief to one of actively prescribing drugs to end life. When challenged by a medical student about the care of a man with terminal lung disease and brain damage, he affirms his intention to "give him morphine and allow him to die peacefully. Without the intense terror and agonizing distress of progressive asphyxia." The bold student tells him that his action would be tantamount to "physician-assisted execution." Murray demurs, arguing that "the key point is that our intent is to relieve Mr. Caughey's suffering, not to cause his death, although I agree with you that morphine may quicken it." These distinctions may seem slight, and they are often rejected as spurious by advocates of physician-assisted suicide,[13] but for many doctors, including myself, the difference between an intention to diminish symptoms of suffering and an intention to kill means a great deal.

Murray's point is that we should take these decisions out of the crucible of technological excess either by not sending patients who are "irrefutably doomed to die" to the ICU or by removing them from the ICU once it becomes clear that a fatal outcome is imminent. There are more humane places—home or hospice, for example—for these patients to go. To some degree, Murray's pleas are already being heeded. In American ICUs that train critical care specialists, a third of patients who died had life support withdrawn, and a tenth had life support withheld. Only 23 percent had full ICU care, including attempts at resuscitation.[14] Although there was variation in practice between ICUs, limits to care are now accepted and commonplace.

There is an omission in Murray's argument, however, which ultimately distorts the choices he presents. He does not provide a more nuanced discussion of end-of-life care. It is here that substantial conceptual and clinical advances have been made to remove the agony encountered by some patients on ICUs and to draw back from what is beginning to be seen as the far from straightforward practice of physician-assisted suicide.

End-of-life care is poorly taught, if taught at all, to American and British medical students, and almost nothing is included in standard medical textbooks recommended to students either before or after graduation.[15] And yet a great deal of research has been done to understand exactly what "end-of-life care" means. The American physician Marion Danis, for example, has brought together doctors who work in intensive care and palliative medicine, experts in medical ethics and education, and consumer advocates to set reasonable professional goals for managing the end of a person's life.[16] They emphasize that care, agreed on jointly with patient or surrogate, must guide technology and not vice versa. (Murray gives several examples of technological imperatives governing care.) Clear decisions about treatment withholding and withdrawal must be made; trust among those taking part in these decisions, based on honest discussion, even in the face of paralyzing uncertainty, should underpin all end-of-life care; cultural diversity must be respected; and the principles of relieving pain and making people more comfortable—palliative care—should occupy a central place in the ICU.

There is a gap, however, between the wishes of professionals and those of patients. When patients are asked what they conceive to be high-quality end-of-life care, the committee jargon of consensus panels is shed in favor of humbling clarity. Patients wish for good measures to relieve pain and symptoms; an end to unnecessary prolongation of dying; a sense of control over their destiny; relief of the burden of physical care and decision-making that rests on family members or friends; and strengthening of relationships with the people closest to them.[17] These contrasting views show that physicians prefer to select only aims they can quantify or qualities they can measure, few of which may be uppermost in their patients' minds.

These matters now demand renewed scrutiny. The hope that assisted suicide might offer a solution to the problem of undignified and costly end-of-life care has recently been proven to be illusory. The Oregon experience, after two years, showed that twelve of twenty-nine patients given supposedly lethal medications did not die. Eleven subsequently died of other causes, and one was still alive when the research was conducted. The conclusion must be that physician-assisted suicide often fails. There are likely damaging physical and psychological consequences of that failure for patients, their families, and the health care team. It is a pity that these complications of unexpected failure were not anticipated by the Oregon researchers.

Worse still, experience from the Netherlands, the country with the most mature system for provision of assisted suicide and euthanasia services, indicates serious unforeseen adverse effects.[18] With 15 percent of patients undergoing physician-assisted suicide, there were "problems with completion," meaning that there was a longer than acceptable time between giving the lethal drug and death. Two patients woke up from their "terminal" coma. For 10 percent of patients, there were technical impediments to assisted suicide, such as difficulties in finding a vein to inject the drug or difficulties with giving drugs by mouth, such as irritation to the throat. And 7 percent of patients experienced complications, including nausea, vomiting, "extreme gasping," and muscle spasms. The brutal reality of physician-assisted suicide is that it can frequently diminish the quality of end-of-life care, not enhance it.

Experience in Oregon is hardly more reassuring. Doctors have reported unwanted publicity surrounding their decisions, difficulties obtaining lethal medications and second opinions, confusion about the state's legal requirements, "not knowing the patient," and troubling issues about protecting patients' privacy. A further, and potentially more serious, concern is the admission that Oregonian doctors may not have considered a diagnosis of depression among those who were dying. After five years of experience with the Oregon act, 198 people took lethal medications to end their lives legally, and 129 were successful in doing so. But only 28 of these 129 were referred for psychiatric evaluation.[19] The motivation of patients making decisions about assisted suicide in Oregon, and possibly elsewhere, is a further anxiety. There seems to be an increasing tendency for patients who opt for lethal medication to do so out of their concern to avoid being a burden to others. From 1998 to 2000, the proportion of those who died after receiving prescriptions or lethal medications and who felt they were a burden to family, friends, or other caregivers rose from two out of sixteen (12 percent) to seven out of twenty-seven (26 percent) to seventeen out of twenty-seven (63 percent) for each successive year. The importance of the context in which these decisions are made is revealed most explicitly among those who died with the assistance of Jack Kevorkian. His patients were more likely to be female, divorced or never married, and suffering a recent but nonterminal decline in their health. These concerns have been underlined by the UN Human Rights Committee. Its rapporteur, Eckart Klein, has commented about the Dutch law that "the main worry is not only the actual practice, but also the fact that this new law could create precedents that dilute the importance and trivialize this act."

There is no quick fix to alleviate suffering at the end of life. The challenges for people giving health care are formidable. And yet when palliative measures are offered—effective pain control, a hospice referral, or treatment for depression—almost half of patients who originally seek assisted suicide change their minds.[20] And when medical personnel know that palliative care services are available, their early willingness to give a lethal drug seems to diminish.[21]

If end-of-life, especially palliative, care is neglected in settings in which decisions about physician-assisted suicide or euthanasia arise, there might also be deficiencies in understanding what patients are truly telling their physicians when they feel all hope is lost. Doctors are good at treating physical symptoms. But they are generally less skilled in addressing their patients' expressions of suffering. When a patient says that he or she wants to die, there is evidence to suggest that this statement paradoxically might indicate loss of autonomy rather than a dignified expression of self-determination. In a study of patients with terminal cancer, Ingrid Bolmsjö quotes one individual as follows: "I'm afraid of ending up just lying there, not being able to do anything, and just waiting to die. In that case, I'd rather take an overdose." Her conclusion is that "loss of autonomy may also give rise to suicidal thoughts."[22]

A doctor's aim should surely be, as far as is reasonably possible, to restore dignity and autonomy, not simply to end a life. In any case, autonomy, important though it is, is not inviolable. My natural rights are circumscribed by the consequences of my actions for others. Ending a person's life—by direct lethal injection or indirect lethal prescription—is an extreme interpretation of the doctor's duty to relieve suffering. One must consider how the benefits of respecting autonomy (satisfying a patient's stated wishes) might be counterbalanced by potential harm (threatening the trust that the larger community puts in doctors to restore health). If the calculus is that greater societal damage might be inflicted by incorporating active euthanasia or physician-assisted suicide into a physician's routine practice, thereby diminishing public trust, then patient autonomy might not be the only source of moral authority for a doctor to take into account.

Before the public debate about who should receive intensive care, what constitutes medical futility, and what place physician-assisted suicide might have in either setting goes any further, the end of a person's life deserves a less reductive analysis by physicians and philosophers and the public alike.

# 17

# THE HEALTH OF PEOPLES

HOW MIGHT NATIONS cooperate to improve the health of their least advantaged people? There is, presently, no coherent political, social, or ethical framework for answering this question. Take the case of Tanzania. The immense difficulties this country's government faces as it tries to build an effective health system for its 35 million citizens were clearly uppermost in the mind of its vice-president, Dr. Ali Mohamed Shein, when he opened a conference of the Global Forum for Health Research in November 2002. He spoke bluntly of the myriad health problems that weigh down Africa: the unfairness of a "skewed system" that damages the most vulnerable peoples of the world; the way that "economies are continuously retarded by poor health"; and the historical inequity of contributions made by cheap labor and raw materials, with such little return, to the wealth of developed countries. He underlined the obligation of rich nations "to assist the developing countries to get out of the vicious cycle of ill health, low productivity, and poverty." But he also emphasized the reciprocal obligation on his own government "to lead the fight against diseases which are weighing us down... to develop our capacities and alternative ways for solving our own problems in agreeable ways and manner." Tanzania's health system is evolving as a partnership between the national government and foreign donors. What principles might a government follow to guide this evolution?

The first strategy in constructing a health system in the modern developing nation-state is to reduce levels of poverty. Tanzania is no exception. One-party rule ended there in 1995 with the election of President Benjamin Mkapa, who made good governance the main goal of his administration and condemned the corruption and financial mismanagement of the past while committing himself to a multiparty political system. However, since 1995, there has been evidence of voting irregularities in Tanzanian elections. Better governance remains a challenge. Meanwhile poverty is deep and pervasive: over half of Tanzania's people are unable to meet their basic food and other requirements, many of the poor remain dependent on subsistence agriculture, and young and old alike are extremely vulnerable to environmental and economic shocks.

Still, Tanzania's long-term vision is clear.[1] Its leaders aim to move the country from its present least-developed status to a middle-income nation by 2025. This enormous social transformation will require improvements in governance, economic management, and education. The nation must reduce its dependence on donors and foster a culture in which reforms can be implemented. The health gains that will follow these policies are defined in terms that apply to many other developing countries, and include food self-sufficiency and security; universal primary education and eradication of illiteracy; gender equality; access to quality primary health care for all and to quality reproductive health services for all who need them; reduction in infant and maternal mortality rates by 75 percent; universal access to safe water; life expectancy consistent with typical middle-income countries; and absence of abject poverty.

When grassroots views were sought at the village level for priorities in poverty-reduction efforts, health ranked third after agriculture and education. Poor health education, weak service provision, lack of involvement of the poor in the design of health programs, and alarm at the threat of HIV/AIDS were the main concerns of those consulted.

In response to these views, together with epidemiological data defining the national burden of disease, the government set targets to be reached by 2003 in infant mortality (from 99 per 1,000 to 85 per 1,000), under-five mortality (from 158 to 127 per 1,000), maternal mortality (from 529 to 450 per 100,000), and malaria-related deaths among under-fives (from 12.8 percent to 10 percent). To achieve these goals, the government focused on expanding immunization coverage, improving the availability of drugs and medical supplies, and increasing the coverage of births by trained birth attendants.

But the chief difficulty for Tanzanian officials can be summed up in one word: money. The government plans to focus its efforts on primary health care services and rigorous analysis of the cost-effectiveness of poverty-reduction initiatives. Its own analysis indicates that "acceptable levels of health care"[2] would cost $9 per person. Two thirds of that sum would cover recurrent expenditures (salaries, drugs, and supplies). That leaves $3 for development spending, a figure that would double present health budgets—an unsustainable increase.

How can the Tanzanian Ministry of Health plan its policies without adequate funding? One approach has been to create a national sentinel surveillance system to collect evidence on indicators of poverty, and national participatory networks to help refine the government's policies. Burden of disease information is communicated to village groups and discussions are then held to balance perceived demands among communities with needs as defined by national surveillance data. The community input comes from groups of adult men and women, adolescents, traditional healers, community health workers, and private and nongovernmental providers. These groups ranked their health priorities as malaria, HIV/AIDS, diarrheal disease, pneumonia, and heart disease.[3] National mortality burden estimates have now been collected and linked to health policy recommendations.[4] Gathering and interpreting reliable information about the burden of disease is key here. For example, the 2003 target for infant mortality is 85 per 1,000. According to the latest data, this target has been achieved: the rate is 60 per 1,000 in urban areas and 83 in poorer rural regions.[5] It remains high and inequitably distributed, but infant mortality rates are showing measurable improvements. Yet how can the government know whether to judge these gains a success given the vast inequalities that remain?

Sentinel data indicate that ten million years of life are lost annually in Tanzania because of premature mortality. For example, almost nine out of ten children die from causes that demand a rapid response from the health system. Half of years lost in those individuals requiring acute care are attributable to malaria. Among older children and adults, a majority require more long-term care, especially for tuberculosis and AIDS, which together account for two thirds of years of life lost for those who need this long-term assistance. Cardiovascular disease, cancer, and anemia account for a quarter of the remaining disease burden share. When these data are translated into policy, it becomes clear that at present it is not cost-effective to treat cancer, diabetes, or neurological, renal, or liver disease, despite evidence that these diseases will present substantial future burdens to the Tanzanian people.

A vision has been established, a strategy articulated, evidence collected, and a program laid out. Can the Tanzanian health system sustain this tribute to rational health care planning? Almost certainly not. Over two thirds of Tanzanians live in rural areas. There are only 409 government health centers, fifty-five district hospitals, seventeen regional hospitals, and four specialized hospitals. Village health and dispensary services do provide a simple but effective preventive network. Each village usually has two health workers and each government dispensary serves about 15,000 people. But Tanzania has difficulty retaining its trained medical staff, who frequently migrate to Namibia, Botswana, and South Africa, while a high population-growth rate and a rising burden of disease and poverty have outstripped what limited progress had been made in the 1960s and

1970s in health-system development. To be sure, the government has a strategy, but it does not yet have a set of political principles by which to guide the improvement of the health of its people.

The question that the Tanzanian government is trying to answer is this: How can it construct a just health system? A further question follows: What principle or set of principles governs the definition of "just"? The past twenty-five years of academic policy analysis and debate about health systems have yielded little consensus about what constitutes the ideal just health system. Indeed, the rancorous controversy surrounding WHO's study of health systems, *World Health Report 2000*,[6] suggests that opinions are more fractured than ever.[7]

Yet efforts to create a single cohesive theory of health systems, based on a systematic appraisal of evidence, have been a recurrent goal of health policymakers. WHO defines a health system as "all the organisations, institutions, and resources that are devoted to producing health actions"—that is, any efforts to improve health. Policy analyses of health systems have progressed in two broad directions. Microanalyses, the more common approach, look in great detail at particular aspects of a health system (for example, patients, small groups of individuals, professions, or other single variables) in one country or between countries. Macroanalyses examine populations, structures, processes, institutions, and political, social, and economic trends that influence health systems. Comparative research on these macro influences is rare, perhaps for logistical reasons. And yet if we are to look at what makes the conditions for a just health system possible in an era of globalization, it is to this category of investigation that we must turn.

Macroanalyses have tended to fall into one of two types. First, policy analysts have tried to classify health systems according to a theoretical or empirical foundation. Milton I. Roemer, for example, described the components of and a model for a national health system twenty years ago as part of WHO's Health for All strategy.[8] Originally, he categorized health systems into nine types, according to whether national economies were affluent, transitional, or poor and the health system modestly, moderately, or highly organized. Oil-producing nations were later added to the list of resource-rich countries, and the health system categories were changed to emphasize government policies toward health—entrepreneurial and permissive (US), welfare-oriented (West Germany), universal and comprehensive (UK), and socialist and centrally planned (the former USSR).[9] There are many other examples of health system taxonomies.[10] Only Roemer's was designed to be put to practical use in the design and organization of national health systems.

A second avenue for health system thinkers is to attempt to turn these descriptive efforts into a single causal model for health systems. J. M. De Miguel, for example, systematically reviewed comparative health systems research[11] to develop such a model, which included individual variables (health status), variables related to institutions (health services), influences from global society (political, economic, social, and demographic patterns), and variables that depend on even larger systems (environment). The point of creating a causal model is to define the present and predict the future. But the oversimplification inherent in a single theory inevitably failed to capture anything but the barest and most obvious of health system components.

The limitations of a purely descriptive and of a totalizing approach are all too clear. The main objection to both methods is that there is no reproducible way to measure the performance of a health system and so create a means of continuously improving it. The culmination of a decade of tentative work in health systems performance came with publication of the *World Health Report 2000*. This analysis has been severely criticized to the point where some of its more original ideas and arguments have been lost amid acrimony. The main accusations against WHO's lead authors, Julio Frenk and Chris J. L. Murray, were these: that many of the published measures of health system funding were guessed at and not collected empirically; that new analytic methods and the assumptions behind them had undergone insufficient external scrutiny; that inequity, an absolutely central idea in understanding the effects of poverty, was excluded from performance measurement; that country rankings were not robust; and that the language used about health systems dominated by government intervention was abusive. This last point is important since it displays the political context of this entire project, which continues to occupy discussion about the legacy of WHO's director-general from 1998 to 2003, Gro Harlem Brundtland.[12]

An external peer review group was charged with investigating the assumptions and data that underpinned the 2000 report findings. Its recommendations, presented to and discussed by WHO's executive board in 2003, called for substantial revisions to WHO's approach. The agency must widen regional participation in its scientific work on health systems performance; individual country rankings must be abandoned; national capacity for data collection and analysis must be strengthened; and all figures to be reported by WHO will in the future have gone through a consultative process with the relevant member state and contain their own explicit audit trails. The original report promised that its health system performance index would be a "regular feature" of future reports. In fact, the index has been quietly dropped.

Critics argue that WHO adopted a politically conservative agenda in its analysis of health systems, too quickly advocating private provision of care to match consumer demand. WHO, it was said, had become supine in the face of the free market ideology of its largest donor, the US government. More seriously still, the 2000 report was seen as a radical and undebated retreat from WHO's policy of Health for All, expressed through the goal of developing primary care services to match population needs. The unpredictability of the market had replaced rational planning of health services.

The conceptual goals of WHO's analysis do deserve further discussion, however, since they try to answer, in part at least, the question of what a just health system actually is. A key idea WHO used was that of fairness:

> The health system also has the responsibility to try to reduce inequalities by preferentially improving the health of the worse-off, wherever these inequalities are caused by conditions amenable to intervention. The objective of good health is really twofold: the best attainable average level—*goodness*—and the smallest feasible differences among individuals and groups—*fairness*. (WHO's emphasis)

The notion of fairness is applied in a narrow sense by WHO—namely, fairness in how the financial burden of supporting a health system is shared. Indeed, WHO's concept of fairness

> says nothing about whether the *utilization* of health services is fair, which is an equally crucial issue in the overall fairness of the system. Fair financing is concerned with the principle of *from each according to ability*, but not with the principle of *to each according to need*. (WHO's emphasis)

WHO judges fair financing in a nonprogressive way—that is, perfect fairness is when "the ratio of total health contribution to total non-food spending is identical for all households, independently of their income, their health status, or their use of the health system." The notion that richer households should pay more—a progressive financing system—is rejected by WHO. The ranking system for fairness runs from 0 (extreme inequality) to 1 (perfect equality). Colombia tops the equality list with an index of 0.992. But the index is not especially sensitive. Sixty-one countries have a financial fairness index greater than 0.950; for 147 nations it is greater than 0.900. The results throw up some surprises. Brazil, for example, is ranked 189 out of 191 countries, with an index of 0.623 (the lowest is Sierra Leone: 0.468). The Brazilian government was furious with WHO, and with Brundtland especially, for what it saw as this very public humiliation.

There was a great deal of immediate criticism of this approach,[13] which was compounded when it was revealed that data on financial fairness were only available and used for 21 out of 191 nations—an index was guessed at (the technical word used was "imputed") for 170 remaining countries.[14] It was also shown that a measure of financial fairness which ranked Columbia first was proof of its flawed nature. Writing from the World Bank, Adam Wagstaff argued that the WHO approach to fairness for financing was no advance on past methods, was based on a misreading of previous research, and was especially flawed because of its lack of progressivity.[15] Given these problems, he concluded, "The concerns that several health ministers and governments have expressed about the [*World Health Report*] rankings are, in such circumstances, entirely understandable."

However, a more nuanced discussion of fairness was published in the *Bulletin of the WHO*, an issue of which was devoted to health systems in 2000.[16] Norbert Daniels and his colleagues set out nine benchmarks of fairness derived and tested in four countries. Their work is based on a clear moral conception of a just society and is opposed to orthodox economic approaches that commonly exclude notions of fairness.[17] They argue that although fairness and equity are often used interchangeably, fairness is a far broader concept, incorporating not only equity (access to all forms of care) but also efficiency (wasted resources deprive others), accountability (the public's ability to influence health care), and patient and provider autonomy. While there are dangers that a liberally conceived approach to fairness might be culture-bound to Western societies, Daniels and his colleagues found "wide agreement" on their benchmarks in countries as diverse as

Colombia, Mexico, Pakistan, and Thailand. They also found that these benchmarks helped to evaluate competing health reform policies and to make comparisons possible across nations. They wryly concluded that their analysis could only be supplemented and not replaced by an index of financial fairness, such as that adopted by WHO.

A difficulty with these abstract definitions and benchmarks of fairness is that they all fail to take account of the historical development of the nation-state in which health systems exist. In the modern era of globalization, the sovereignty of the nation-state appears threatened by the continued creation of international political, judicial, and financial institutions, regional alliances, and transnational businesses. Human rights are increasingly recognized as global norms, regardless of national laws. State defenses may be unable to protect citizens from political violence, terrorism, and weapons of mass destruction. Health and environmental threats transcend national borders. Capital flows in the world economy prevent nations from effectively managing their own financial affairs. And global communications undermine languages and cultures. If the nation-state is unable to fulfill its promise to increase the well-being of its people, it will lose its legitimacy as a result.[18]

Individual nation-states are likely to develop in different ways. Tanzania, for example, only achieved nation-statehood forty years ago. Whereas the US has the capacity to cushion itself against disease, environmental threats, and global economic fluxes, Tanzania is less resilient. These differences between nation-states indicate that instead of studying health systems in isolation from their political, economic, and social context, they can only be viewed as part of the prevailing political culture.

The value of a historical approach comes when one considers health sector reform. A health system cannot be reengineered in a vacuum, and any efforts to change it must be done through existing political structures. This exposes the greatest, and largely ignored, weakness of WHO's approach to health systems. In the *World Health*

*Report 2000*, they are abstracted from their day-to-day existence within a nation-state. The same criticism applies to benchmarks of fairness that do not take account of the wider political context. Tanzania is an example of a country whose development from a health perspective has been strongly influenced by its political environment. There was neither a long-term health vision nor a poverty-reduction strategy before a new government was elected in 1995.[19]

Yet the orthodox position in the mainstream of health systems research is to ignore politics. Julio Frenk, a prime mover behind the *World Health Report 2000* and an influential thinker on global health issues (he was Mexico's nominee for WHO director-general in 2003), avoided the issue of governance entirely in his appraisal of globalization's impact on health systems.[20] In a technical paper reviewing the conceptual framework behind WHO's analysis, Frenk and Chris Murray acknowledge that "general attributes of government, such as ethical codes of conduct and the tolerance of corruption, can also influence the performance of stewardship [of the health system] and other functions."[21] But they do not build this idea into their performance evaluation. What they offer is the concept of stewardship—namely, a duty of government to take explicit responsibility for the health of its population.[22] This notion of stewardship is stripped of its political content and reduced to little more than a plea for ministries of health to, at the very least, do no harm.

The predicament for the modern nation-state, regardless of its level of development, is how it can defend and advance the health of its people at a time when global, demographic, economic, and political forces are undermining its ability to sustain a welfare policy. To meet its goals, those responsible for creating the conditions that make a just health system possible need a framework that goes beyond health, into the core of a nation-state's political and cultural history. Successful health system reform therefore requires a bridge between health and politics, with a coherent theory of justice linking the two.

Such a project has long been a goal of public health scientists. The present uncertain future of health systems in globalized nation-states brings new urgency to this work.

The question that I am attempting to answer is this: Under what conditions might reasonable peoples cooperate to improve the health of their nation's citizens? There is good reason to be cynical about any reply that displays optimism. John Rawls, the twentieth-century's most influential writer about political justice, once quoted Robert Gilpin's assessment of the realpolitik of efforts to reach global accords:

> The fundamental nature of international relations has not changed over the millennia. International relations continue to be a recurring struggle for wealth and power among independent actors in a state of anarchy.[23]

The nation-state puts national interests before global responsibilities. Despite globalization, this is as true today as ever. Negotiations over European Union enlargement to the east have laid out a plan that is profoundly inequitable to new member states.[24] And America's perceived retreat—its peaceful retreat at any rate—from global commitments has caused anguish among many US diplomats committed to a constructive role for the US overseas.[25] The challenge, therefore, is to find a way of thinking about the health of peoples which offers opportunities for building consensus among and cooperation between nations.

In *A Theory of Justice*, Rawls set out two principles.[26] First, that every person in a society has an equal claim to a basic set of rights and liberties compatible with a similar set of rights and liberties for all (the liberty principle). Second, and this principle has two parts, that social and economic inequalities can only be tolerated provided that offices and positions are open to all (the equal opportunity principle) and that these inequalities bring the greatest possible benefit to the least advantaged members of society (the difference principle). The difference principle reveals Rawls to be neither an egalitarian nor a free-market purist. Inequalities are not by themselves unjust. But they are not to be tolerated simply because the market produces them. Governments must work to eradicate inequalities, Rawls argued, unless they benefit the least well off.

In *The Law of Peoples*, a neglected work in Rawls's canon, he takes these principles further by investigating how people "might live together peacefully in a just world." He defines the law of peoples as "a family of political concepts with principles of right, justice, and the common good, that specify the content of a liberal conception of justice worked up to extend to and to apply to international law."[27] The goal of his inquiry is a "realistic utopia"—that is, an achievable world that offers justice for what Rawls called "liberal and decent peoples." Rawls was not a practicing politician. His aim was not to write a manifesto, stand for election, or put into practice all that he wrote about. Instead, he wanted to clarify the principles that would allow people to live free from evil and political injustice.

J. M. Bryant was the first to describe how much Rawls's ideas offer to public health. Taking his cue from Rawls's *A Theory of Justice*, he argued that the

> Rawlsian concept of justice can immediately be seen to have implications for health care. Its language can be translated directly into a principle of justice applicable to health care: whatever health services are available should be equally available to all unless an unequal distribution would be to the advantage of the least favored.[28]

Bryant applied this notion of equality to health care systems with varying scarcity of resources. He argued that, despite inequalities, a health system could provide a firm floor for health services to all, while also distributing resources above that floor, albeit unevenly, so as to ultimately benefit the least favored.

Rawls's notion of a law of peoples, as he called it, which he first published in 1993 as an Oxford Amnesty lecture, is based on a reinvigorated notion of the social contract. His concern is how a society should relate to other societies and how it should conduct itself toward them; how far liberal societies should tolerate nonliberal societies; how notions of individual obligation derived from collective benefit can be fostered and used in forming a coherent idea of justice, and how one can apply the idea that a social contract demands that "fair representation is given to each individual as a moral person."[29] If one applies these ideas to global public health—the notion of a health of peoples—the goal, following Rawls, becomes to define a set of principles for improving the health of the least advantaged.

But this idea cannot be applied to every society at all times. Societies differ in their political makeup—the issue elided by agencies such as WHO—and any strategy to improve the health of peoples must take account of these differences. Rawls's thinking ties in with modern evolving notions of the nation-state since the powers of the state must be revised so as to satisfy his law of peoples. Thus, states have neither traditional rights to war nor unrestricted internal autonomy. There are limits to their sovereignty. Moreover, liberal peoples freely grant respect and recognition to other peoples. One nation is not superior to another. Liberal peoples are free and independent, they observe international treaties, they have a right to self-defense but not to go to war unless in self-defense, they respect human rights, and they have an obligation to help other peoples who live in unfavorable conditions.

For what Rawls calls liberal peoples, one important principle of justice is that all citizens have sufficient "primary goods to enable them to make intelligent and effective use of their freedoms." Although

Rawls does not specify it as such, health must surely be one of these primary goods. An essential adjunct to these principles is an institutional structure to support them, to negotiate relations between peoples. The UN system is the only legitimate body to take responsibility for this regulation, although it has now been added to, in health at least, by the World Bank and WTO.

A law of peoples therefore creates arrangements to protect not only the liberty but also, I argue, the health of peoples. The conditions needed to improve global public health also depend on two further factors identified by Rawls. The first is stability. People will only subscribe to a law of peoples if, by adhering to these principles, they see that society is demonstrably better off—in standards of living, civic culture, and social justice. Second, improved health systems depend on democratic peace, reflected in notions such as equality of opportunity, a reasonably fair distribution of income, "basic health care assured for all citizens," and regular publicly financed elections. These, in turn, require reasoned public debate and a free press, political decisions made by taking account of peoples elsewhere, the elimination of the rhetoric of national exceptionalism, and the existence of truly democratic global institutions.

These principles are all well and good. But what about nonliberal peoples? Rawls argues that liberal societies should assist all peoples. Mutual respect is central to Rawls's vision of cooperation among peoples. If respect is denied, the result will be bitterness and resentment. A problem arises with outlaw states. In Rawls's view, well-ordered societies "simply do not tolerate outlaw states.... [They] are aggressive and dangerous; all peoples are safer and more secure if such states change, or are forced to change, their ways." The goal of well-ordered societies is to bring outlaw states within the umbrella of well-ordered peoples. Burdened societies are another special case. Well-ordered peoples, according to Rawls, "have a *duty* to assist burdened societies." The goal is to build social cohesion among peoples based on their common sympathies. These are questions of foreign, not health, policy, and WHO is an important instrument in achieving these foreign policy objectives and regulating cooperation between nation-states.

Rawls offers a policy framework that can be applied to public health. While he wants to identify the conditions necessary for peoples to live together for their greatest collective advantage, I want to clarify the principles that might apply in the sphere of health—to create the conditions to improve the health of these same peoples. A similarly broad approach to health sector reform has been a decade in the making. In 1994, arguing against the tendency to depoliticize health policy and portray it as a purely technical matter, Gill Walt wrote that "the traditional focus on the content of policy neglects the other dimensions of process, actors and context which can make the difference between effective and ineffective policy choice and implementation."[30] It is here that Rawls, although never writing directly about health or health policy—in his original essay, he does, however, briefly refer to health as a problem of justice—brings a moral as well as a political perspective to health systems. Applied to health systems, five propositions follow from Rawls's arguments.

*1. A culture of recognition, respect, reciprocity, and research will assist the political process of creating mutually caring peoples.*

Rawls wishes to expand the present "relatively narrow circle" of mutually caring peoples. This narrowness also distorts priorities for global public health. A truly global program to tackle the diseases that affect most of the world's peoples does not exist. The creation of transnational communities among health professionals could be a powerful means of fostering a global conversation about dealing with these health issues; sharing, discussing, and agreeing on norms; and giving groups some incentive to bring about change without disrupting the political organization of society. Christopher Hill calls these professional elites "epistemic communities." Scientists, doctors, lawyers, diplomats, and engineers have replaced, in modern society, the church and the aristocracy. According to Hill,

> On occasions epistemic communities are capable of mobilising themselves to become temporary international actors, with the aim of changing public policy. International media campaigns are not unknown on relatively "soft" subjects such as famine relief.... Effective humanitarian action is more likely to be mobilised by ad hoc coalitions of specialists, preferably with wide reputations and operating out of universities.[31]

Responsibility for creating these associations lies largely with existing professional groups—for example, specialist medical societies that presently only concern themselves with a circumscribed regional interest. There are signs that these groups are changing. The European Society of Cardiology has embraced Eastern Europe as a new audience. But it has also, for the past two years, held a symposium on global cardiology, especially focusing on Africa and Asia.

A reasonable criticism of this route to mutual recognition and respect among peoples is that it only appeals to a very small number of individuals—a specialist elite. How much benefit accrues to society as a whole? Holding a symposium without any long-term strategy is crude tokenism. A measure of the success of such transnational collaborations in fostering capacity for knowledge might be the number of scientific papers produced and citations to those papers received per unit of population. These figures are not routinely reported in the UN Development Program's *Human Development Report* or the World Bank's *World Development Report*. However, measures of scientific output were described in the *Arab Human Development Report 2002*.[32] For example, the US had forty-three frequently cited papers (articles with forty or more citations) per million people in 1987. The figures for Saudi Arabia, Egypt, and India were 0.07, 0.02, and 0.04, respectively. UNDP concludes that without national science and technology systems, the domestic economic performance and external economic relations of Arab nations will "suffer considerably." Collaborations to build and sustain such capacities are part of Rawls's notion of recognition and respect.

2. *Aid is part of a well-ordered peoples' duty of assistance, but its goals and limits need to be redefined.*

Rawls argues the case for limits in assisting burdened nations. He sets out three guidelines for aid. First, that a well-ordered society need not be a wealthy society. A donor's goal ought to be to help create and preserve institutions, not maximize levels of wealth. Second, the political culture into which aid is given is all-important. Money alone will not relieve social injustice. Rawls sees no easy solution here. All that can be recommended is the provision of good technical advice, and, he points out, a focus on the particular needs of women. Third, donors should aim to help burdened societies manage their own affairs. Once this has been achieved, aid can and should be gradually withdrawn. The ultimate goal of assistance is a liberal or decent government. He defines the success of aid in institutional, not personal terms, arguing that there is "no reason to narrow the gap between the average wealth of different peoples." Aid is only a way to help a people move from zero self-determination to a well-ordered state. Thus, Rawls specifies a target (a liberal or decent society) and a cut-off point when a duty of assistance ceases.

Concepts of aid became much more complex during the past decade. The mix of donor arrangements—through bilateral and multilateral government accords, international agency mandates, the emergence of powerful new actors (such as the World Bank), and nongovernmental organizations—made coordination necessary if health systems were not to be damaged by duplication and multiple conflicting demands. This policy environment required more careful definition of the goals of aid—namely, to bring efficiency, effectiveness, and equity to health sector reform—together with ways of measuring the success of coordination.[33]

These notions of coordination gave way to issues of resource management by the late 1990s. How was aid to be given? Good governance became the orthodoxy for influential donors, such as the World Bank. For example, a 1998 World Bank report concluded that "when donor-financed projects fail, it is often because of weak institutions and public organisations."[34] Aid coordination requires an overall view of how society should evolve. James D. Wolfensohn, president of the World Bank, has led efforts to harmonize aid policies between developing nations and donors. In advance of a 2003 meeting in Rome to better coordinate poverty-reduction efforts, he pointed out that the consultancy industry that aid has spawned was worth a grotesque $4 billion in Africa alone.[35] This is Rawls's argument too.

None of these qualifications obviates the need for more generous aid spending. Anne C. Richard, a former director of resources and policy at the US State Department between 1999 and 2001, has railed against US "stinginess" in foreign spending. She notes the self-delusion among many in the US:

> Despite the slide in funding, Americans continue to believe that theirs is the most generous nation. The United States does provide more foreign aid, in absolute terms, than any other country and is the No. 1 donor of food aid and refugee assistance. But in terms of ability to pay—development aid measured as a percentage of national wealth—the United States comes last among donor nations.[36]

3. *An important aim of development is to move nation-states toward the ideal of well-ordered peoples.*

In keeping with many of today's political commentators, Rawls assigns liberal democratic governments a special place as the ultimate political arrangement for securing justice for peoples.[37] The characteristics of these arrangements are clear—respect for basic rights and liberties, provision of "requisite primary goods" to enable effective use of these freedoms, creating institutions free from corruption and honored by citizens, limiting the influence of corporate power, and restricting rights to war and unfettered internal autonomy. These are contingent on a state of peace and stability, and Rawls sets out the determinants of that stability as equality of opportunity (notably in education and training); decent distribution of income; society as an employer of last resort; provision of basic health care for all citizens; and public financing of information and elections.

To provide basic health care as a foundation for democratic peace requires a strategy for how the health care system will evolve. The priority Rawls gives to health reflects its importance to the overall political development of the country, as well as its intrinsic value. He has a special interest in institution building, and so a reasonable question is: What is a model Ministry of Health and what are the ideal characteristics of a health minister? They are obviously broad: a commitment to public health; an activist for equity; the ability to create and control policy, build coalitions, communicate with and involve the public, protect health budgets, influence other ministers and ministries, and be interested in evaluation.[38]

A reciprocal obligation exists at the global level. If one is inviting democratic reform within a country, what are global institutions doing to enhance their democratic legitimacy? For example, at the World Bank and the International Monetary Fund, almost half of all voting power rests with just seven countries—the US, UK, Japan, France, Saudi Arabia, China, and the Russian Federation. The *Human Development Report 2002* concluded that "the old rules about representation are no longer viable or desirable. Put bluntly, the IMF and World Bank will not be able to do their jobs effectively if they remain tied to structures that reflect the balance of power at the end of the Second World War."

4. *Human rights must be promoted and protected, but perhaps not all rights, and not all of the time.*

Rawls classes the human rights necessary for a law of peoples as "urgent rights." This class of rights reflects the view that war is no longer a legitimate extension of government policymaking and that the authority of government over its own people is now heavily circumscribed. Human rights set limits on state sovereignty. But these rights are not identical to those we take for granted in liberal democracies. Rawls writes:

> Some think of human rights as roughly the same rights that citizens have in a reasonable constitutional democratic regime; this view simply expands the class of human rights to include all the rights that liberal governments guarantee. Human rights in the Law of Peoples, by contrast, express a special class of urgent rights.

Critics of Rawls—and even Rawls himself—see this limit on rights as a serious objection to his argument. Human rights that make up this special class—Rawls does not define these rights, although he does refer to "freedom from slavery and serfdom, liberty (but not equal liberty) of conscience, and security of ethnic groups from mass murder and genocide"—are a "necessary condition" of a society's decency. In his earlier essay on a law of peoples, his definition of this minimum set of rights is slightly more expansive. He writes about "means of subsistence and security (the right to life), to liberty (freedom from slavery, serfdom, and forced occupations) and (personal) property, as well as to formal equality as expressed by the rules of natural justice...."

Rawls insists that human rights be set free from claims that they are ethnocentric, originating from and applying to Western society only. They are not, he argues, defined by some special characteristics of human beings as free citizens, who are assigned either special moral worth or intellectual powers. Human rights are generalizable across peoples because the only assumption is that persons are "responsible and cooperating members of society who can recognize and act in accordance with their moral duties and obligations."

*5. Foster a deliberative culture of public reason.*

Rawls added to his long essay on the law of peoples a further reworking of an earlier idea central to his understanding of constitutional democracy—namely, public reason. He views public reason as the fundamental political questions of a society. But he confines public reason to the deliberations of specific groups in that society: judges, government officials, and candidates for public office. These three groups all take part in a public conversation about the deepest moral and political values of society. Their contributions to public debate are accorded a special importance.

Rawls also distinguished a larger "background culture" into which this conversation extends. This is civil society, whose deliberations are not part of his conception of public reason. He recognizes that critics may want to include civil society as part of a fuller and more open public forum, but he resists this. He attaches special importance to judges, government officials, and candidates for public office, but he also bestows special responsibilities on these groups. They must explain and justify their positions to other citizens—what he calls a "duty of civility." The moral duty of civil society is to hold these special groups, together with their explanations and justifications, to account.

The creation of well-ordered peoples requires a space in which the voices of public reason can be expressed—newspapers, books, radio, television—and through which civil society can hold them accountable. Rawls calls this system a deliberative democracy. He demands that the public be informed about "pressing problems." There must be "public occasions of orderly and serious discussion of fundamental questions and issues of public policy. Public deliberation must be made possible, recognized as a basic feature of democracy, and set free from the curse of money."

There are at least three aspects of Rawls's position on public reason relevant to the health of peoples. First, for truly participatory self-government, a nation's citizens must be sufficiently healthy to take part in the debate that holds public reason to account. If disease is not checked and controlled, democracy will be diminished, even threatened. Disease imperils the long-term stability of the nation-state to debate and decide its own future.

Second, there must be sufficient capacity within a country to generate, analyze, publish, distribute, and debate information about the health of the population. Without a system of public health surveillance and communication, public reason will be incomplete. There is substantial evidence that such systems are weak and fragile.[39] And third, the duties of assistance between countries can only be realized if health issues that matter to the poorest nations of the world are accurately reported in those countries that have the greatest responsibility for providing assistance.

If, as I have argued, improving the health of peoples depends upon adopting an explicitly political perspective like Rawls's toward health systems, why has such a perspective hitherto been largely excluded from health policy analysis? Within international agencies, such as WHO, senior administrators repeatedly underline the fact that their organizations are intergovernmental bodies, restrained from doing or saying anything that is not mandated by member governments. An explicit political dimension to WHO's health system work might therefore seem impossible to many sensitive bureaucrats, especially given that over a fifth of staff salaries are paid for by a single government, that of the US. A similar fear of losing funding may explain why investigators omit political analysis from their work. Nevertheless, politics cannot be ignored. And the margins of the debate about politics and public health have been moving, albeit, until recently, slowly.[40]

A substantial change in the contours of debate about politics, development, and health has taken place during the past decade. With Amartya Sen's *Development as Freedom*,[41] based on a series of lectures he gave at the World Bank in 1996, came a shift in the way global agencies and institutions approached the politics of human development. Sen's main argument was that "expansion of freedom is...the primary end and...the principal means of development." Strengthening democratic systems became an essential part of development. The individual was now seen as the active agent of change rather than the passive recipient of aid. Health became a vital component of this new development process. Sen cites one intercountry analysis that showed how life expectancy depended on public expenditure for health and poverty reduction, not on any measure of economic performance.

WHO's Commission on Macroeconomics and Health took this argument about freedom and development directly into the health sector. The commission set out clear functions for the state in what its authors called a close-to-client (that is, community-based) health delivery system. First, to define a set of essential, locally specific health interventions. Second, to guarantee financing for universal access to these interventions. Third, to act as both provider of and contractor for health services. And finally, to be the guarantor of quality in the health service. But to be an effective steward requires the elimination of constraints, such as government bureaucracy, corruption, lack of a free press, and political instability. The commission was clear in its linkage of health to politics:

> National governance that is marked by corruption, a lack of planning, and a lack of concern for long-term development will undermine the health sector as well as the rest of the economy. Countries in violent conflict, or that repress ethnic or racial minorities, or that discriminate against girls and women, will find it difficult or impossible to make sustained improvements in health sector capacity.[42]

The most explicit statement emphasizing the value of political analysis in debate about human development, especially in the context of the health-dominated Millennium Development Goals, came with the *Human Development Report 2002*.[43] Entitled *Deepening Democracy in a Fragmented World*, this report put politics—or at least one type of political system—center stage. Various subjective indicators of governance were cited—a polity score based on civil liberties, political rights, press freedom, voice and accountability, political stability and lack of violence, law and order, government effectiveness, and corruption. These were reported next to more objective indicators, such as the date of the most recent election, trade union membership, numbers of nongovernmental organizations, and ratification of international agreements on political rights. Figures were cited for 173 countries. Tanzania, for example, is ranked number 151 by the Human Development Index. It had a polity score in 2000 of 2 (range −10 to +10). The polity score measures the degree to which laws and institutions allow democratic participation. A score of −10 indicates an authoritarian regime, of +10 a democratic one. Tanzania is designated as only partly free, according to measures of civil liberties, political rights, and press freedom.

The *Human Development Report 2002* is a landmark document in the political history of human development. It not only describes the present situation of democratic accountability among nation-states but also advocates reforms needed to strengthen participatory democratic processes. If a criticism can be leveled against the report, it is this: that it only reports preliminary work in progress. Many of the subjective measures of democracy must be qualified with a high margin of error. There are so many indicators, so many ways of dissecting and measuring a democracy, that it sometimes seems hard to see precisely what needs to be done next to further democratize a country. Moreover, the exclusive focus on democracy looks at a single end point. The *Human Development Report* does not look at starting points—the stability of existing governments, for example—for the thirty-six countries listed in the category of low human development. The report is lacking the detail needed to help governments and their peoples devise reasonable and practical plans for creating conditions not only for a law of peoples but also for a health of peoples. Finally, there is a serious flaw in this analysis, one oddly acknowledged by the report itself. It is that there is no automatic link between democracy and either equity or human development. Democracy alone does not guarantee anything.

In sum, considerable theoretical and empirical work is required before a coherent approach to the politics of development and health can be claimed. This Rawlsian analysis goes beyond either free-market or egalitarian ideologies and helps, I think, to define, from a clear set of philosophical principles, the components that enable just and stable societies to exist, societies in which health systems, once these conditions are met, can be realistically sustained. Could these components—working toward a wider circle of mutually-caring peoples, redefining aid, moving nation-states along a path to well-ordered peoples, protecting a more limited set of human rights, and fostering a culture of public reason—reasonably constitute a quantitative Rawlsian index for a health of peoples, perhaps akin to the Human Development Index?

Rawls concludes *The Law of Peoples* by looking at why his model of political justice might fail. The two most vulnerable principles, he argues, are the norms of conduct of war against aggressive outlaw states and the duty of assistance to burdened societies. These are fragile because both principles demand courage and foresight from political leaders who have to convince their own, most likely skeptical, people of their importance. The entire project for political justice comes down to the quality of political leadership. Physicians have an important part to play in shaping public debate about improving the health of their own and other peoples. The fact that few adopt such a role leaves medicine increasingly disengaged from some of the global issues that matter most to the least-advantaged people. Doctors continue to fail the world's peoples most burdened by disease.

# 18

## TAKING DIGNITY SERIOUSLY

THE ADDIS ABABA Fistula Hospital, protected by locked gates, sits behind the Swiss embassy in one of the Ethiopian capital's quieter neighborhoods. Its buildings are clean and modern. As one enters the main ward, there are two rows of perfectly made beds stretching back toward four operating rooms. In each a woman lies still beneath the turquoise covers. About two thirds of the 120 or so patients are younger than twenty, and some are only fourteen. All are recovering from fistula repairs.

Fistulas—abnormal passageways, usually between the vagina and the bladder in these young women—are a natural complication of prolonged labor, which in places with few obstetric services can last up to a week. In many cases Ethiopian women are married well before puberty, and are kept from their husbands until their first menstrual bleed. The man may then have sex with his wife. Of those who conceive, one in twenty has an obstructed labor. In rural areas with few or no medical facilities, the outcome is predictable. Once the dead child has eventually been delivered, the woman may lie in bed for months or even years, waiting for her fistula to heal. Without proper care it will not, and one in seven women develops permanent and disabling muscle or nerve damage.

The Fistula Hospital admits nine hundred women each year. A few are so physically injured that they will never be well enough to return home. Those who do leave are given new clothes to signify a fresh start to their lives. The hospital was founded by Reginald and Catherine Hamlin, obstetricians from New Zealand and Australia. They moved to Addis Ababa in 1954, and set up the hospital in 1975 because women with fistulas, soaked as they were in urine and feces, were being turned away from local clinics.

This kind of medical assistance seems an ideal to be replicated—humane, skilled, practicable, a mix of charitable and government aid, meeting an urgent clinical need, and enabling new knowledge to be passed on to locally trained medical staff. But the contrast with care outside Addis Ababa is stark. In the mud and wood *tukuls* several miles' walk into the forest near Jima, layers of carefully aligned newsprint are used as colorful wall coverings. The headlines are a mix of Finnish (the nearest health center was, until recently, run by a Finnish mission) and English. One page reads, "Pay no cash for up to $240,000 of medical protection." The irony is heartbreaking. The nearby health center at Shebe includes rudimentary (and always full) wards, a laboratory (with a centrifuge, two microscopes, and basic diagnostic facilities), a clinic, and a pharmacy. One doctor and several nurses struggle to keep the center going. The Finns handed it over and left a year ago, and the government can no longer sustain the same level of support, a disaster for local people who lead, along with 80 percent of the Ethiopian population, a mainly rural subsistence life.

Within the urban bustle of Addis Ababa, the Fistula Hospital seems a wonderful yet perverse luxury. The greatest good for the greatest number of Ethiopians would come from sustainable primary care, but that is a long way off. In 2003, Meles Zenawi, Ethiopia's prime minister, castigated the West for its "slackening... pace of delivery" of aid. During a visit to the UK, he spoke of the "hypocrisy" of Western governments that subsidized their own businesses while enforcing crippling deregulated markets on economically weaker nations. The result was, inescapably, a "human tragedy." It is easy to say that poverty is the greatest threat to the people of Ethiopia, and to human survival and development more generally, given the international consensus surrounding this proposition. But although poverty is the central material indicator of human deprivation, it is an inadequate and reductive concept for understanding the lives and health of the poor.

With the growing awareness that disease takes a disproportionate toll on the poor, the year 2000 saw important shifts in thinking across several major UN agencies concerned with global health and development. The World Health Organization's *World Health Report 2000*[1] tried to establish a new basis for setting health standards by seeking evidence about the performance of national health systems. After much reflection on resources and stewardship, WHO concluded, "The denial of access to basic health care is fundamentally linked to poverty, the greatest blight on humanity's landscape." The impact of the failure of health systems, WHO went on, "is undoubtedly most severe on the poor, who are driven deeper into poverty by lack of financial protection against ill-health."

The United Nations Development Program's *Human Development Report 2002*[2] adopted a strongly human rights–based approach in its analysis of human progress, one heavily influenced by Amartya Sen, whose idea of development as freedom[3] has also been highly influential at the World Bank. In his opening chapter to the UNDP report, Sen writes, "Human development and human rights are close enough in motivation and concern to be compatible and congruous, and they are different enough in strategy and design to supplement each other fruitfully." This new direction is provocative. But in the end, UNDP's aim is the same as WHO's: "Poverty eradication is not only a developmental goal—it is the central challenge for human rights in the twenty-first century."

The most striking convert to the poverty agenda is the World Bank, whose sudden policy revision took many critics by surprise.[4] The Bank's *World Development Report 2000–2001*[5] opened with the claim that "poverty amid plenty is the world's greatest challenge." The Bank put a figure on those in income poverty: 2.8 billion of the world's six billion people live on less than $2 per day, a number that is growing. Yet the Bank took a broader view of poverty than any other international agency:

> The report accepts the now established view of poverty as encompassing not only low income and consumption but also low achievement in education, health, nutrition, and other areas of human development. And based on what people say poverty means to them, it expands this definition to include powerlessness and voicelessness, and vulnerability and fear.

This approach was radically new for the Bank. Not only would it encourage market reform, as it always had with unremitting compulsion: "But we now also recognise the need for much more emphasis on laying the institutional and social foundations for the development process and on managing vulnerability and encouraging participation to ensure inclusive growth." The agreement about an antipoverty human disease and development agenda is shared by most experts, especially those who work in health settings.[6] Indeed, health is often one standard for judging the success of these antipoverty policies.

Yet poverty remains hard to define. The World Bank argues passionately for multidimensional measures. But in the Bank's technical notes buried at the back of its reports, poverty is still defined only in terms of income and consumption. UNDP calculates a "human poverty index" (HPI). For developing countries, the HPI—called HPI-1—is a composite measure of human survival (the proportion of people not expected to live to fifty years of age), knowledge (the proportion of adults who are illiterate), and standard of living (a combination of proportions reflecting those without access to clean water and health services, and children under five who are underweight). The HPI for industrialized nations (HPI-2) measures survival (age sixty is the threshold in this measure), knowledge, standard of living (the proportion of people living below the poverty line), and social inclusion (the rate of long-term unemployment). While there is agreement that poverty is the number-one enemy of human life in the world today, there seems to be no agreement about exactly what poverty means.

Yet I would contend that examining the erosion of dignity is a fuller, and in some ways better, means of assessing the threat to human health and development. Dignity is not entirely set aside by either WHO or UNDP. But the current application of dignity as a useful idea in public health policy is, for the most part, largely ignored or rhetorical at best. WHO, for example, throws in dignity as a well-intentioned afterthought: "Health systems have a responsibility not just to improve people's health but to protect them against the financial cost of illness—and to treat them with dignity." Ill-health, WHO argues, undermines an individual's dignity, which is included with autonomy and confidentiality as three elements in the concept of "respect for persons." These components of respect "show no relation to health system spending"—they are "costless"—except for "some training of providers and administrators." Yet for all this attention, dignity is defined only negatively by WHO. It is violated if basic human rights are ignored and "it means not humiliating or demeaning patients."

Like WHO, the UNDP includes in its report many pages of numerical data, from measures of gender empowerment (seats in parliament held by women) to personal distress (suicides, divorces, numbers of internally displaced people and refugees). Dignity is invisible in all these calculations because it has no positive definition that can be converted into a measurable variable. But the UNDP report acknowledges that "the mark of all civilizations is the respect they accord to human dignity and freedom." These emblems of progress are damaged by authoritarianism, racism, sexism, and xenophobia. More positive attributes of dignity are given by UNDP in its discussion of the rights empowering people in its antipoverty policies:

> A decent standard of living, adequate nutrition, health care and other social and economic achievements are not just development goals. They are human rights inherent in human freedom and dignity.

NB In all these analyses, dignity is deployed as a sentimental gesture, evoked across pages of figures in vague, ill-defined ways. Can a coherent theory of human dignity be worked out, one that has some practical value to health and development—one that might mean something to the women of the Addis Ababa Fistula Hospital or the families of Shebe?

A survey of dignity's history as an idea reveals aspects that echo in today's debates about both individual and global health. Early writers on medicine paid little attention to the notion. Hippocrates and his collaborators were more concerned to establish the scientific credentials of medicine. They underlined a doctor's responsibility to help the sick, but warned that the science of medicine would not advance by seeking to discover "what man is." That role led inevitably—and damagingly, they implied—to philosophy, a discipline that had "more to do with painting than medicine." A good doctor required only a "thorough mastery" of science.

Galen, some six hundred years later, adopted a broader view. He insisted on a medicine that went beyond science, one that included "the logical, the physical, and the ethical."[7] The goods of the body, according to Galen, were health, the perfection of its functions, and beauty. Medicine, an art as much as a Hippocratic science, must have "health as its primary aim." But dignity, either as an individual or a social end, was a concept outside the realm of Roman medicine.

Medieval philosopher-monks ignored their medical forebears and investigated the nature of human worth by asking the obvious, if unscientific, question: What is man? They concluded that the soul and body were combined as the supreme product of God's creation.[8] The human condition, in all its constituent elements, was a blessed microcosm of the universe. Medicine and a theory of human dignity eventually converged in the writings of Marius of Salerno, a medical commentator, who, according to his translator Richard Dales, argued that it was "man's rational soul that makes him the most excellent of animals." In this view reason lay at the root of any claim to human dignity.

Dignity finally became a respectable concept when the Italian philosopher Giovanni Pico della Mirandola (1463–1494) wrote an oration (never delivered) entitled *On the Dignity of Man*. Pico was an eclectic pluralist who bridged the medieval and Renaissance eras, and fused theology with an early natural philosophy. His great theme was to claim man as "the moulder and maker of thyself." Sitting at the center of the world, "it is given to [man] to have that which he chooses and to be that which he wills." The inspiration is deeply religious but passed through a humanist lens: "Moses gives us these direct commands, and in giving them he advises us, arouses us, urges us to make ready our way through philosophy to future celestial glory, while we can." As Paul Miller points out in his essay on Pico,[9] this freedom of the human will is a "moral freedom, the ability to give oneself the character or set of moral habits that one chooses.... Man selects his own moral nature." Pico is graphic on the options open to this version of man: "Thou canst grow downward into the lower nature which are brutes. Thou canst again grow upward from thy soul's reason into the higher natures which are divine." Dignity, he says, means not merely the possession of a rational mind but the exercise of moral choice.

Thomas Hobbes introduced a radically different view of dignity in his *Leviathan*.[10] In a discussion of power, worth, dignity, and honor, Hobbes wrote:

> The public worth of a man, which is the value set on him by the commonwealth, is that which men commonly call DIGNITY. And this value of him by the commonwealth, is understood, by offices of command, judicature, public employment; or by names and titles, introduced for distinction of such value.

This was very different from the notion of dignity judged according to inner reason and moral choice. Dignity was something conferred by others, the result of an evaluation by one's fellows. Hobbes's secular definition says nothing about the human dispositions to be judged "dignified." They are presumably open to manipulation by the one being judged. Only the end—the final judgment of one's peers—seems to matter.

After the high-minded probity of medieval and Renaissance writers, this seventeenth-century attitude emphasized dignity as a shallow adornment, bestowed by others and to be shown off. La Rochefoucauld, in his aphorisms and moral maxims, claimed that dignity was not intrinsic to the human condition. It was merely a secondary and rather superficial attribute: "Dignity is to merit what fine clothes are to natural beauty."[11]

David Hume later reflected on these contrasts in his essay on the dignity of human nature.[12] Hume divided the disputants on dignity into two camps. First, there were pious declaimers who saw "man as a kind of human demigod, who derives his origin from heaven." Second, there were those who ridiculed the notion of human dignity by exposing the vanity of anyone who made such an ambitious claim for humanity. Neither position was correct, according to Hume. He saw dignity as an intrinsic feature of human nature, but one that could be measured only by comparing one person with another. Cynics might argue, Hume concluded, that since there are few genuinely wise and virtuous men in the world, the human species is largely contemptible, but he dismissed such an extreme interpretation. Difference does not prove depravity. Human virtues may vary between individuals but, Hume insisted, each person should be judged comparatively according to the sincere expression of his or her natural stock of virtue.

But the most significant break in the history of dignity, and the one most relevant to dignity in medicine, came with Mary Wollstonecraft's publication of two treatises on the rights of men and women in 1790 and 1792, respectively.[13] In her letter to Edmund Burke, she declared that "the birthright of man . . . is such a degree of liberty, civil and religious, as is compatible with the liberty of every other individual with whom he is united in a social compact." Violation of these rights was a negation of "the native dignity of man." Her polemic on behalf of "English liberty" was a devastating rebuke to those who saw dignity as contingent on the judgment, benevolence, or whim of others: "The aversion which men feel to accept a right as a favour, should rather be extolled as a vestige of native dignity, than stigmatised as the odious offspring of ingratitude." Wollstonecraft submitted herself to reason and the result was an "enlightened self-love" that reflected the respect she had for a human being's natural rights. Recognition of these rights indicated a resilience in the face of adversity—"conscious dignity may make us rise superior to calumny, and sternly brave the winds of adverse fortune."

In *A Vindication of the Rights of Woman*, Wollstonecraft developed and slightly adjusted her case:

> My own sex, I hope, will excuse me, if I treat them like rational creatures. . . . I earnestly wish to point out in what true dignity and human happiness consists—I wish to persuade women to endeavour to acquire strength, both of mind and body, and to convince them that the soft phrases, susceptibility of heart, delicacy of sentiment, and refinement of taste, are almost synonymous with epithets of weakness.

Here she goes beyond natural rights as the foundation for human dignity. Dignity now became a powerful transforming force that could be acquired through reason, virtue, and knowledge. To rely on natural rights alone would not change the way women were seen in society. The active pursuit of dignity by penetrating the intellectual world —"speaking of women at large, their first duty is to themselves as rational creatures"—is a revolutionary call to overcome the degrading treatment women had thus far received and to find "rational fellowship [with men] instead of slavish obedience."

Yet the most developed and robust theory of dignity was worked out by Immanuel Kant, in two complementary tracts—*Grounding for the Metaphysics of Morals* (1785) and *The Metaphysics of Morals* (1797).[14] In *Grounding*, Kant extended the approach of Marius and Pico. Dignity lay in the rational human being who had the ability to exercise the categorical imperative. In Kant's ideal moral community —the Kingdom of Ends—dignity had no price. It simply existed as an intrinsic "unconditional and incomparable worth."

> Morality and humanity, insofar as it is capable of morality, alone have dignity.... This estimation ... puts it infinitely beyond all price, with which it cannot in the least be brought into competition or comparison without, as it were, violating its sanctity.

The basis of this dignity was autonomy—"the ground of the dignity of human nature and of every rational creature." But Kant, in *Grounding*, was ambiguous, for he seemed to suggest that dignity was a quality that could also be acquired: "We thereby ascribe a certain dignity and sublimity to the person who fulfils all his duties." Dignity was an extrinsic as well as an intrinsic element of human nature.

Kant resolved this uncertainty in *The Metaphysics*:

> But a human being regarded as a *person*... is not to be valued merely as a means to the ends of others or even to his own ends, but as an end in himself, that is, he possesses a *dignity* (an absolute inner worth) by which he exacts *respect* for himself from all other rational beings in the world. He can measure himself with every other being of this kind and value himself on a footing of equality with them.

Personhood, an end in oneself, inner worth, all justifying respect and equality. Here was a dramatic extension of the concept of dignity, to which Kant added two important details. First, the "dignity of a citizen," although inalienable, could be lost by a person becoming "a mere tool of another's choice." Second, dignity was not simply a quality possessed by the individual. "Humanity itself is a dignity," Kant wrote. It had social as well as personal meaning.

The history of dignity, therefore, displays two distinct lines of emphasis that persist today in modern medicine and global health policy. Dignity as an external quality of the human condition was first conceived as something endowed by God's creation. A secular reinterpretation of this idea was developed by Hobbes, and, in part, by Hume. In today's clinical and development settings, the dignity of people can be strengthened, these writers might have argued, through assistance and aid. But it is the intrinsic nature of dignity that has been most fully conceived, first and tentatively by Marius, more powerfully and in the moral setting by Pico, and finally, and in parallel, by Wollstonecraft and Kant. Kant's contribution is well known, but Wollstonecraft's has languished at the margins of dignity studies. It is their philosophical legacy that deserves further scrutiny in the brutally mortal environment of human health.

What has become of the notion of dignity since Kant and Wollstonecraft? The most important political result of philosophical inquiries into dignity is surely the installation of this idea as the intellectual spine of the Universal Declaration of Human Rights. Dignity is mentioned no less than five times in the Declaration. It first appears in the opening line of the preamble: "*Whereas* recognition of the inherent dignity and of the equal and inalienable rights of all members of the human family is the foundation of freedom, justice, and peace in the world...." It appears again in the fifth paragraph, where "The peoples of the United Nations have in their Charter reaffirmed their faith in fundamental human rights, in the dignity and worth of the human person and in the equal rights of men and women and have determined to promote social progress and better standards of life in larger freedom."

In Article 1, dignity is closely linked to rights as the basis on which all humans are born free and equal. The importance of the rational human mind as a means for expression of these principles is also stressed: "All human beings are born free and equal in dignity and rights. They are endowed with reason and conscience and should act towards one another in a spirit of brotherhood." Dignity is also mentioned in Article 22 as an end in itself for a set of economic, social, and cultural rights. And finally, in Article 23, the protection of human dignity is predicated on a "just and favourable remuneration... supplemented, if necessary, by other means of social protection." Dignity is further enshrined in UN declarations concerning independence for colonial peoples (1960), protection from torture (1975), and elimination of religious intolerance and discrimination (1981), as well as the convention on the rights of the child (1989).

Given that a central aim of the Universal Declaration is to establish rights that enable the protection of human dignity and the full expression of human potential, health is clearly one necessary if not sufficient quality if the Universal Declaration is to be fulfilled. But the idea that health itself is a human right has been slow in coming. Health is included only by implication in Article 25: "Everyone has the right to a standard of living adequate for the health and well-being of himself and of his family, including food, clothing, housing, and medical care...." There is no explicit statement that health itself is a human right. That milestone did not come until 1966, with the International Covenant on Economic, Social, and Cultural Rights, which entered into force in 1976. Article 12 of this covenant describes "the right of everyone to the enjoyment of the highest attainable standard of physical and mental health."

Yet it is only in the past decade that there has been a noticeable acceleration in the appreciation of health as a separate human right and, more important, as a tool in the struggle for human development and poverty reduction. There is new ground to find between the territory of dignity—a still imprecise product of Enlightenment thought—and that of health as an explicit right in human development. The most important figure in this new conjunction of disciplines was Jonathan Mann, who died in the Swissair 111 crash on September 2, 1998.[15] In a pivotal article in the journal *Health and Human Rights*, which he helped to found, Mann and his colleagues set out a new agenda for medicine, public health, and human development in the context of human rights.[16]

First, after reviewing the effects of health policy on human rights, Mann developed the heuristic that "it may be useful to adopt the maxim that health policies and programs should be considered discriminatory and burdensome on human rights until proven otherwise." He offered no evidence to support this assumption but he found the maxim a valuable foil for his subsequent argument. Second, Mann considered the influence of human rights violations on health. His entirely original conclusion was that "all rights violations, particularly when severe, widespread and sustained, engender important health effects, which must be recognised and assessed." Finally, in looking at the relation between health and human rights, Mann suggested new standards for judging health. He asked whether "the extent to which human rights are realised may represent a better and more comprehensive index of well-being than traditional health status indicators." In this early article, dignity was still something of a puzzle:

> A related, yet even more complex problem involves the potential health impact associated with violating individual and collective dignity.... While important dignity-related health impacts may include such problems as the poor health status of many indigenous peoples, a coherent vocabulary and framework to characterize dignity and different forms of dignity violations are lacking. A taxonomy and an epidemiology of violations of dignity may uncover an enormous field of previously suspected, yet thus far unnamed and therefore undocumented damage to physical, mental and social well-being.

No one seemed to take up this challenge and it was left to Mann himself, in a paper that remained incomplete at the time of his death,[17] to return to dignity as a health and human rights issue. He approached the concept of human dignity empirically, by asking what it is to have one's dignity violated. He set out the steps that would be needed to take this early work to the bedside or the clinic—naming and classifying violations of dignity more precisely, taking a wide social rather than a narrow biomedical approach to dignity studies, and seeking practical ways to strengthen the dignity of others. In answer to the question "What is dignity?," Mann described four dimensions that existed between two axes, one internal ("how I see myself") and one external ("how others see me"). This "provisional taxonomy" included not being seen (being ignored or insufficiently acknowledged); being seen, but only as a member of a group and not as an individual; violations of personal space, including rape; and humiliation. If health is defined, as it is by WHO, as a state of complete mental, physical, and social well-being, then Mann was surely correct to write that there is "a potentially profound relationship between dignity and health."

The future of this line of inquiry depended, according to Mann the epidemiologist, on solidifying dignity as a concept that could be measured. But in advance of this work, which has yet to take place,[18] Mann was prepared to make a strong prediction: "Injuries to individual and collective dignity may represent a hitherto unrecognized pathogenic force with a destructive capacity towards physical, mental and social well-being at least equal to that of viruses or bacteria."

I began this examination of dignity by juxtaposing the lives of the poor in rural Ethiopia with the World Bank's new commitment, in its words, to "attacking poverty." The Bank's willingness to seek solutions to development questions beyond its usual market preoccupations was a welcome sign of deeper thought about the effects of its policies in the field. But the expansion of poverty's meaning to include health, education, vulnerability, voicelessness, and powerlessness takes a necessary spotlight off the savage effects of poverty defined simply in terms of income. That root problem still needs to be tackled by a combination of unfettered external aid, debt relief, and wealth creation, and it is easy to see why the Bank may wish to discourage enthusiasm for either of these first two policies. Widening the definition of poverty makes the alleviation of economic disadvantages seem less urgent, or at least makes the problem appear to be one that money alone cannot solve. Poverty is thus too important a measure to dilute. The concept of dignity, however, provides a means of bringing together various disparate indicators of development, including health, water, pollution, food, crime, employment, political stability, gender equity, and access to information. Dignity also provides the bridge, as Mann showed, between human rights and health.

If dignity is a useful complementary concept to poverty when discussing global human health, what of the dignity of individuals afflicted by illness? If only we could agree on what dignity is! Perhaps I am expecting too much from this one word. In doing so, it could easily become everything and nothing all at once. Mann's conception of dignity, defined according to its violations—being ignored, being grouped, having control over one's personal space undermined, or being humiliated—was the first attempt to translate dignity into experiences we can all understand, and therefore measure.[19] But although valuable as a taxonomy of transgression, it fails to grasp the positive essence of what dignity is, or how one could enhance or protect it.

A similar constraint exists in the most common contemporary invocation of dignity—namely, death with dignity. But in death, dignity is merely a weapon of persuasion.[20] Nowhere in Senate Bill 491—the 1999 revision of Oregon's Death with Dignity law—is dignity defined. For all practical purposes, "Death with Dignity" means "Death with Humane Intent." But it also, and importantly, refers to the autonomy of those seeking an end to their lives. Yet dignity is not equivalent to autonomy, in the sense of a wish backed up by an action. I can be free to express a desire for a particular course of action but I might be unable to realize that desire. Autonomy demands freedom of choice *and* the capacity to put that choice into effect. But autonomy by itself seems to me to lack something essential to the meaning of dignity.

While a purely medical approach to dignity has often produced complex and rather clouded definitions,[21] nursing studies have been a far richer source of thinking. For instance, Jane Haddock, after conducting a wide-ranging analysis of the concept of dignity, concluded that "dignity is the ability to feel important and valuable in relation to others, communicate this to others, and be treated as such by others, in contexts which are perceived as threatening."[22] Nursing research has emphasized dignity as an indication of human capabilities matching personal circumstances. If capabilities are lacking, or if circumstances limit the effective application of capabilities, human dignity is diminished.

From this idea, the notion emerges of dignity as the ability to control the circumstances of the situation (or predicament) one is in. This concept of control implicitly includes the idea of free moral choice, but it also, and crucially, includes the ability to make good on those expressed choices. Dignity, in this sense, is a virtue that can be exercised personally and strengthened externally. To equate dignity with control has its dangers, of course. A despot can control those around him, but it would be foolish to claim that he had more dignity by doing so. Dignity might better be thought of, after Wollstonecraft, as the capacity to control one's environment while preserving the dignity of others—a virtuous control, by which I wish to imply the notion of arranging, organizing, or influencing. Virtuous control has nothing to do with forcing, commanding, compelling, dictating, or coercing. This makes the notion of personal dignity dependent not only on one's inner worth but also on one's actions. At a person's core, there still remains an irreducible dignity that reflects the fact that every human being has the potential for conscious moral choice, even if that choice and control cannot always be exercised.

The importance of claiming virtuous control as the concept underlying notions of dignity is that a loss of control is directly linked to measures of human potential, such as ill-health. Lack of control over one's environment—in Western populations, at work, for example—seems to produce not only personal dissatisfaction but also higher rates of heart disease,[23] increased blood pressure, poorer mental health, and reduced immunity to infection. Control over one's life can be shown to have a precise and direct biological correlate. Here may lie the elusive connection between dignity, conceived as virtuous control, and health, the connection that Mann was searching for shortly before he died.

Nevertheless, in the clinical setting, this positive definition of dignity seems equivalent to the notion of autonomy—a choice made, backed up by an action. Dignity, as I have tried to indicate, is surely more than this; it is autonomy plus something else. But what exactly?

The most detailed analysis of what dignity might encompass, fusing many of the ideas of Mann, nursing studies, and even philosophers, comes from Harvey Max Chochinov, a psychiatrist at the University of Manitoba in Canada.[24] He derived his framework from interviews with patients who were living with terminal cancer. He wanted to understand their interpretations of dignity as they awaited death. But his ideas seem relevant beyond end-of-life care, although Chochinov makes one important caveat—namely, that his approach is inevitably culture-bound, relying as it does on the exclusive experiences of Canadians. Whether it can be generalized to other peoples must remain open to study.

Chochinov divides questions of dignity into three areas. First, there are illness-related concerns. Symptom distress is clearly a significant aspect of any illness, including as it does physical and psychological distress, together with anxiety over one's future. The illness is also likely to raise questions about a person's level of independence—physical, mental, and functional. Second, there is a dignity-conserving repertoire of attitudes and behaviors that shape a person's overall sense of individual dignity. For example, dignity-conserving practices include living for the moment, focusing on the things a person can do regularly for themselves (for example, going out or reading), and finding a source of spiritual comfort. Perspectives are as important as practices. So a person's dignity will be protected, Chochinov argues, if he can maintain pride in what he does, retain autonomy over his life, and feel hopeful about the future. The third area in Chochinov's conception of dignity is what he calls the social-dignity inventory. What social support is the person receiving? Is appropriate care being provided? Is the person made to feel a burden to others? Issues of privacy also arise.

What are the implications of this integrated view of dignity at the personal level and for improving global health? First, dignity cannot be conferred directly by the development process itself, as something materializing out of donor benevolence. This was Wollstonecraft's claim when she wrote of the rich man's response to the poor: "If the poor are in distress, [the rich] will make some *benevolent* exertions to assist them; they will confer obligations, but not do justice. Benevolence is a very amiable specious quality." Indeed, people may be poor in material terms, without that having any direct bearing on their dignity. Likewise, compromised dignity, unlike income poverty, cannot be resolved by economic aid alone. Aid can only go so far in helping to create the conditions for human dignity.

Second, the goal of development must be to create settings that foster the conscious awareness and expression of dignity in an individual. Taking control of one's environment by asserting a sense of oneself as a human being, exerting the right to dignity, is likely to open new worlds of interest and influence, much as Wollstonecraft predicted it would do for women. In Shebe, for example, there is no safe water, no safe sanitation, few health services, only one doctor, no obstetric or pediatric facilities, and no electricity. It is a subsistence life—but families and communities have strong ties. They have dignity.

And here is the third factor in creating the conditions for individual dignity—namely, social capital. This term is relatively new to development studies, but the World Bank, to its credit, is now paying serious attention to it.[25] The phenomenon of social capital currently provokes extremely polarized debate. First of all, no uniform definition of social capital exists. The term has been used to mean "social reserve"—namely, if you have given more time to others than they have given to you, that reserve can be drawn on to protect your own social networks if you hit a crisis. An alternative definition is that social capital includes those parts of social organizations that foster cooperation for the common good. Trust, mutual aid, and participation in civic activities fall into this category. Such a view of social capital is a prevalent one right now—although the World Bank defines social capital broadly as "social institutions"—and its erosion is linked to higher death rates from heart disease and cancer, as well as higher rates of violent crime.[26]

Social capital may exert its influence on human dignity through individuals (tolerance, cooperation), family (trust, reciprocity), communities (where inequalities in power or competition between groups may produce harm as well as benefit in Rawlsian terms), or institutions (protection of human rights by governments and the courts). Social capital emphasizes the dignity (and development) gains that can be made through collective action or by supporting social institutions—for example, in providing shelter, health services, food security, water supply, and education; and protection from violence, epidemics, and the extreme effects of climate. The introduction of this concept into the development debate challenges past policies at the World Bank. The Bank's packages for economic renewal tied to loans have frequently harmed social networks and human dignity. These networks can be measured, again giving weight to the notion that dignity is a quantifiable goal of development. Family structures; membership in local associations, schools, youth clubs, trades unions, churches, or political parties; doing unpaid work for these groups; and self-reported feelings of trust in these settings—all of these measures reflect the expression of dignity in civil society, which Kant drew attention to by noting that the sum total of humanity itself possesses dignity.

A problem remains over how individual human beings conceive dignity—in Ethiopia, Canada, or elsewhere. There has been a serious global effort in recent years to give voice to the voiceless. The World Bank report makes much of its Voices of the Poor project, which drew on the testimonies of 60,000 men and women from sixty countries. Before quoting from these studies, the authors of the 2000/2001 Bank report comment that their findings show "that poor people are active agents in their lives, but are often powerless to influence the social and economic factors that determine their well-being." But this risks implying that the poor, by definition, possess less dignity.

And yet here we remain caught out by Clifford Geertz's troubling insight, delivered over a quarter of a century ago, that listening to and interpreting these voices is not a moral but an epistemological issue. Geertz insisted that "the ethnographer does not, and, in my opinion, largely cannot, perceive what his informants perceive." All the observer can try to do is take part in "a continuous dialectical tacking between the most local of local detail and the most global of global structure in such a way as to bring them into simultaneous view." Geertz's warning reverberates in development circles. Modern measures of human development, as used by UNDP, are based on life expectancy, educational attainment, and standard of living. But many critics take issue with these highly contrived Western models. Vincent Tucker, a respected development analyst, questioned the entire project of human development on the grounds that its quantification required a method in which "all that defines [a people's] identity and existence is destroyed."[27] To identity and existence, one might add dignity.

Another way of viewing dignity is to see it as a kind of freedom: a freedom from distress and anxiety, a freedom that confers independence, capability, pride, hope, autonomy, living in the moment, and the means to secure privacy. Amartya Sen has done more than anyone to make the case that development is a process of acquiring freedoms. These freedoms, whether they be political, economic, or social, together "advance the general capability of a person." In this "agent-oriented view," Sen seems to come near to notions of dignity as virtuous control. By focusing on individual agency, Sen largely sets to one side the groups that make up social capital.[28] Yet it is the interplay between the individual and the group—dialectical tacking once again—that creates the conditions for dignity to be protected and fostered.

Dignity is an idea that is at the core of what it is to be human. It represents the dynamic potential of the human mind to alter the world for one's own and others' benefit. Dignity embraces ideas of liberty, moral choice, knowledge, and virtuous action. The notion of dignity that runs through the Universal Declaration of Human Rights is not an expression of sublime idealism, but rather an urgent call for social justice among the least advantaged peoples of the world.

Medicine is an important lever for restoring human dignity, at the bedsides of the sick as well as among the world's threatened peoples. The role of the doctor must be to alleviate dis-ease as well as disease, to have the quiet humility to listen when faced with pervasive anxiety, to have the strength to give sustenance when faced with despair, and to have the confidence to act as the voice of one's patient or people, through advocacy, when faced with vulnerability and powerlessness. The restoration of dignity is the end common to all of these endeavors. Amid the many exaggerated scientific claims and harsh political debates that characterize much of modern medicine, this simple idea, so easily overlooked, is the fundamental reason why medicine matters, and why we need to take human dignity a great deal more seriously than we do today.

# A NOTE ON ORIGINS

The preface, introduction, epilogue to chapters 1 to 3, and chapters 15, 17, and 18—a little over a third of the present volume—have not been published previously. The rest of the book consists of extensively revised and updated versions of essays that first appeared in *The New York Review of Books*, *The Lancet*, *The Times Literary Supplement*, and *London Review of Books*, to whose editors or publishers I owe thanks for allowing me to reproduce these articles in part or whole.

In a review published in the *The Times Literary Supplement*, David Wootton, a historian at Queen Mary College, London, rather severely took Quentin Skinner to task for rewriting articles covering some forty years of work, which were reissued in three new volumes in 2003. Wootton wrote that Skinner

> revises as if, through sheer effort, he could not only make his argument irrefutable and his meaning inescapable, but could render his work impervious to time's assault. I am sure I will not be alone in preferring the occasionally imperfect original essays.[1]

The trouble with medicine is that it can never be "impervious to time's assault." Our understanding of health and disease seems to change almost daily. Yet I was, like Wootton, uneasy as I reread, deleted from, and added to many of these chapters, the earliest of which was published in 1992 (although all except two have been published mostly within the past five years). What once seemed straightforward, even a few years ago, has now become more complicated. What were once deemed facts are now fictions. I have updated news as well as numbers. In many cases I have added either epilogues or lengthy additional sections woven into what were the ends of the original essays. Whatever the literary, if that word can be applied to medicine, vandalism I have delivered, these chapters are at least more timely and accurate. At any rate, after this lengthy excuse here are my debts.

Versions of chapters 1 and 2 were first published in *The New York Review of Books* of April 16, 1995, and August 9, 2001, respectively.

A version of chapter 3 was first published in *Global Public Health*, edited by Robert Beaglehole (Oxford University Press, 2003).

Chapter 4 was published as two articles in *The Lancet* of June 19, 1999, and June 26, 1999.

Chapter 5 was published in *The Lancet* of December 22–29, 2001.

Part of the Epilogue to chapters 4 and 5 was published in *The Lancet* of August 24, 2002.

Parts of chapter 6 were published in the *London Review of Books* of October 8, 1992, and *The Times Literary Supplement* of May 17, 2002.

Chapter 7 first appeared in *The New York Review of Books* of May 25, 2000.

Parts of chapters 8 and 9 were first published in *The New York Review of Books* of May 23, 1996, and May 17, 2001, respectively. Part of chapter 8 also appeared in *The Times Literary Supplement* on August 4, 2000.

Part of chapter 10 was published in *The Times Literary Supplement* of November 12, 1999.

Part of chapter 11 was first published in *The Lancet* of May 4, 2002.

A version of chapter 12 was first published in *The New York Review of Books* of November 2, 2000, and draws on ideas originally published in *Controlled Clinical Trials*,Vol. 22 (2001), pp. 593–604.

Chapter 13 is based on articles published in *The New York Review of Books* of July 13, 1995, and *The Times Literary Supplement* of March 9, 2001.

A version of chapter 14 first appeared in *The Times Literary Supplement* of September 13, 2002.

The ideas discussed in chapter 15 were first presented in the British Journal of Surgery Lecture, delivered in Utrecht, the Netherlands, in November 2002.

A version of chapter 16 was first published in *The New York Review of Books* of August 10, 2000.

Early ideas that form the basis for chapter 18 were first presented at a seminar in the Department of Anthropology, University College London, in 2002.

## NOTES TO THE PREFACE

1. *The News About the News: American Journalism in Peril* (Vintage, 2003). To be fair, even medicine's own journals and magazines do a poor job of covering the diseases that matter most. See my "Medical Journals: Evidence of Bias Against the Diseases of Poverty," *The Lancet*, Vol. 361 (2003), pp. 712–713.

2. See *World Heath Report 2002: Reducing Risks, Promoting Healthy Life* (Geneva: World Health Organization, 2002).

3. For example, see Mark Neuman, Asaf Bitton, and Stanton Glantz, "Tobacco Industry Strategies for Influencing European Community Tobacco Advertising Legislation," *The Lancet*, Vol. 359 (2002), pp. 1323–1330.

4. "The Pharmaceutical Industry as a Political Player," *The Lancet*, Vol. 360 (2002), pp. 1498–1502.

5. Arnold S. Relman and Marcia Angell, "America's Other Drug Problem: How the Drug Industry Distorts Medicine and Politics," *The New Republic*, December 16, 2002, pp. 27–41.

6. Anne Buvé, Kizito Bishikwabo-Nsarhaza, and Gladys Mutangadura, "The Spread and Effect of HIV-1 Infection in Sub-Saharan Africa," *The Lancet*, Vol. 359 (2002), pp. 2011–2017; and François Dabis and Ehounou René Ekpini, "HIV-1/AIDS and Maternal and Child Health in Africa," *The Lancet*, Vol. 359 (2002), pp. 2097–2104.

7. Robert Hogg et al., "Time to Act: Global Apathy Towards HIV/AIDS Is a Crime Against Humanity," *The Lancet*, Vol. 360 (2002), pp. 1710–1711.

8. Haile Yemaneberhan et al., "Prevalence of Wheeze and Asthma and Relation to Atopy in Urban and Rural Ethiopia," *The Lancet*, Vol. 350 (1997), pp. 85–90.

9. Salim Yusuf et al., "Global Burden of Cardiovascular Diseases," *Circulation*, Vol. 104 (2001), pp. 2746–2753, and Vol. 104 (2001) pp. 2855–2864.

10. Lawrence K. Altman and Keith Bradshaw, "Warning Issued on Mystery Illness," *International Herald Tribune*, March 17, 2003, p. 1.

11. Michael R. Phillips et al., "Suicide Rates in China, 1995–99," *The Lancet*, Vol. 359 (2002), pp. 835–840; and "Risk Factors for Suicide in China," *The Lancet*, Vol. 360 (2002), pp. 1728–1736.

12. William L. Parish et al., "Population-Based Study of Chlamydial Infection in China," *JAMA*, Vol. 289 (2003), pp. 1265–1273.

13. Hua Shan et al., "Blood Banking in China," *The Lancet*, Vol. 360

(2002), pp. 1770– 1775.

14. "The World's Forgotten Children," *The Lancet*, Vol. 361 (2003), p. 1.

15. Cara B. Ebbeling et al., "Childhood Obesity: Public-Health Crisis, Common Sense Cure," *The Lancet*, Vol. 360 (2002), pp. 473–482.

16. Carl Zimmer, "Tinker, Tailor: Can Venter Stitch Together a Genome from Scratch?" *Science*, Vol. 299 (2003), pp. 1006–1007.

17. The full quotation is: "There is no doubt that all these doctors sought fame by means of some innovation, and irresponsibly trafficked with our lives. This accounts for those wretched arguments at the sick-bed when no two doctors gave the same opinion for fear that a colleague's diagnosis might appear to carry more weight." See Pliny the Elder, *Natural History* (Penguin, 1991), p. 263. Here are some more of my favorite Pliny lines, all true to this day: "Doctors learn by exposing us to risks, and conduct experiments at the expense of our lives"; "Only a doctor can kill a man with impunity. Indeed, the blame is transferred to the deceased, who is criticised for want of moderation, and it is thus the dead who are censured"; "One is instantly reminded of the malign influence of fashion on medicine, more than on any other science. Even nowadays it is subject to fads, although no science is actually more profitable"; and "Assuredly, there is no greater reason for the decay of morals than medicine." Pliny the Elder was the Ivan Illich of the Roman era.

## NOTES TO THE INTRODUCTION

1. This painting was, until 1997, classified as "whereabouts unknown." It now hangs in London's National Gallery. *Alexander and His Doctor* was painted around 1648–1649 for Jérôme de Nouveau, the superintendent-general of posts—hence, presumably, the selection of a scene in which a letter plays an important part. The painting was bought by an English aristocrat at the end of the nineteenth century, in whose house it remained unrecognized and in "total oblivion" until recently. Eustache Le Sueur (1616–1655) was known as "Le Raphael Français." See A. Merot and H. Wine, "'Alexander and His Doctor': A Rediscovered Masterpiece by Eustache Le Sueur," *Burlington Magazine*, May 2000, pp. 292–296.

2. *The Age of Alexander* (Penguin, 1973), pp. 252–334.

3. Alexander had the capacity to be extraordinarily unforgiving in the

face of alleged medical negligence. When his friend Hephaestion developed a fever, the physician Glaucus advised a strict diet and promptly left for the theater. Hephaestion chose to disregard his doctor's advice and gorged himself on boiled fowl and copious wine, whereupon he died. Alexander ordered the "unlucky physician" to be crucified. See Plutarch, *The Age of Alexander*, p. 329.

4. *Hippocratic Writings* (Penguin, 1983), p. 67.

5. *Confessions of a Medicine Man* (MIT Press, 2000), pp. 114–116.

6. *Harold Shipman's Clinical Practice* (Norwich: The Stationery Office, 2001).

7. T.A. Brennan, L.L. Leape, N.M. Laird, et al., "Incidence of Adverse Events and Negligence in Hospitalized Patients," *New England Journal of Medicine*, Vol. 324 (1991), pp. 370–376; and, by the same authors, "The Nature of Adverse Events in Hospitalized Patients," *New England Journal of Medicine*, Vol. 324 (1991), pp. 377–384.

8. *To Err Is Human* (Washington, D.C.: National Academy of Sciences, 2000).

9. Error was defined by the Institute of Medicine "as the failure of a planned action to be completed as intended or the use of a wrong plan to achieve an aim." Safety was defined "as freedom from accidental injury."

10. C.J. McDonald, M. Weiner, and S.L. Hui, "Deaths Due to Medical Errors are Exaggerated in Institute of Medicine Report," *JAMA*, Vol. 284 (2000), pp. 93–95.

11. L.L. Leape, "Institute of Medicine Medical Error Figures Are Not Exaggerated," *JAMA*, Vol. 284 (2000), pp. 95–97. In any case, most American physicians seem to believe that errors in medicine have been exaggerated, and that there is no need for a national agency to provide leadership and research into medical error. See Andrew R. Robinson et al., "Physician and Public Opinions on Quality of Health Care and the Problem of Medical Errors," *Archives of Internal Medicine*, Vol. 162 (2002), pp. 2186–2190; and Robert J. Blendon et al., "Views of Practicing Physicians and the Public on Medical Errors," *New England Journal of Medicine*, Vol. 347 (2002), pp. 1933–1940.

12. *Hippocratic Writings*.

13. A.A. Gawande, E.J. Thomas, M.J. Zinner, and T.A. Brennan, "The Incidence and Nature of Surgical Adverse Events in Colorado and Utah in 1992," *Surgery*, Vol. 126 (1999), pp. 66–75.

14. M.R. de Leval, J. Carthey, D.J. Wright, V.T. Farewell, and J.T. Reason,

"Human Factors and Cardiac Surgery: A Multicenter Study," *Journal of Thoracic and Cardiovascular Surgery*, Vol. 119 (2000), pp. 661–672.

15. I once made a tiny effort to help this cultural change along. I wrote about an error I had made while still working as a doctor, one that led to the death of a patient I had admitted to the hospital. I asked whether doctors might like to begin a debate about the uses of error in medicine. Nothing much happened. Two years later, I invited readers of *The Lancet* once again to share their mistakes with us—in print. There now seemed to be a desire to do so, and "The Uses of Error" has become a regular section of the journal. See "The Uses of Error," *The Lancet*, Vol. 353 (1999), pp. 422–423; and "We All Make Mistakes: Tell Us Yours," *The Lancet*, Vol. 357 (2001), p. 88. A more scholarly appraisal of human error and systems approaches in medicine can be found in Charles Vincent, "Understanding and Responding to Adverse Events," *New England Journal of Medicine*, Vol. 348 (2003), pp. 1051–1056.

16. *Selected Works* (Penguin, 1997), pp. 202–289.

17. *The World and Other Writings* (Cambridge University Press, 1998), pp. 99–169.

18. *Cellular Pathology* (London: Classics of Medicine, 1978).

19. D. Botstein et al., "Molecular Portraits of Human Breast Tumours," *Nature*, Vol. 406 (2000), pp. 747–752; and Marc J. Van de Vijver et al., "A Gene Expression Signature as a Predictor of Survival in Breast Cancer," *New England Journal of Medicine*, Vol. 347 (2002), pp. 1999–2009.

20. L. K. F. Temple, R. S. McLeod, S. Gallinger, and J. G. Wright, "Defining Disease in the Genomics Era," *Science*, Vol. 293 (2001), pp. 807–808.

21. Zone, 1991.

22. *Science, Society, and the Perplexed Physician* (Royal College of Physicians, 2000).

23. "Doctor Discontent," *New England Journal of Medicine*, Vol. 339 (1998), pp. 1543–1545.

24. *British Medical Journal*, Vol. 322 (2001), pp. 1073–1074.

25. Yale University Press, 1996.

26. Oxford University Press, 1995.

27. *The Lost Art of Healing* (Houghton Mifflin, 1996).

28. *Caring for Patients* (Stanford University Press, 1995).

29. The notion of a personal medicine was raised most eloquently by Theodore Fox, a former editor of *The Lancet*, in "Personal Medicine," *Bulletin of the New York Academy of Medicine*, Vol. 38 (1962), pp. 527–534.

30. David L. Sackett et al., *Evidence-Based Medicine* (Churchill Livingstone, 2000).

31. *Rational Diagnosis and Treatment* (Blackwell, 2000).

32. F. S. Bagenal et al., "Survival of Patients with Breast Cancer Attending Bristol Cancer Help Centre," *The Lancet*, Vol. 336 (1990), pp. 606–610.

33. Heather Goodare, editor, *Fighting Spirit: The Stories of Women in the Bristol Breast Cancer Survey* (Scarlet, 1996).

34. "Bristol Cancer Help Centre," *The Lancet*, Vol. 338 (1991), pp. 1401–1402.

35. The Database of Patients' Experiences (DIPEX) aims to link evidence-based information about disease with patients' experiences of illness. The intention is to identify questions that matter to patients, rather than to doctors. See Andrew Herxheimer, "Database of Patients' Experiences: A Multimedia Approach to Sharing Experiences and Information," *The Lancet*, Vol. 355 (2000), pp. 1540–1543.

36. See, for example, Martin Hollis, *Trust within Reason* (Cambridge University Press, 1998); Piotr Sztompka, *Trust: A Sociological Theory* (Cambridge University Press, 1999); Adam B. Seligman, *The Problem of Trust* (Princeton, 1997); and Onora O'Neill, *A Question of Trust* (Cambridge University Press, 2002).

37. Polity, 1991.

38. Gretchen K. Berland et al., "Health Information on the Internet," *JAMA*, Vol. 285 (2001), pp. 2612–2621.

39. Marion Boyars, 1975.

40. David Weatherall, for example, called *Medical Nemesis* a "not always balanced outburst." He concluded that "it seems unlikely that we should take such an emotional and completely one-sided attack too seriously."

41. See the results of the UK's National Survey of Sexual Attitudes and Lifestyles. Overall, for example, 6 percent of Britons reported being drunk as the main reason for their first sexual encounter; "Sexual Behaviour in Britain," *The Lancet*, Vol. 358 (2001), pp. 1835–1854.

42. Illich acknowledges the epistemological issue, but with a different emphasis than mine. He identifies "a new crisis in the concept of disease." He writes of "medical ideology" and he concludes that "disease is a socially created reality." Illich is not interested, as far as I can see, in the detail of how the patient and the doctor share their experiences to construct a consensual space of knowing within which the patient's predicament can be faced.

43. David A. Wood, "Clinical Reality of Coronary Prevention Guidelines," *The Lancet*, Vol. 357 (2001), pp. 995–1001.

44. Mark H. Drazner et al., "Prognostic Importance of Elevated Jugular Venous Pressure and a Third Heart Sound in Patients with Heart Failure," *New England Journal of Medicine*, Vol. 345 (2001), pp. 574–581.

45. "Concordancing: Use of Language-Based Research in Medical Communication," *The Lancet*, Vol. 353 (1999), pp. 108–111.

46. In the recent redefinition of heart attack—called by doctors an acute myocardial infarction—the inexactness of the patient's story was underlined: "These complaints may go unrecognised or may be erroneously labelled as another disease entity, such as indigestion or a viral syndrome." See *European Heart Journal*, Vol. 21 (2000), pp. 1502–1513.

47. *Doctor's Stories* (Princeton University Press, 1991).

48. Roberto Grilli et al., "Practice Guidelines Developed by Specialty Societies: The Need for a Critical Appraisal," *The Lancet*, Vol. 355 (2000), pp. 103–106.

49. See, for example, C. Thompson et al., "Effects of a Clinical-Practice Guideline and Practice-Based Education on Detection and Outcome of Depression in Primary Care," *The Lancet*, Vol. 355 (2000), pp. 85–91.

50. *How We Think* (Prometheus, 1991).

51. "Judgment under Uncertainty: Heuristics and Biases," *Science*, Vol. 185 (1974), pp. 1124–1131.

52. Mary Dixon-Woods et al., "Parents' Accounts of Obtaining a Diagnosis of Childhood Cancer," *The Lancet*, Vol. 357 (2001), pp. 670–674.

53. Kate Hunt et al., "Lay Constructions of a Family History of Heart Disease: Potential for Misunderstandings in the Clinical Encounter?," *The Lancet*, Vol. 357 (2001), pp. 1168–1171.

54. Zelda di Blasi et al., "Influence of Context Effects on Health Outcomes," *The Lancet*, Vol. 357 (2001), pp. 757–762.

## NOTES TO CHAPTER 1
## INFECTION: THE GLOBAL THREAT

1. Paul W. Ewald, "The Evolution of Virulence," *Scientific American*, April 1993, pp. 86–93.

2. Random House, 1995.

3. Farrar, Straus and Giroux, 1995.

4. The rapid progress of the global AIDS pandemic led to the merger of six United Nations AIDS organizations into one: WHO's Global Program on AIDS, World Bank, UNICEF, UN Development Program, UNESCO, and the UN Population Fund. The work of the International Labour Organisation and the UN Office of Drug Control and Crime Prevention has been added to these initial collaborations.

5. P. B. Jahrling et al., "Preliminary Report: Isolation of Ebola Virus from Monkeys Imported to USA," *The Lancet*, Vol. 335 (1990), pp. 502–505.

6. *History of the Peloponnesian War* (Penguin, 1954; revised edition, 1972), Book II, chapter 51.

7. Since 1977, when the first rabid raccoon was documented, almost four thousand infected raccoons were identified through 1991. By 1992, rabid raccoons had reached Massachusetts; over nine hundred infected animals were found there during the first half of 1994. See Robin E. Kirby, "Rabies: An Old Disease of New Importance," *Clinical Microbiology Newsletter*, January 1, 1995, pp. 1–4.

8. Danny A. Brass, *Rabies in Bats* (Livia Press, 1994).

9. "Tuberculosis Morbidity Among US-Born and Foreign-Born Populations—US, 2000," *Morbidity and Mortality Weekly Report*, February 8, 2002, www.cdc.gov/mmwr.

10. The risk of producing multidrug-resistant tuberculosis after incomplete antibiotic therapy can be largely eliminated with "directly observed therapy" (DOTS). In this technique, each patient is supervised by a member of the health care team when they take their medications. The frequency of drug resistance and relapse of disease is strikingly reduced in such programs. See Stephen E. Weis et al., "The Effect of Directly Observed Therapy on the Rates of Drug Resistance and Relapse in Tuberculosis," *New England Journal of Medicine*, Vol. 330 (1994), pp. 1179–1184. Since DOTS was widely introduced in 1991, over ten million people have undergone treatment with cure rates of over 90 percent, although the African epidemic continues unabated.

11. In the US between 1980 and 1992, physicians increasingly prescribed antibiotics that killed a wider range of bacteria. Although this practice might seem intuitively reasonable (even sensible), a less specific drug is far more likely to encourage an organism to escape its actions and go on to develop resistance. The trend to use drugs in a way that will facilitate the emergence of resistant bacteria is an ominous sign. See L. F. McCaig and J. M. Hughes,

"Trends in Anti-microbial Drug Prescribing Among Office-Based Physicians in the United States," *JAMA*, Vol. 273 (1995), pp. 214–219.

12. Steve Sternberg, "The Emerging Fungal Threat," *Science*, Vol. 266 (1994), pp. 1632–1634.

13. "The U-Shaped Curve of Concern," *American Review of Respiratory Disease*, Vol. 144 (1991), pp. 741–742.

14. The origin of HIV remains a moot point. Preston oversimplifies a complex issue. As Garrett notes, there is clear evidence that HIV caused deaths from AIDS as far back as 1959. Moreover, it seems that, at least in central Africa, there was low-level exposure to HIV for some time before the epidemic began in earnest. The explosion of cases on two continents—Africa and North America—almost simultaneously in the late 1970s argues against central Africa being the origin of HIV. Indeed, genetic typing of HIV confirms that six different groups ("clades") of the virus exist. Type A is found in central Africa and India, while type B dominates North America and Europe.

15. Hyperion, 2000.

16. Lawrence K. Altman, "Yale Accepts Blame for Safety Lapses Linked to Lab Accident," *The New York Times*, December 13, 1994, p. C7.

17. Grant L. Campbell and James M. Hughes, "Plague in India: A New Warning from an Old Nemesis," *Annals of Internal Medicine*, Vol. 122 (1995), pp. 151–153.

18. Bernard Roizman and James M. Hughes, *Infectious Disease in an Age of Change* (National Academy of Sciences, 1995), pp. iv–v.

19. Richard Horton, "Suitable Cases for Treatment," *The Times Literary Supplement*, May 17, 2002, p. 8.

20. William Muraskin, professor of urban studies at Queens College, CUNY, argues that one important success in the use of vaccines is in controlling infection by the hepatitis B virus (HBV). This agent is more contagious than HIV and infects up to 300,000 people in the Western world annually. More important from an international public health viewpoint, HBV causes 80 percent of cases of primary liver cancer, the major cancer found in the nonindustrialized world. Muraskin writes that current programs to develop and supply a vaccine for children against HBV in order to achieve universal immunization by 1997 will eventually be described as "one of the great scientific achievements of the twentieth century." His conclusion is premature—control of HBV is likely to take fifteen to twenty years—but lack of an animal source for HBV makes eradication a real possibility. See William Muraskin,

*The War Against Hepatitis B* (University of Pennsylvania Press, 1995).

21. Christopher H. Foreman, Jr., *Plagues, Products, and Politics: Emergent Public Health Hazards and National Policy Making* (Brookings Institution, 1994).

22. *Evolutionary Medicine: Rethinking the Origins of Disease* (Sierra Club Books, 1994), p. 8.

## NOTES TO CHAPTER 2
## THE PLAGUES ARE FLYING

1. *The Diary of Elizabeth Drinker*, edited and abridged by Elaine Forman Crane (Northeastern University Press, 1994).

2. *Yellow Fever and the South* (Rutgers University Press, 1992). In *Malaria: Poverty, Race, and Public Health in the United States* (Johns Hopkins University Press, 2001), Humphreys traces the influence of malaria, another mosquito-borne disease, on American life.

3. *Letters on Yellow Fever Addressed to Dr. William Currie* (Johns Hopkins University Press, 1947).

4. Alastair Hay, "A Magic Sword or a Big Itch: An Historical Look at the United States Biological Weapons Programme," *Medicine, Conflict and Survival*, Vol. 15 (1999), pp. 215–234.

5. Andrew Spielman and Michael D'Antonio, *Mosquito: A Natural History of Our Most Persistent and Deadly Foe* (Hyperion, 2001).

6. *Prevention and Control of Yellow Fever in Africa* (Geneva: World Health Organization, 1986).

7. Eduard J. Sanders et al., "First Recorded Outbreak of Yellow Fever in Kenya, 1992–1993," *American Journal of Tropical Medicine and Hygiene*, Vol. 459 (1998), pp. 644–649.

8. P. van der Stuyft et al., "Urbanisation of Yellow Fever in Santa Cruz, Bolivia," *The Lancet*, Vol. 353 (1999), pp. 1558–1562.

9. Pedro F.C. Vasconcelos et al., "Serious Adverse Events Associated with Yellow Fever 17DD Vaccine in Brazil," *The Lancet*, Vol. 357 (2001), pp. 91–97; and Michael Martin et al., "Fever and Multisystem Organ Failure Possibly Associated with 17D Yellow Fever Vaccine," *The Lancet*, Vol. 357 (2001), pp. 98–104.

10. Spielman has sounded this warning before. In 1991, together with

colleagues, he wrote that "changes in recreational behavior and residential placement have exposed people to a diverse array of novel . . . infectious agents, and travel practices have increased this diversity still further by introducing exotic 'tropical' infectious agents and vectors into sites in which they thrive." See Sam R. Telford, Richard J. Pollack, and Andrew Spielman, "Emerging Vector-Borne Infections," *Infectious Disease Clinics of North America*, Vol. 5 (March 1991), pp. 7–17.

11. Denis Nash et al., "The Outbreak of West Nile Virus Infection in the New York City Area in 1999," *New England Journal of Medicine*, Vol. 344 (2001), pp. 1807–1814.

12. Xi-Yu Jia et al., "Genetic Analysis of West Nile New York 1999 Encephalitis Virus," *The Lancet*, Vol. 354 (1999), pp. 1971–1972.

13. Martin Enserink, "West Nile Researchers Get Ready for Round Three," *Science*, Vol. 292 (2001), pp. 1289–1290.

14. "Pa. Officials Expect W. Nile Virus to Spread Despite Measures," *The Philadelphia Inquirer*, May 10, 2001, p. B3.

15. For example, see Jennifer Huget, "It's Okay to DEET Responsibly," *The Washington Post*, June 12, 2001, p. HE6.

16. One of these experts was Fred Soper. He became the main proponent of worldwide eradication after winning stunning battles against malaria in Brazil and Sardinia. See Malcolm Gladwell, "The Mosquito Killer," *The New Yorker*, July 2, 2001, pp. 42–51.

17. Awareness of the world's malaria crisis has certainly risen. Johns Hopkins University, for example, was the recent beneficiary of a $100 million gift to build an institute devoted solely to malaria research.

18. Andrew Spielman et al., "Time Limitation and the Role of Research in the Worldwide Attempt to Eradicate Malaria," *Journal of Medical Entomology*, Vol. 30 (1993), pp. 6–19.

19. Raymond S. Bradley, "Many Citations Support Global Warming Trend," *Science*, Vol. 292 (2001), p. 2011.

20. "Malaria and Global Warming in Perspective?," *Emerging Infectious Diseases*, www.cdc.gov/ncidod/eid/vol6no4/reiter_letter.htm.

21. Jonathan A. Patz et al., "The Potential Health Impacts of Climate Variability and Change for the United States," *Environmental Health Perspectives*, Vol. 108 (2000), pp. 367–376.

22. "The Global Spread of Malaria in a Future, Warmer World," *Science*, Vol. 289 (2000), pp. 1763–1766.

23. R. Sari Kovats, "El Niño and Human Health," *Bulletin of the World Health Organization*, Vol. 78 (2000), pp. 1127–1135.

24. Simon Hales et al., "The Potential Global Distribution of Dengue Fever," *The Lancet*, E-print 01Let/4163, www.thelancet.com.

25. "Research Priorities for Managing the Transmission of Vector-Borne Disease," *Preventive Medicine*, Vol. 23 (1994), pp. 693–699.

26. "A Forgotten Suggestion," *The Lancet*, Vol. 1 (1900), pp. 1400–1401.

## NOTES TO CHAPTER 3
## WAITING FOR THE BIOWAR

1. H. Studd, "MOD Carried Out Bio-warfare Test on Tube Travellers," *The Times*, February 22, 2002, p. 13.

2. L. M. Bush, B. H. Abrams, A. Beall, and C. C. Johnson, "Index Case of Fatal Inhalational Anthrax Due to Bioterrorism in the US," *New England Journal of Medicine*, Vol. 345 (2001), pp. 1607–1610.

3. L. Borio, D. Frank, V. Mani, et al., "Death Due to Bioterrorism-Related Inhalational Anthrax," *JAMA*, No. 286 (2001), pp. 2554–2559; and T. A. Mayer, S. Bersoff-Matcha, C. Murphy, et al., "Clinical Presentation of Inhalational Anthrax Following Bioterrorism Exposure," *JAMA*, Vol. 286 (2001), pp. 2549–2553.

4. "Bioterrorism on the Home Front," *JAMA*, Vol. 286 (2001), pp. 2595–2597. New guidance on management of bioweapons-related anthrax was eventually published in 2002. See Thomas V. Inglesby et al., "Anthrax as a Biological Weapon, 2002," *JAMA*, Vol. 287 (2002), pp. 2236–2252. The experts who drew up this guidance emphasized the need for a better vaccine, more rapid diagnostic tests, new treatments, and a greater understanding of the virulence of anthrax. There were significant gaps in our knowledge if we were to face down this threat successfully.

5. M. A. Schuster, B. D. Stein, L. H. Jaycox, et al., "A National Survey of Stress Reactions after the September 11, 2001, Terrorist Attacks," *New England Journal of Medicine*, Vol. 345 (2001), pp. 1507–1512.

6. D. Malakoff, "Scientists Pan Plans for New US Agency," *Science*, Vol. 297 (2002), pp. 27–28.

7. "A European Centre to Respond to Threats of Bioterrorism and Major Epidemics," *Bulletin of the World Health Organization*, Vol. 79 (2001), p. 1044.

8. "How to Protect the Homeland," *The New York Times*, September 25, 2001, p. A29.

9. A. Caffrey and R. Gold, "Before Federal Security Office Forms, States Get a Jump on Defenses," *The Wall Street Journal*, September 25, 2001, p. A6.

10. J. Miller, "The 27 Whose Assets Will Be Frozen Are Just the First of Many, a US Official Says," *The New York Times*, September 25, 2001, p. B4.

11. Daniel Benjamin and Steven Simon, "A Failure of Intelligence?," *The New York Review of Books*, December 20, 2001, pp. 76–80.

12. B. Balmer, *Britain and Biological Warfare* (Palgrave, 2001).

13. The Royal Society, *Measures for Controlling the Threat from Biological Weapons* (London: Royal Society, 2000).

14. *The Threat from Terrorism*, Vols. I and II (London: Stationery Office, 2001).

15. *The Anti-Terrorism, Crime and Security Bill 2001* (London: The Stationery Office, 2001).

16. *Anti-Terrorism, Crime and Security Act 2001* (London: The Stationery Office, 2001).

17. *Getting Ahead of the Curve: A Strategy for Combating Infectious Diseases* (London: Department of Health, 2001).

18. "Biological Security in a Changed World," *Science*, Vol. 293 (2001), p. 2349.

19. N. Lightfoot, M. Wale, R. Spencer, and A. Nicoll, "Appropriate Responses to Bioterrorist Threats," *British Medical Journal*, Vol. 323 (2001), pp. 877–878.

20. J. D. Simon, "Biological Terrorism: Preparing to Meet the Threat," *JAMA*, Vol. 278 (1997), pp. 428–430.

21. S. H. Silber, N. Oster, B. Simmons, and C. Garrett, "Y2K Medical Disaster Preparedness in New York City," *Journal of Prehospital and Disaster Medicine*, Vol. 16 (2001), pp. 88–95.

22. R. Pear, "In Anthrax Crisis, Health Secretary Finds Unsteady Going," *The New York Times*, October 25, 2001.

23. T. V. Inglesby, D. A. Henderson, J. G. Bartlett, et al., "Anthrax as a Biological Weapon: Medical and Public Health Management," *JAMA*, Vol. 281 (1999), pp. 1735–1745.

24. D. A. Henderson, T. V. Inglesby, J. G. Bartlett, et al., "Smallpox as a Biological Weapon: Medical and Public Health Management," *JAMA*, Vol. 281 (1999), pp. 2127–2137.

25. T. V. Inglesby, D. A. Henderson, J. G. Bartlett, et al., "Plague as a Biological Weapon: Medical and Public Health Management," *JAMA*, Vol. 281 (1999), pp. 2281–2290.

26. S. S. Arnon, R. Schechter, T. V. Inglesby, et al., "Botulinum Toxin as a Biological Weapon: Medical and Public Health Management," *JAMA*, Vol. 285 (2001), pp. 1059–1070.

27. D. T. Dennis, T. V. Inglesby, D. A. Henderson, et al., "Tularemia as a Biological Weapon: Medical and Public Health Management," *JAMA*, Vol. 285 (2001), pp. 2763–2773.

28. A. S. Khan, S. Morse, and S. Lillibridge, "Public-Health Preparedness for Biological Terrorism in the USA," *The Lancet*, Vol. 356 (2000), pp. 1179–1182.

29. T. O'Toole and T. V. Inglesby, "Facing the Biological Weapons Threat," *The Lancet*, Vol. 356 (2000), pp. 1128–1129.

30. "The Specter of Biological Terror," *The New York Times*, September 26, 2001.

31. C. Denny, "Rules Relaxed in Rush for New Smallpox Vaccine," *The Guardian*, October 25, 2001.

32. "Infectious Disease and Biological Weapons: Prophylaxis and Mitigation," *JAMA*, Vol. 278 (1997), pp. 435–436.

33. Editorial, "A World War Against Terrorism," *The Lancet*, Vol. 358 (2001), pp. 937–938.

34. R. Horton, "Public Health: A Neglected Counterterrorist Measure," *The Lancet*, Vol. 358 (2001), pp. 1112–1113.

35. R. Horton, "Violence and Medicine: The Necessary Politics of Public Health," *The Lancet*, Vol. 358 (2001), pp. 1472–1473.

36. G. MacQueen, J. Santa-Barbara, V. Neufeld, S. Yusuf, and R. Horton, "Health and Peace: Time for a New Discipline," *The Lancet*, Vol. 357 (2001), pp. 1460–1461.

37. *Macroeconomics and Health: Investing in Health for Economic Development* (Geneva: World Health Organization, 2001).

38. S. Wesseley, K. C. Hyams, and R. Bartholomew, "Psychological Implications of Chemical and Biological Weapons," *British Medical Journal*, Vol. 323 (2001), pp. 878–879.

39. M. Maselson, J. Guillemin, M. Hugh-Jones, et al., "The Sverdlovsk Anthrax Outbreak of 1979," *Science*, Vol. 266 (1994), pp. 1202–1208.

40. R. E. LaPorte, F. Sauer, S. Dearwater, et al., "Towards an Internet

Civil Defence Against Bioterrorism," *The Lancet Infectious Diseases*, Vol. 1 (2001), pp. 125–127.

41. L. K. Altman and G. Kolata, "Anthrax Missteps Offer Guide to Fight Next Bioterror Battle," *The New York Times*, January 6, 2002.

## NOTES TO THE EPILOGUE TO CHAPTERS 1, 2, AND 3

1. An immediate qualification is needed. A report published in 2002 claimed to provide evidence for "a spontaneously assembled 'artificial' bacterium." What scientists had actually created was a membrane closely linked to protein filaments—a primitive cellular skeleton. This structure was, they believed, "reminiscent" of a bacterial cell wall. It was more a piece of whimsy than concrete creation. See Gerard C. L. Wong et al., "Hierarchical Self-Assembly of F-Actin and Cationic Lipid Complexes: Stacked Three-Layer Tubule Networks," *Science*, Vol. 288 (2000), pp. 2035–2039.

2. Jeronimo Cello et al., "Chemical Synthesis of Poliovirus cDNA: Generation of Infectious Virus in the Absence of Natural Template," *Science*, Vol. 297 (2002), pp. 1016–1018. The publication of this research paper provoked a strong debate about the responsibility of scientific journals in an era of bioterrorism. Politicians argued that scientists and editors should self-censor material that might help those intending to design weapons of mass destruction. Many scientists objected that censorship of any sort was against the spirit of free inquiry. The upshot of this discussion was a statement written by scientists and editors, including editors of prestigious journals such as *Science*, *Nature*, and the *New England Journal of Medicine*, pledging to take account of the potential costs as well as benefits of research. They wrote:

> We recognize that on occasions an editor may conclude that the potential harm of publication outweighs the potential societal benefits. Under such circumstances, the paper should be modified, or not be published.

I believe this principle is misguided. It suggests that some editors think that they are a little more influential than they really are. The lesson of science is that one can never quite predict the impact of a piece of research once it is published. A finding that seemed interesting at the time of publication might lead nowhere. A report that once seemed mundane can occasionally open up a fresh field of study. Science is predictably unpredictable. We editors are not going to be an effective front-line defense against those intent on developing weapons of mass destruction. A pity. See "Statement on the Consideration of Biodefence and Biosecurity," *Nature*, Vol. 421 (2003), p. 771.

3. Steven M. Block, "A Not-So-Cheap Stunt," *Science*, Vol. 297 (2002), p. 769.

4. *World Health Report 2001* (Geneva: World Health Organization, 2001).

5. *HIV/AIDS: Awareness and Behavior* (Geneva: World Health Organization, 2002).

6. Martin Enserink and Elizabeth Pennisi, "Researchers Crack Malaria Genome," *Science*, Vol. 295 (2002), p. 1207.

7. Junitsu Ito et al., "Transgenic Anopheline Mosquitoes Impaired in Transmission of a Malaria Parasite," *Nature*, Vol. 417 (2002), pp. 452–455.

8. Gareth J. Lycett and Fotis C. Kafatos, "Anti-Malarial Mosquitoes?," *Nature*, Vol. 417 (2002), pp. 387–388.

9. Kalifa A. Bojang et al., "Efficacy of RTS, S/AS02 Malaria Vaccine Against *Plasmodium falciparum* Infection in Semi-immune Adult Men in the Gambia," *The Lancet*, Vol. 358 (2001), pp. 1927–1934; Louis Schofield et al., "Synthetic GPI as a Candidate Antitoxic Vaccine in a Model of Malaria," *Nature*, Vol. 418 (2002), pp. 785–789; and John Schutzer-Weissmann and Lorraine Fraser, "British Vaccine Breakthrough Will Save Millions from Malaria," *The Sunday Telegraph*, August 18, 2002, p. 10.

10. "Imperfect Vaccines and the Evolution of Pathogen Virulence," *Nature*, Vol. 414 (2001), pp. 751–756.

11. Philippe J. Guerin et al., "Malaria: Current Status of Control, Diagnosis, Treatment, and a Proposed Agenda for Research and Development," *The Lancet Infectious Diseases*, Vol. 2 (2002), pp. 564–573.

12. MIT Press, 2002.

## NOTES TO CHAPTER 4
## SURVIVING CONFLICT

1. Z. Lovric, M. Martinac, and J. Mihaljevic, "Mobile Surgical Teams of Croatian Special Police Forces: Analysis of Casualties During Combat," *Military Medicine*, Vol. 162 (1997), pp. 360–362.

2. S. Soldo and D. Puntaric, "Injuries in Croatian Army Brigade Soldiers Inflicted in an Offensive Action During the 1991–1992 War in Croatia," *Military Medicine*, Vol. 163 (1998), pp. 420–422.

3. K. Janosi and Z. Lovric, "War Surgery in Osijek During the 1991–1992 War in Croatia," *Croatian Medical Journal*, Vol. 36 (1995), pp. 104–107.

4. I. Balen, D. Danic, D. Prgomet, and D. Puntaric, "Work of the Slavonski Brod General Hospital During the War in Croatia and Bosnia and Herzegovina in 1991–1992," *Military Medicine*, Vol. 160 (1995), pp. 588–592.

5. D. Mijatovic, N. Henigsberg, M. Judas, and I. Kostovic, "Use of Digital Wireless Communications System for Rapid and Efficient Communication Between Croatian Medical Centres in War," *Croatian Medical Journal*, Vol. 37 (1996), pp. 71–74.

6. B. Ljubic and B. Hrabac, "Priority Setting and Scarce Resources: Case of the Federation of Bosnia and Herzegovina," *Croatian Medical Journal*, Vol. 39 (1998), pp. 276–280.

7. M. Definis-Gojanovic, S. Andelinovic, and J. Ivanovic, "Forensic Data on 874 Victims of War Autopsied in Split, 1991–1994," *Croatian Medical Journal*, Vol. 36 (1995), pp. 282–286.

8. D. Puntaric, A. Brkljacic, D. Krajcar, et al., "Sanitation of the Liberated Territories in Croatia After the Storm Campaign: The Example of Lika-Senj County," *Military Medicine*, Vol. 162 (1997), pp. 333–337.

9. E. Halilovic, "Cardiovascular Diseases Recorded in Bosnian Refugees in Kruge Outpatients Medical Office for Refugees, Zagreb, Croatia," *Croatian Medical Journal*, Vol. 36 (1995), pp. 65–66.

10. "Kosovo's Refugees: From Crisis to Catastrophe," *The Lancet*, Vol. 353 (1999), p. 1199.

11. Z. Lovric, B. Wertheimer, K. Candrlic, S. Markic, and O. Rubin, "The Reconstruction of Major Femoral Vessels in a Four-year-old Girl Wounded with Shrapnel," *Journal of Cardiovascular Surgery*, Vol. 34 (1993), pp. 267–269.

12. Z. Lovric, "Reconstruction of Major Arteries of Extremities After War Injuries," *Journal of Cardiovascular Surgery*, Vol. 34 (1993), pp. 33–37.

13. Z. Lovric, B. Wertheimer, K. Candrlic, et al., "War Injuries of Major Extremity Vessels," *Journal of Trauma*, Vol. 36 (1994), pp. 248–251.

14. Z. Lovric, V. Lehner, L. Kosic-Lovric, and B. Wertheimer, "Reconstruction of Major Arteries of Lower Extremities After War Injuries: Long-Term Follow Up," *Journal of Cardiovascular Surgery*, Vol. 37 (1996), pp. 223–227.

15. D. Kozaric-Kovacic, A. Marusic, and T. Ljubin, "Combat-Experienced Soldiers and Tortured Prisoners of War Differ in the Clinical Presentation of Post-traumatic Stress Disorder," *Nordic Journal of Psychiatry*, Vol. 53 (1999), pp. 11–15.

16. G.T. Simunkovic-Tocilj and I. Urlic, "War Trauma: Emotional Responses and Psychological Defences of Displaced Persons," *Croatian Medical Journal*, Vol. 36 (1995), pp. 253–261.

17. C.H. Gray, *Postmodern War: The New Politics of Conflict* (Guilford, 1997).

18. D. Kozaric-Kovacic and V. Folnegovic-Smalc, "Systematic Raping of Women in Croatia and Bosnia and Herzegovina: A Preliminary Psychiatric Report," *Croatian Medical Journal*, Vol. 34 (1993), pp. 86–87.

19. D. Kozaric-Kovacic, V. Folnegovic-Smalc, J. Skrinjaric, N.M. Szajnberg, and A. Marusic, "Rape, Torture, and Traumatization of Bosnian and Croatian Women: Psychological Sequelae," *American Journal of Orthopsychiatry*, Vol. 65 (1995), pp. 428–433.

20. L.T. Arcel, "Sexual Torture of Women as a Weapon of War: The Case of Bosnia-Herzegovina," in *War Violence, Trauma, and the Coping Process*, edited by Libby Arcel (Copenhagen: International Rehabilitation Council for Torture Victims, 1998), pp. 183–211.

21. Children's Rights Commission, *On Violation of the Convention on the Rights of the Child During the War in the Republic of Croatia* (Zagreb: UNICEF, 1994).

22. D. Kocijan-Hercigonja, M. Rijavec, A. Marusic, and V. Hercigonja, "Coping Strategies of Refugee, Displaced, and Nondisplaced Children in a War Area," *Nordic Journal of Psychiatry*, Vol. 52 (1998), pp. 45–50.

23. M. Pibernik-Okanovic and Z. Metelko, "War-Induced Prolonged Stress and Metabolic Control in Type 2 Diabetic Patients," *Diabetologia Croatica*, Vol. 20 (1991), pp. 175–177.

24. S. Lang, N. Javornik, K. Bakalic, et al., "'Save Lives' Operation in Liberated Parts of Croatia in 1995: An Emergency Public Health Action to Assist Abandoned Elderly Populations," *Croatian Medical Journal*, Vol. 38 (1997), pp. 265–270.

25. S. Soldo, Z. Petrovecki, D. Puntaric, and D. Prgomet, "Injuries Caused by Antipersonnel Mines in Croatian Army Soldiers on the East Slavonia Front During the 1991–1992 War in Croatia," *Military Medicine*, Vol. 164 (1999), pp. 141–144.

26. Letter in possession of Dr. Ivan Bagaric, translated by Vladimir Mikulic.

27. B. Ljubic, B. Hrabac, and Z. Rebac, "Reform of Health Insurance in the Federation of Bosnia and Herzegovina," *Croatian Medical Journal*, Vol. 40 (1999), pp. 160–165.

28. "Financing of Dental Health Care in the Federation of Bosnia and Herzegovina," *Croatian Medical Journal*, Vol. 40 (1999), pp. 166–174.

29. G. F. Pyle, C. R. Thompson, S. Oreskovic, and I. Bagaric, "Rebuilding the Healthcare System in Mostar: Challenge and Opportunity," *Croatian Medical Journal*, Vol. 39 (1998), pp. 281–284.

30. B. Ljubic and B. Hrabac, "Priority Setting and Scarce Resources: Case of the Federation of Bosnia and Herzegovina," *Croatian Medical Journal*, Vol. 39 (1998), pp. 276–280.

31. Z. Puvacic, B. Hrabac, N. Jaganjac, A. Gabrielli, N. Charez, and S. Puvacic, "Vaccination Coverage in Bosnia and Herzegovina During the 1992–1995 War," *Croatian Medical Journal*, Vol. 38 (1997), pp. 140–142.

32. I. Sarac, I. Bagaric, S. Oreskovic, J. Reamy, V. J. Simunovic, and S. Lang, "Physician Requirements for the Croat Population in Bosnia and Herzegovina," *Croatian Medical Journal*, Vol. 38 (1997), pp. 83–87.

33. L. Kovacic and Z. Susic, "Organisation of Health Care in Croatia: Needs and Priorities," *Croatian Medical Journal*, Vol. 39 (1998), pp. 249–255.

34. Z. Rajic and B. Gorski, "Zagreb Hospitals at a Turning Point," *Croatian Medical Journal*, Vol. 35 (1994), pp. 203–213.

35. "A Critique of Seven Assumptions Behind Psychological Trauma Programmes in War-affected Areas," *Social Science and Medicine*, Vol. 48 (1999), pp. 1449–1462.

36. M. Marusic, "On the Advancement of Science in Developing Countries: An Example of 70 Croatian Young Scientists Educated in Germany and USA," *Croatian Medical Journal*, Vol. 37 (1996), pp. 73–82.

37. D. Eterovic, L. Juretic-Kuscic, V. Capkin, and Z. Dujic, "Pyelolithotomy Improves While Extracorporeal Lithotripsy Impairs Kidney Function," *Journal of Urology*, Vol. 161 (1999), pp. 39–44; and D. Eterovic, T. Strinic, and Z. Dujic, "Blood Gasses and Sex Hormones in Women with and without Genital Descensus," *Respiration*, Vol. 66 (1999), pp. 400–406.

38. D. Primorac, S. Andelinovic, M. Definis-Gojanovic, et al., "Identification of War Victims from Mass Graves in Croatia, Bosnia, and Herzegovina by the Use of Standard Forensic Methods and DNA Typing," *Journal of*

*Forensic Science*, Vol. 41 (1996), pp. 891–894.

39. M. Marusic, "Scientific Editing Around the Globe: Croatia," CBE *Views*, Vol. 21 (1998), pp. 12–13.

40. S.M. Jankovic, D.R. Milovanovic, and S.V. Jankovic, "Schild's Equation and the Best Estimate of PA2 Value and Dissociation Constant of an Antagonist," *Croatian Medical Journal*, Vol. 40 (1999), pp. 67–70.

41. N. Cikes, "The Role of *Lijecnicki vjesnik* in the Education of Croatian Physicians," *Lijecnicki vjesnik*, Vol. 121 (1999), pp. 1–3.

42. "The Third Balkan War: Red Cross Bleeding," *Croatian Medical Journal*, Vol. 34 (1993), pp. 5–20; "Human Rights, Medicine and Health: Tragic Symbols of Eastern Slavonia That Became a Reality," *Croatian Medical Journal*, Vol. 36 (1995), pp. 3–6; and "Challenge of Goodness: Twelve Humanitarian Proposals Based on the Experience of 1991–1995 Wars in Croatia and Bosnia and Herzegovina," *Croatian Medical Journal*, Vol. 39 (1998), pp. 72–76.

43. "Intervention," *Medicine, Conflict and Survival*, Vol. 15 (1999), pp. 115–125.

44. S. Zizek, "Against the Double Blackmail," *New Left Review*, Vol. 234 (1999), pp. 6–82.

45. "The Demolition of World Order," *Harper's*, June 1999, pp. 15–18.

46. Z. Reiner, "WHO and the EU: United Will They Stand," *Eurohealth*, Vol. 4 (1998–1999), pp. 2–4.

47. "Foreign Aid, International Organisations, and the World's Children," *Pediatrics*, Vol. 103 (1999), pp. 646–654.

48. L. Kostovic, M. Judas, and N. Henigsberg, "Medical Documentation of Human Rights Violations and War Crimes on the Territory of Croatia During the 1991/1993 War," *Croatian Medical Journal*, Vol. 34 (1993), pp. 285–293.

49. J. Leaning, L. Vollen, and C. Palmer, "PHR Documents Systematic Abuse Against Ethnic Albanian Physicians and Patients," *The Lancet*, Vol. 353 (1999), pp. 921–922.

50. My thanks to Matko and Ana Marusic for encouraging my visit to Croatia and Bosnia-Herzegovina and for giving me unlimited assistance in learning about Croatian and Bosnian medicine and science.

## NOTES TO CHAPTER 5
## THE AFRICAN CHALLENGE

1. Oxford University Press, 2002.

2. *The Scramble for Africa* (Random House, 1991).

3. *Kwame Nkrumah: The Anatomy of an African Dictatorship* (Accra: Sankofa, 2000).

4. F.I.D. Konotey-Ahulu, "First Graduates of Ghana Medical School," *Ghana Medical Journal*, Vol. 8 (1969), p. 172.

5. "Training of Doctors in Ghana," *Ghana Medical Journal*, Vol. 8 (1969), pp. 208–217.

6. "Fellowship Awards 2000," *Ghana Medical Journal*, Vol. 35 (2001), p. 4.

7. WHO/CHD Immunisation-Linked Vitamin A Supplementation Study Group, "Randomised Trial to Assess Benefits and Safety of Vitamin A Supplementation Linked to Immunisation in Early Infancy," *The Lancet*, Vol. 352 (1998), pp. 1257–1263.

8. S. Owusu-Agyei, K.A. Koram, J.K. Baird, et al., "Incidence of Symptomatic and Asymptomatic Plasmodium Falciparum Infection Following Curative Therapy in Adult Residents of Northern Ghana," *American Journal of Tropical Medicine and Hygiene*, Vol. 65 (2001), pp. 197–203; A. Hodgson, J. Smith, S. Gagneux, et al., "Risk Factors for Meningococcal Meningitis in Northern Ghana," *Transactions of the Royal Society of Tropical Medicine and Hygiene*, Vol. 95 (2001), pp. 477–480.

9. N. Unwin, P. Setel, S. Rashid, et al., "Non-communicable Diseases in Sub-Saharan Africa: Where Do They Feature in the Health Research Agenda?" *Bulletin of the World Health Organization*, Vol. 79 (2001), pp. 947–953.

10. F.P. Cappuccio, J. Plange-Rhule, R.O. Phillips, and J.B. Eastwood, "Prevention of Hypertension and Stroke in Africa," *The Lancet*, Vol. 356 (2000), pp. 677–678.

11. J.B. Eastwood, J. Plange-Rhule, V. Parry, and S. Tomlinson, "Medical Collaboration Between Developed and Developing Countries," *Quarterly Journal of Medicine*, Vol. 94 (2001), pp. 637–641.

12. "Educating Doctors for World Health," *The Lancet*, Vol. 358 (2001), p. 1471.

13. "Message to the Ghana Medical Association," *Ghana Medical Journal*, Vol. 1 (1962), p. 1.

14. R.C. Crook and J. Manor, *Democracy and Decentralisation in South*

*Asia and West Africa* (Cambridge University Press, 1998).

15. *The Health of the Nation* (Ghana: Ministry of Health, 2001).

16. T. Ensor, G. Dakpallah, and D. Osei, "Geographical Resource Allocation in Health Sector of Ghana" (September 2001).

17. "Neoliberalism, the World Bank and the New Politics of Development," in Uma Kothari and Martin Minogue, *Development Theory and Practice: Critical Perspectives* (London: Palgrave, 2001), pp. 157–178.

18. *World Development Report 2002: Building Institutions for Markets* (Oxford University Press, 2002).

19. *The Myth of Development* (London: Zed, 2001).

20. A. Fentiman, A. Hall, and D. Bundy, "Health and Cultural Factors Associated with Enrollment in Basic Education: A Study in Rural Ghana," *Social Science and Medicine*, Vol. 52 (2001), pp. 429–439.

21. "The Ghana Medical School," *Ghana Medical Journal*, Vol. 3 (1964), pp. 183–184.

22. I owe a debt of thanks to Professor Eldryd Parry, former dean of the School of Medical Sciences at Kumasi (1980–1985) and presently chairman of the Tropical Health and Education Trust, for introducing me to Ghana, being a perspicacious traveling companion, and for long conversations on the road.

## NOTES TO THE EPILOGUE TO CHAPTERS 4 AND 5

1. The 2002 *Human Development Report* (Oxford University Press) built on the intellectual framework set out by Amartya Sen in his book *Development as Freedom* (Oxford University Press, 1999). Sen wrote:

> Development consists of the removal of various types of unfreedoms that leave people with little choice and little opportunity of exercising their reasoned agency. The removal of substantial unfreedoms . . . is *constitutive* of development.

His arguments have slowly seeped into the mainstream of the development debate, especially given the return of terrorism to the political center stage; the 2002 *Human Development Report* concluded:

> Globalisation is forging greater interdependence, yet the world seems more fragmented—between rich and poor, between the powerful and

> the powerless, and between those who welcome the new global economy and those who demand a different course. The September 11, 2001, terrorist attacks on the United States cast new light on those divisions.... For politics and political institutions to promote human development and safeguard the freedom and dignity of all people, democracy must widen and deepen.

2. See S. V. Subramanian, P. Belli, and I. Kawachi, "The Macroeconomic Determinants of Health," *Annual Review of Public Health*, Vol. 23 (2002), pp. 287–302. The most influential report linking health to development came from the 2001 Commission on Macroeconomics and Health, chaired by Jeffery Sachs, a respected development economist who now directs not only the Earth Institute at Columbia University but also the Millennium Project. This UN-led project aims to devise the best strategies for meeting the Millennium Development Goals, although its work is, so far, shrouded in secrecy. Sachs's earlier commission concluded that health investment in the world's poorest countries in the short term (an additional $22 billion per year by 2007, above a current baseline of $6 billion per year) would yield eight million lives saved each year by 2010 and $360 billion per year in extra revenues between 2015 and 2020. See *Macroeconomics and Health: Investing in Health for Economic Development* (Geneva: World Health Organization, 2001).

3. Other observers would disagree with me here. For example, the World Bank believes that markets and market institutions are the best routes for achieving development goals. As James Wolfensohn writes in his introduction to the *2002 World Development Report*, "Markets are central to the lives of poor people," and "institutions can promote inclusive and integrated markets, and ensure stable growth and thus dramatically improve peoples' incomes and reduce poverty." Meanwhile, the Millennium Project aims to devise policies, but not to implement them.

4. In some ways, it is unfair to criticize the UN directly. As the embodiment of the "international community," it is little more than a reflection of its member states. Its failures are those not only of its own leadership and administrative bureaucracy, but also those of its member states. One consequence of globalization is that injustice is ever more transparent. But as William Shawcross writes in *Deliver Us from Evil* (Simon and Schuster, 2001), his perceptive analysis of the UN role in global conflict, "We want more to be put right, but we are prepared to sacrifice less." We who live in Western democracies may cry for action to be taken in the face of the latest

humanitarian crisis. Yet we are frequently unwilling to accept the consequences of that action: loss of life among our own people, or a heavy financial cost. The failure to make progress on human development is collectively ours.

5. *Globalization and its Discontents* (Norton, 2002).

6. There is a historical irony here. The two most influential thinkers about global capital were Karl Marx and Adam Smith. Both writers emphasized the interdependence between capital and globalization. Marx, for example, together with Engels, argued in the *Communist Manifesto* of 1848 that when domestic capitalism had reached its limit of progress, or a crisis, the response of industrialists would be the "conquest of new markets, and... more thorough exploitation of the old ones." They predicted an "industrial war of extermination between nations." Smith saw that capital acquired in one particular setting had no inherent reason to remain where it had been created. The vicissitudes of the global market were more powerful forces than sentiments of national allegiance. In Book III of *The Wealth of Nations* (1776), Smith wrote:

> A merchant, it has been said very properly, is not necessarily the citizen of any particular country. It is in a great measure indifferent to him from what place he carries on his trade; and a very trifling disgust will make him remove his capital, and together with it all the industry which it supports, from one country to another. No part of it can be said to belong to any particular country, till it has been spread as it were over the face of that country, either in buildings, or in the lasting improvement of lands.

These are the truths that the World Bank and IMF still face today. But their economists have done little to study the implications of their impact for the poor despite the passage of four centuries.

7. One UN body that transcends the UN straightjacket but which officially lies within its umbrella is UNAIDS, the Joint United Nations Programme on HIV/AIDS. UNAIDS was created in 1995 as a successor to WHO's failing Global Program on AIDS. It links the work of UNICEF, UNDP, WHO, the World Bank, UNESCO, UNFPA, UNDCP, and the ILO. It has been extremely successful in its global advocacy for HIV/AIDS.

8. Available at www.worldbank.org.

9. Institute of Economic Affairs, 2002.

10. *A Globalist Manifesto for Public Policy* (Institute of Economic Affairs, 2002).

11. *Development Theory and Practice*, edited by Uma Kothari and Martin Minogue (Palgrave, 2002).

12. Graeme McQueen et al., "Health and Peace: Time for a New Discipline," *The Lancet*, Vol. 357 (2001), pp. 1460–1461.

13. See my two essays "Public Health: A Neglected Counterterrorist Measure," *The Lancet*, Vol. 358 (2001), pp. 1112–1113; and "Violence and Medicine: The Necessary Politics of Public Health," *The Lancet*, Vol. 358 (2001), pp. 1472–1473.

14. G. Massera et al., "North-South Twinning in Paediatric Haemato-oncology: The La Mascota Programme, Nicaragua," *The Lancet*, Vol. 352 (1998), pp. 1923–1926; and Robert L. Broadhead and Adamson S. Muula, "Creating a Medical School for Malawi: Problems and Achievements," *British Medical Journal*, Vol. 325 (2002), pp. 384–387.

## NOTES TO CHAPTER 6
## VACCINE MYTHS

1. Deutsch, 1991.

2. Sarah Boseley, *The Guardian*, February 27, 1998, p. 5.

3. Andrew Wakefield et al., "Ileal-lymphoid Nodular Hyperplasia, Non-specific Colitis, and Pervasive Developmental Disorder in Children," *The Lancet*, Vol. 351 (1998), pp. 637–641.

4. "Vaccine Adverse Events: Causal or Coincidental?," *The Lancet*, Vol. 351 (1998), pp. 611–612.

5. *World Health Report 2002* (Geneva: World Health Organization, 2002).

6. Philip J. Hilts, "House Panel Asks for Study of a Vaccine," *The New York Times*, April 7, 2000.

7. J. W. Lee et al., "Autism, Inflammatory Bowel Disease, and MMR Vaccine," *The Lancet*, Vol. 351 (1998), pp. 905–909.

8. One notable feature of news reports describing Wakefield's results was its sober nature. His findings were repeatedly qualified, and the enormous importance of continuing MMR vaccination programs was underlined. It seemed that the critics of the report were reacting less to the tone and content of the coverage than to the fact of the coverage itself. To me, at the sharp end of much of this debate, such responses simply proved the point that the safety of vaccines could never be debated fairly, regardless of the evidence or care

with which that evidence was brought to public attention. But I know that such an interpretation also smacks of self-justification for my decision to publish.

9. B. A. Hendricksen and J. R. Turner, "MMR Vaccination, Ileal-lymphoid-nodular Hyperplasia, and Possible Developmental Disorder," *The Lancet*, Vol. 359 (2002), pp. 2051–2052.

10. *Enduring Memories of a Paediatric Gastroenterolgist* (Durham: Memoir Club, 2003).

11. Sophie Petit-Zeman, "Most MMR Studies Are Meaningless, Investigation Claims," *The Observer*, October 6, 2002. Our lack of understanding about how vaccines exert their effects is reflected in an intriguing debate about the benefits and risks of vaccines in developing countries. Peter Aaby has shown that measles vaccination in Bangladesh, Benin, Burundi, Guinea-Bissau, Haiti, Senegal, and Zaire provides a beneficial effect that seems unrelated to the protection against measles alone. The vaccine seems to be doing something else that benefits the child. But what? See Peter Aaby et al., "Non-specific Beneficial Effect of Measles Immunisation: Analysis of Mortality Studies from Developing Countries," *British Medical Journal*, Vol. 331 (1995), pp. 481–485; and Ines Kristensen et al., "Routine Vaccinations and Child Survival," *British Medical Journal*, Vol. 321 (2000), pp. 1435–1438.

12. *The Interpretation of Cultures* (Basic Books, 1973).

13. *Report on the Investigation into the Cause of the 1978 Birmingham Smallpox Occurrence* (London: The Stationery Office, 1980).

14. The currently available smallpox vaccine consists of a live virus called vaccinia. Complications include encephalitis, severe skin damage, and progressive vaccinia, an uncontrollable and frequently fatal systemic infection. New and safer vaccines are being designed. Some of these new vaccines will contain weakened strains of vaccinia, while others will be genetically engineered variants.

15. See Jim Koopman, "Controlling Smallpox," *Science*, Vol. 298 (2002), pp. 1342–1344; M. Elizabeth Halloran et al., "Containing Bioterrorist Smallpox," *Science*, Vol. 298 (2002), pp. 1428–1432; and Samuel A. Bozzette et al., "A Model for a Smallpox-Vaccination Policy," *New England Journal of Medicine*, Vol. 348 (2003), pp. 416–425.

16. Robert J. Blendon et al., "The Public and the Smallpox Threat," *New England Journal of Medicine*, Vol. 348 (2003), pp. 426–432.

17. Helen L. Collins and Stefan H. E. Kaufmann, "Prospects for Better Tuberculosis Vaccines," *The Lancet Infectious Diseases*, Vol. 1 (2001), pp. 21–28.

18. *State of the World's Vaccines and Immunisation* (Geneva: World Health Organization, 2002).

19. So enormous is the task that critics argue that GAVI is pushing ahead too fast, ignoring practical difficulties, such as poor staffing levels in countries where vaccines are being distributed, weak vaccine delivery networks, and inadequate means to store vaccines safely. See Ruairi Brugha et al., "GAVI, the First Steps," *The Lancet*, Vol. 359 (2002), pp. 435–438; and Sarah Boseley, "Charity Attacks Vaccine Alliance," *The Guardian*, January 16, 2002, p. 15.

## NOTES TO CHAPTER 7
## AN AUTOPSY OF DR. OSLER

1. Harvey Cushing, *Life of Sir William Osler* (Clarendon Press, 1925), Vol. 1, pp. 264–266, and Vol. 2, p. 666. This biography won a Pulitzer Prize in 1926.

2. Oxford University Press, 2000.

3. Appleton, 1892.

4. Osler's "Pathological Report of the Montreal General Hospital for the Year Ending May 1st, 1877," was praised in *The Lancet* of June 22, 1878, as "a careful and elaborate analysis... which will bear comparison with any similar report published in the mother country."

5. William Osler, "On the Brains of Criminals, with a Description of the Brains of Two Murderers," *Canada Medical & Surgical Journal*, February 1882, pp. 385–398.

6. The spectacle provoked wry disapproval of the American public scene by some correspondents. An anonymous New York reporter took pleasure in noting that "as many of the medical journals were to point out, the Americans are somewhat deficient in a sense of humour when they themselves are directly concerned" (*The Lancet*, March 25, 1905, p. 829).

7. W. Bruce Fye, "William Osler's Departure from North America," *New England Journal of Medicine*, Vol. 320 (1989), pp. 1425–1431. Fye concludes that in Oxford "the pace was slower, and he had more time for his son and his historical and literary interests."

8. Bliss misleadingly quotes only part of what Osler has to say about the struggle for acceptance of a new finding—"We are better prepared today"—leaving the impression that he was optimistic about the future "growth of

truth." In fact, Osler goes on to comment:

> We may have become more plastic and receptive, but I doubt it; even our generation—that great generation of the last quarter of the nineteenth century—had a practical demonstration of the slowness of the acceptation of an obvious truth in the long fight for the aseptic treatment of wounds. ... [It was] a long and grievous battle, as many of us well know who had to contend in hospitals with the opposition of men who could not—not who would not—see the truth.

9. *The Lancet*, October 9, 1915, pp. 795–801.

10. Sherwin B. Nuland, "The Saint," *The New Republic*, December 13, 1999, pp. 27–33.

11. "The Osler Magic Revisited," *Nature*, Vol. 403 (2000), pp. 249–250.

12. The most recent piece of hagiography, which concluded that "Osler is the quintessential physician of our time because of his literary legacy, scientific and clinical accomplishments, educational contributions, and influence on intraprofessional relationships," was published, unadorned by critical reflection, in *JAMA*, Vol. 282 (December 15, 1999), pp. 2252–2258.

13. Norman B. Gwyn, "The Letters of a Devoted Father to an Unresponsive Son," *Bulletin of the History of Medicine*, Vol. 7 (1939), pp. 335–351.

## NOTES TO CHAPTER 8
## TRUTH AND HERESY ABOUT AIDS

1. Regnery, 1996.

2. "À Duesberg, Adieu," *Nature*, Vol. 380 (1996), pp. 293–294.

3. North Atlantic, 1996.

4. Kluwer Academic, 1996.

5. *The Molecular Biology of HIV/AIDS* (Wiley, 1996), pp. 22, 53, 57, respectively.

6. William A. Paxton et al., "Relative Resistance to HIV-1 Infection of CD4 Lymphocytes from Persons Who Remain Uninfected Despite Multiple High-Risk Sexual Exposures," *Nature Medicine*, Vol. 2 (1996), pp. 412–417.

7. Perhaps the best evidence that HIV is sufficient by itself to cause AIDS came from the elimination of virus-infected blood from the US transfusion service. Screening of blood for HIV began in 1985. By 1995, Eve Lackritz

estimated that no more than twenty-seven blood donations out of 12 million annually were infected with HIV. The exclusion of HIV from the blood supply was accompanied by the removal of HIV disease from the recipients of blood. See Eve M. Lackritz et al., "Estimated Risk of Transmission of the HIV by Screened Blood in the US," *New England Journal of Medicine*, Vol. 333 (1995), pp. 1721–1725.

8. Jon Cohen, "Controversy: Is KS Really Caused by New Herpes-virus?," *Science*, Vol. 268 (1995), pp. 1847–1848.

9. Lever, *The Molecular Biology of HIV/AIDS*, p. 98.

10. Sarah C. Darby et al., "Mortality Before and After HIV Infection in the Complete UK Population of Haemophiliacs," *Nature*, Volume 377 (1995), pp. 79–82.

11. Martin T. Schechter et al., "HIV-1 and the Aetiology of AIDS," *The Lancet*, Vol. 341 (1993), pp. 658–659.

12. "Time to Hit HIV, Early and Hard," *New England Journal of Medicine*, Vol. 333 (1995), pp. 450–451.

13. Matthias Egger et al., "Prognosis of HIV-1-Infected Patients Starting Highly Active Antiretroviral Therapy," *The Lancet*, Vol. 360 (2002), pp. 119–129.

14. Paul Cotton, "Many Clues, Few Conclusions on AIDS," *JAMA*, Vol. 272 (1994), pp. 753–756.

15. The observation that a chimpanzee developed AIDS ten years after being inoculated with HIV raised the prospect that vaccines may be testable in laboratory animal models. See Lawrence K. Altman, "Infected with Human Virus, a Chimpanzee Develops AIDS," *The New York Times*, January 31, 1996, p. A14.

16. "Has Duesberg a Right of Reply?," *Nature*, Vol. 363 (1993), p. 109.

17. Maddox wrote, somewhat tendentiously, that Duesberg's reply "will be eagerly awaited and will be published with the usual provisos—that it is not libelous or needlessly rude, that it pertains to the new results and that it should not be longer than it needs to be."

18. Patricia A. Yusingco, editorial, *American Journal of Continuing Education in Nursing*, No. 7 (1995), p. 1. *Science* also conducted its own investigation into Duesberg's beliefs, giving arguments for and against his views. See Jon Cohen, "The Duesberg Phenomenon," *Science*, Vol. 266 (1994), pp. 1642–1644.

19. *Practices of Freedom: Selected Writings on HIV/AIDS* (Duke, 1994), pp. 244–245.

20. "The Unbeliever," *The New York Times Book Review*, April 7, 1996, pp. 8–9.

21. *The Gravest Show on Earth: America in the Age of* AIDS (Houghton Mifflin, 1995), p. 60ff.

22. Concorde Coordinating Committee, "CONCORDE: MRC/ARNS Randomised Double-blind Controlled Trial of Immediate and Deferred Zidovudine in Symptom-Free HIV Infection," *The Lancet*, Vol. 343 (1994), pp. 871–881.

23. *Quantification and the Quest for Medical Certainty* (Princeton University Press, 1995).

24. Edward H. Ahrens Jr., *The Crisis in Clinical Research: Overcoming Institutional Obstacles* (Oxford University Press, 1992).

25. Editorial, "Evidence-Based Medicine, in Its Place," *The Lancet*, Vol. 346 (1995), p. 785.

26. "More Conviction on HIV and AIDS," *Nature*, Vol. 337 (1995), p. 1.

27. Michael S. Ascher et al., "Paradox Remains," *Nature*, Vol. 375 (1995), p. 196.

28. "Researchers Air Alternative Views on How HIV Kills Cells," *Science*, Vol. 269 (1995), pp. 1044–1045.

29. J. Marx, "Debate Surges over the Origins of Genomic Defects in Cancer," *Science*, Vol. 297 (2002), pp. 544–546.

30. Serge Lang, *Challenges* (Springer, 1998).

31. See David Gisselquist et al., "Let It Be Sexual: How Health Care Transmission of AIDS in Africa Was Ignored," *International Journal of* STD *and* AIDS, Vol. 14 (2003), pp. 148–161. Subsequent work has shown that Gisselquist's case is weak, although Polly Walker and her colleagues agree that "it is important to highlight the issue of pathogen transmission by unsafe injection." See Polly R. Walker et al., "Sexual Transmission of HIV in Africa," *Nature*, Vol. 422 (2003), p. 679.

## NOTES TO CHAPTER 9
## A FATAL EROSION OF INTEGRITY

1. The documents from which I have extracted quotations can be found on the FDA's Web site, www.fda.gov.

2. Perseus, 2001.

3. G.F. Somers, "Pharmacological Properties of Thalidomide, a New

Sedative Hypnotic Drug," *British Journal of Pharmacology*, Vol. 15 (1960), pp. 111–116.

4. Editorial, "Thalidomide Neuropathy," *British Medical Journal*, September 30, 1961, pp. 876–877.

5. Thalidomide was not withdrawn so quickly elsewhere. In Canada, for example, thalidomide remained available until March 1962, and in Japan until May 1962.

6. "Thalidomide and Congenital Abnormalities," *The Lancet*, December 16, 1961, p. 1358. As the current editor of *The Lancet*, I should declare a potential conflict here. McBride has alleged, and Stephens and Brynner repeat his claim, that *The Lancet* rejected an earlier paper, submitted in June 1961, describing the link between thalidomide and birth defects. To my knowledge, there is no record of this submission, and McBride has never produced any evidence to back his claim. If what he says is true, however, Stephens and Brynner are right to caution that "had such a paper been published in July 1961, much suffering would have been prevented." In the original version of this essay, I invited McBride to submit a copy of this letter of rejection to *The New York Review* for independent verification. On August 7, 2002, he wrote to me listing many inaccuracies in *Dark Remedy*. For example, he claimed that Lenz had conceded that it was McBride who was the first to link thalidomide with malformations. He alleged that the legal costs of the complaints unit that sought his exclusion from medical practice in 1989 were paid, in part, by a drug company that presumably saw him as an irritant that needed to be removed. As for the rejection letter, he told me that he had not kept a copy—"being rejected is not something that cheers me," he wrote.

7. In 1993, McBride was found guilty of scientific fraud in a case unrelated to his work on thalidomide. He was barred from medical practice, only returning to the Australian medical registry in 1998. Stephens and Brynner call McBride's later career "a study in hubris." He was continuing to publish papers on thalidomide up to 2003, when he sadly suffered a brain hemorrhage at age seventy-five.

8. "Thalidomide and Congenital Abnormalities," *The Lancet*, April 28, 1962, pp. 912–913.

9. Quoted in Elizabeth Whatley, "Thalidomide-Damaged Babies," *The Lancet*, July 7, 1962, p. 46.

10. "Thalidomide and Congenital Abnormalities," *The Lancet*, March 31, 1962, p. 691. A later editorial, entitled "Another Chance for Thalidomide?,"

argued that the drug should not be "relegated to the 'lumber room of medical history'" (see *The Lancet*, November 20, 1965, p. 1059).

11. Signature, 2001.

12. Trent D. Stephens and Bradley J. Fillmore, "Thalidomide Embryopathy—Proposed Mechanism of Action," *Teratology*, Vol. 61 (2000), pp. 189–195.

13. Robert J. D'Amato et al., "Thalidomide Is an Inhibitor of Angiogenesis," *Proceedings of the National Academy of Sciences USA*, April 1994, pp. 4082–4085.

14. Seema Singhal et al., "Antitumor Activity of Thalidomide in Refractory Multiple Myeloma," *New England Journal of Medicine*, Vol. 341 (1999), pp. 1565–1571. The efficacy of thalidomide for patients newly diagnosed with multiple myeloma has now been established. The results were reported in the *Journal of Clinical Oncology*, November 1, 2002.

15. "Thalidomide Update: Regulatory Aspects," *Teratology*, Vol. 38 (1998), pp. 221–226.

16. Michael Camilleri et al., "Efficacy and Safety of Alosetron in Women with Irritable Bowel Syndrome," *The Lancet*, Vol. 355 (2000), pp. 1035–1040. This study was later criticized by Ralph Nader's Public Citizen Health Research Group as exaggerated, misleading, and in danger of causing overprescription.

17. Drummond Rennie, "Thyroid Storm," *JAMA*, Vol. 277 (1997), pp. 1238–1243; and Catherine DeAngelis, "Conflict of Interest and the Public Trust," *JAMA*, Vol. 284 (2000), pp. 2237–2238.

18. Elizabeth A. Boyd and Lisa A. Bero, "Assessing Faculty Financial Relationships with Industry," *JAMA*, Vol. 284 (2000), pp. 2209–2214.

19. Henry Thomas Stelfox et al., "Conflict of Interest in the Debate over Calcium-Channel Antagonists," *New England Journal of Medicine*, Vol. 388 (1998), pp. 101–106.

## NOTES TO CHAPTER 10
## SECRET SOCIETY

1. Marie Boas Hall, *Henry Oldenburg: Shaping the Royal Society* (Oxford University Press, 2002).

2. *Philosophical Transactions*, Series B, Vol. 292 (1981), pp. 399–609.

3. Administrative beauty is, of course, in the eye of the skeptical beholder.

Richard Lewontin, in his review of National Research Council pronouncements about genetically modified organisms, called the National Academy of Sciences "a self-perpetuating body of the American scientific elite," which operates by "forced consensus." See his *It Ain't Necessarily So: The Dream of the Human Genome and Other Illusions* (New York Review Books, second edition, 2001).

4. House of Commons Science and Technology Committee, *Government Funding of the Scientific Learned Societies* (London: The Stationery Office, 2002).

5. Editor, "Editorial Note," *Nature*, Vol. 416 (2002), p. 600.

6. Matin Qaim and David Zilberman, "Yield Effects of Genetically Modified Crops in Developing Countries," *Science*, Vol. 299 (2003), pp. 900–902.

7. G. J. V. Nossal and Ross L. Coppel, *Reshaping Life: Key Issues in Genetic Engineering* (Cambridge University Press, 2002).

8. Lizette Alvarez, "As for Modified Foods, Europeans Just Say 'No,'" *International Herald Tribune*, February 11, 2003, p. 1.

9. John Crace, "Peer Trouble," *The Guardian*, February 11, 2003, G2, p. 12. See chapter 6 for a discussion of the MMR vaccine controversy. The Royal Society's more open approach to scientific controversy will be tested still further when the results of farm-scale evaluations of genetically modified crops are published in 2003 and 2004. Presently in the UK there is a ban on commercial planting of genetically modified crops. Only when the results of these farm-scale studies are available will the government consider lifting that ban. The first set of papers reporting the results of these environmental experiments has already been submitted to *Philosophical Transactions of the Royal Society*. When some or all of these papers are published, May has pledged to give details of how the work was peer-reviewed and judged, together with the conflicts of interest of reviewers. May is anxious to distance the Royal Society from the results of this work. The Royal Society's Web site notes that "the decision to accept a paper for publication . . . does not mean that the views expressed in it necessarily reflect those of the Council of the Royal Society." Defensiveness within the Royal Society flourishes three hundred years after Oldenburg. See Bob May, "Moment of Truth for GM Crops," *The Guardian*, April 10, 2003, p. 12.

## NOTES TO CHAPTER 11
## WORLD HEALTH DISORGANIZATION

1. Y. Al-Mazrou, S. Berkley, B. Bloom, et al., "A Vital Opportunity for Global Health: Supporting the World Health Organization at a Critical Juncture," *The Lancet*, Vol. 350 (1997), pp. 750–751.

2. G. Walt, "WHO Under Stress: Implications for Health Policy," *Health Policy*, Vol. 24 (1993), pp. 125–144; F. Godlee, "The World Health Organization: WHO in Crisis," *British Medical Journal*, Vol. 309 (1994), pp. 1424–1428; and A. Lucas, "WHO at Country Level," *The Lancet*, Vol. 351 (1998), pp. 743–747.

3. World Health Organization, *World Health Report 2000: Health Systems—Improving Performance* (Geneva: World Health Organization, 2000).

4. *Macroeconomics and Health: Investing in Health for Economic Development* (Geneva: World Health Organization, 2001).

5. P. Farmer, F. Leandre, J.S. Mukherjee, et al., "Community-Based Approaches to HIV Treatment in Resource-Poor Settings," *The Lancet*, Vol. 358 (2001), pp. 404–409; and A.D. Harries, D.S. Nyangulu, N.J. Hargreaves, O. Kaluwa, and F.M. Salaniponi, "Preventing Antiretroviral Anarchy in Sub-Saharan Africa," *The Lancet*, Vol. 358 (2001), pp. 410–414.

6. J.D. Quick, "Partnerships Need Principles," *Bulletin of the World Health Organization*, Vol. 79 (2001), p. 776; and "Maintaining the Integrity of the Clinical Evidence Base," *Bulletin of the World Health Organization*, Vol. 79 (2001), p. 1093.

7. Bill Clinton, "World Without Walls," *The Guardian*, January 26, 2002, p. 1.

8. J. Frenk and F. Knaul, "Health and the Economy: Empowerment Through Evidence," *Bulletin of the World Health Organization*, Vol. 80 (2002), p. 88.

9. R.F. Brugha, M. Starling, and G. Walt, "GAVI, the First Steps: Lessons for the Global Fund," *The Lancet*, Vol. 359 (2002), pp. 435–440.

10. S. Boseley, "Unhealthy Influence: There Is a Danger that WHO's New Partnership with Drug Companies Will Skew Its Health Policies," *The Guardian*, February 6, 2002, p. 18.

11. C. Kapp, "UN Inspectorate Gives WHO Administration a Mixed Review," *The Lancet*, Vol. 359 (2002), p. 329.

12. *World Health and World Politics* (University of South Carolina Press, 1995).

13. See chapter 5, "The African Challenge."

14. A. M. Pollock and D. Price, "Rewriting the Regulations: How the World Trade Organisation Could Accelerate Privatisation in Health-Care Systems," *The Lancet*, Vol. 356 (2000), pp. 1995–2000.

15. I owe many thanks to staff at WHO, especially those in the director-general's office, for allowing me to have almost unrestricted access to WHO employees, meetings, and documents. Also, I thank those *Lancet* advisers who provided me with valuable background on WHO's recent record.

16. For a review of the issues facing WHO over the next five to ten years, see my "WHO's Mandate: A Damaging Reinterpretation Is Taking Place," *The Lancet*, Vol. 360 (2002), pp. 960–961; and "WHO Cares?," *The Boston Globe*, January 19, 2003, p. D1. See also Richard Horton and Ariel Pablos-Mendez, "WHO's Next Director-General: The Person and the Programme," *The Lancet*, Vol. 360 (2002), pp. 1799–1800.

17. Robert E. Black et al., "How 10 Million Children Will Die This Year," *The Lancet* (2003, in press).

## NOTES TO CHAPTER 12
## HOW SICK IS MODERN MEDICINE?

1. Galen, "My Own Books," in *Selected Works*, translated by P. N. Singer (Oxford University Press, 1997), p. 8.

2. Carroll and Graf, 2000.

3. "Looking Back on the Millennium in Medicine," *New England Journal of Medicine*, Vol. 342 (2000), p. 42.

4. *The Greatest Benefit to Mankind* (HarperCollins, 1997), p. 12.

5. *The Alarming History of Medicine* (Mandarin, 1993), pp. 1–2.

6. *Medicine's 10 Greatest Discoveries* (Yale University Press, 1998), pp. 1, 37.

7. *Healing the Schism: Epidemiology, Medicine, and the Public's Health* (Springer-Verlag, 1991), p. xi.

8. *Morbidity and Mortality Weekly Report*, April 2, 1999, pp. 241–243.

9. "From Genotype to Phenotype: Genetics and Medical Practice in the New Millennium," *Philosophical Transactions of the Royal Society of London*, Vol. 354, B (1999), p. 2008.

10. Paul Lichtenstein et al., "Environmental and Heritable Factors in the

Causation of Cancer," *The New England Journal of Medicine*, Vol. 343 (2000), pp. 78–85.

11. June 23, 2000.

12. W. French Anderson, "The Best of Times, the Worst of Times," *Science*, Vol. 288 (2000), pp. 627–629.

13. Marina Cavazzana-Calvo et al., "Gene Therapy of Human Severe Combined Immunodeficiency (SCID)–X1 Disease," *Science*, Vol. 288 (2000), pp. 669–672. In 2003, gene therapy trials for SCID were halted around the world when two patients from France were reported to have developed leukemia during treatment. Unexpected risks and unintended consequences are likely to blight gene therapy programs for some years to come.

14. See, for example, James Le Fanu, "Scientists Who Should Carry a Health Warning," *The Sunday Telegraph*, July 9, 2000, p. 2.

15. Meir J. Stampfer et al., "Primary Prevention of Coronary Heart Disease in Women Through Diet and Lifestyle," *New England Journal of Medicine*, Vol. 343 (2000), p. 21.

16. Kennedy R. Lees et al., "Glycine Antagonist in Neuroprotection in Patients with Acute Stroke," *The Lancet*, Vol. 355 (2000), pp. 1949–1954.

17. Ash A. Alizadeh et al., "Distinct Types of Diffuse Large B-Cell Lymphoma Identified by Gene Expression Profiling," *Nature*, Vol. 403 (2000), pp. 503–511.

18. Carmen Perez-Casas, *HIV/AIDS Medicines Pricing Report* (Médecins Sans Frontières, 2000).

19. E. J. Meijers-Heijboer et al., "Presymptomatic DNA Testing and Prophylactic Surgery in Families with a BRCA1 or BRCA2 Mutation," *The Lancet*, Vol. 355 (2000), p. 2019.

20. Shanthimala de Silva et al., "Thalassaemia in Sri Lanka," *The Lancet*, Vol. 355 (2000), pp. 786–791.

21. H. Demiroglu, O. I. Ozcebe, I. Barista, S. Dundar, and B. Eldem, "Interferon Alfa-2b, Colchicine, and Benzathine Penicillin versus Colchicine and Benzathine Penicillin in Behçet's Disease," *The Lancet*, Vol. 355 (2000), pp. 605–609.

22. R. B. Weiss, G. G. Gill, and C. A. Hudis, "An On-Site Audit of the South African Trial of High-Dose Chemotherapy for Metastatic Breast Cancer and Associated Publications," *Journal of Clinical Oncology*, Vol. 19 (2001).

23. M. J. Brown, C. R. Palmer, A. Castaigne, et al., "Morbidity and Mortality in Patients Randomized to Double-Blind Treatment with a Long-Acting

Calcium-Channel Blocker or Diuretic in the International Nifedipine GITS Study," *The Lancet*, Vol. 356 (2000), pp. 366–372.

24. *Managing Allegations of Scientific Misconduct: A Guidance Document for Editors* (Washington: Office of Research Integrity, 2000).

25. C.R. Freed, P.E. Greene, R.E. Breeze, et al., "Transplantation of Embryonic Dopamine Neurons for Severe Parkinson's Disease," *New England Journal of Medicine*, Vol. 344 (2001), pp. 710–719.

26. S. Petit-Zeman, "Trial and Error," *The Guardian*, March 15, 2001, pp. 14–15.

27. L. Rogers, "Pumped Back to Life," *The Sunday Times*, September 3, 2000, p. 14.

28. "Uneasy Alliance: Clinical Investigators and the Pharmaceutical Industry," *New England Journal of Medicine*, Vol. 342 (2000), pp. 1539–1544.

29. "Is Academic Medicine for Sale?," *New England Journal of Medicine*, Vol. 342 (2000), pp. 1516–1518.

30. "Discussion Sections in Reports of Controlled Trials Published in General Medical Journals," *JAMA*, Vol. 280 (1998), pp. 280–282.

31. R. Horton, "The Grammar of Interpretive Medicine," *CMAJ*, Vol. 159 (1998), pp. 245–249.

32. R. Horton, "The Unstable Medical Research Paper," *Journal of Clinical Epidemiology*, Vol. 50 (1997), pp. 981–986.

33. R. Horton, "The Rhetoric of Research," *British Medical Journal*, Vol. 310 (1995), pp. 985–988.

34. R. Horton, "Common Sense and Figures: The Rhetoric of Validity in Medicine," *Statistical Medicine*, Vol. 19 (2000), pp. 3149–3164.

35. David J. Rothman, "The Shame of Medical Research," *The New York Review*, November 30, 2000, pp. 60–64.

36. "Protecting Research Subjects—What Must Be Done," *New England Journal of Medicine*, Vol. 343 (2000), pp. 808–810.

37. Washington, D.C.: Institute of Medicine, 2001.

38. W.J. Burman, R.R. Reeves, D.L. Cohn, and R.T. Schooley, "Breaking the Camel's Back: Multicenter Clinical Trials and Local IRBs," *Annals of Internal Medicine*, Vol. 134 (2001), pp. 152–157.

39. "It's Official: Evaluative Research Must Become Part of Routine Care in the NHS," *Journal of the Royal Society of Medicine*, Vol. 93 (2000), pp. 555–556.

40. C. Langley, S. Gray, S. Selley, C. Bowie, and C. Price, "Clinicians'

Attitudes to Recruitment to Randomized Trials in Cancer Care," *Journal of Health Services Research & Policy*, Vol. 5 (2000), pp. 164–169.

41. D. Dazzi, B. Agnetti, L. Bandini, et al., "What Do the People Think (and Know) about Informed Consent for Participation in a Medical Trial," *Archives of Internal Medicine*, Vol. 161 (2001), pp. 768–769. These findings were recently reinforced in surveys of patients who took part in a large clinical trial. Fewer than one in five participants in the trial read the patient information sheet before giving their consent. This information was written at a level that required a high school education; but, again, only one in five patients had been educated beyond secondary school. The investigators who did this work concluded, rather bluntly, that the consent process "was inappropriate for the needs of most patients." This study is probably typical of most research projects in medicine. See Barbara F. Williams et al., "Informed Consent During the Clinical Emergency of Acute Myocardial Infarction," *The Lancet*, Vol. 361 (2003), pp. 918–922.

## NOTES TO CHAPTER 13
## DNA: THE LIFE OF A DEAD MOLECULE

1. "Molecular Structure of Nucleic Acids," *Nature*, Vol. 171 (1953).

2. "The Human Genome," *Nature*, Vol. 409 (2001).

3. University of Chicago Press, 1997.

4. J. C. Venter et al., "The Sequence of the Human Genome," *Science*, Vol. 291 (2001).

5. *The Triple Helix: Gene, Organism, and Environment* (Harvard University Press, 2000).

6. *The Language of the Genes* (London: HarperCollins, 1993).

7. *Consilience: The Unity of Knowledge* (Knopf, 1998).

8. Roland Heilig et al., "The DNA Sequence and Analysis of Human Chromosome 14," *Nature*, Vol. 421 (2003), pp. 601–607.

9. *Perversions: Psychodynamics and Therapy*, edited by Sandor Lorand and Michael Balint (Ortolan Press, 1965; first edition, Random House, 1956), p. 75.

10. Quoted in Kenneth Lewes, *The Psychoanalytic Theory of Male Homosexuality* (Simon and Schuster, 1988), p. 188.

11. *Sexual Deviation in American Society* (College and University Press,

1967), p. 146.

12. Karen de Witt, "Quayle Contends Homosexuality Is a Matter of Choice, Not Biology," *The New York Times*, September 14, 1992, p. A17.

13. Larry Thompson, "Search for a Gay Gene," *Time*, June 12, 1995, pp. 60–61.

14. "Misexpression of the White (*w*) Gene Triggers Male-Male Courtship in *Drosophila*," *Proceedings of the National Academy of Sciences, USA*, Vol. 92 (1995), pp. 5525–5529.

15. "A Difference in Hypothalamic Structure Between Heterosexual and Homosexual Men," *Science*, Vol. 253 (1991), pp. 1034–1037.

16. The suprachiasmatic nucleus, also located in the hypothalamus, is larger in homosexual men than in either heterosexual men or women. The anterior commissure of the corpus callosum (a band of tissue that connects the right and left hemispheres of the brain) is also larger in gay men.

17. MIT Press/A Bradford Book, 1995.

18. Dean H. Hamer et al., "A Linkage Between DNA Markers on the X Chromosome and Male Sexual Orientation," *Science*, Vol. 261 (1993), pp. 321–327.

19. The normal complement of human chromosomes is forty-six per individual, two of which are designated sex chromosomes. In the male, the sex chromosomal makeup is XY, while in the female it is XX. If a gene for homosexuality (Xh) was transmitted through the maternal line, one can see how the subsequent offspring would be affected.

| | X | Xh |
|---|---|---|
| X | XX | XXh |
| Y | XY | XhY |

Suppose the unaffected female carrier for homosexuality (XXh) produced offspring with a non-Xh male (XY). Half of all female children would be carriers of Xh (like their mothers), while half of all male offspring would carry Xh unopposed by another X. The Xh trait—homosexuality—would then be able to express itself.

20. By chance, one would expect each pair of brothers to share half their DNA. So, assuming that there was no gene for homosexuality, one would expect twenty of the forty pairs of brothers to share the X chromosome marker.

21. Simon and Schuster, 1995.

22. LeVay completed a second book in collaboration with Elisabeth

Nonas—*City of Friends*—that surveys gay and lesbian culture. He also wrote *Queer Science*, a study of how scientific research has affected the lives of gays and lesbians.

23. "Genetics and Male Sexual Orientation," *Science*, Vol. 261 (1993), p. 1257.

24. For example, David Weatherall notes that "these findings should not surprise us. Almost every condition . . . reveals a complex mixture of nature and nurture." See his *Science and the Quiet Art* (Norton, 1995), p. 287.

25. R. C. Lewontin, S. Rose, and L. J. Kamin, *Not in Our Genes* (Pantheon, 1984).

26. Lewontin is not a total skeptic about the importance of molecular genetics research in medicine. For instance, he accepts "that some fraction of cancers arise on a background of genetic predisposition." See R. C. Lewontin, "The Dream of the Human Genome," *The New York Review*, May 28, 1992, pp. 31–40.

27. M. W. Feldman and R. C. Lewontin, "The Heritability Hang-up," *Science*, Vol. 190 (1975), pp. 1163–1168.

28. Robert Plomin, "The Role of Inheritance in Behavior," *Science*, Vol. 248 (1990), pp. 183–188.

29. "The Analysis of Variance and the Analysis of Causes," *The American Journal of Human Genetics*, Vol. 26 (1974), pp. 400–411.

30. For example, in a UK study (see Anne M. Johnson, "Sexual Lifestyles and HIV Risks," *Nature*, Vol. 360 (1992), pp. 410–412), although only 1.4 percent of men reported a male partner during the past five years, 6.1 percent of men reported having some same-gender experience.

31. *Sexual Life: A Clinician's Guide* (Plenum, 1992). The Kinsey scale has seven levels ranging from exclusively heterosexual (0) to exclusively gay (6). Hamer applied this scale to four aspects of sexuality: self-identification, attraction, fantasy, and behavior.

32. "The Five Sexes: Why Male and Female Are Not Enough," *The Sciences*, Vol. 33 (1993), pp. 20–24.

33. *The History of Sexuality*, Vols. One and Two (Vintage, 1990).

34. Dr. K. F. O. Westphal became the first modern author to publish an account of what he described as a "contrary sexual feeling" (*Die conträre Sexualempfindung*), although the word "homosexual" was first used in a private letter written by Karl Maria Kertbeny on May 6, 1868. This linguistic history is described in detail by Jonathan Katz (see note 35).

35. *The Invention of Heterosexuality* (Dutton, 1995).

36. Lewontin, "The Analysis of Variance and the Analysis of Causes," pp. 400–411.

37. Plomin, "The Role of Inheritance in Behavior."

38. Stella Hu et al., "Linkage Between Sexual Orientation and Chromosome Xq28 in Males but Not in Females," *Nature Genetics*, Vol. 11 (1995), pp. 248–256.

39. George Rice et al., "Male Homosexuality: Absence of Linkage to Microsatellite Markers at Xq28," *Science*, Vol. 284 (1999), pp. 665–667.

40. Gina Kolata, "Tests to Assess Risks for Cancer Raising Questions," *The New York Times*, March 27, 1995, p. A1.

41. "NIMH's Cowdry Defends Institute's Research Against Appropriations Committee, Watchdog Group Criticism," *The Blue Sheet*, March 29, 1995, pp. 5–6.

42. Hamer's position at NIH came under serious threat in 1995. One of his colleagues accused him of biased data collection, a practice that, if true, would have given him a much better chance of discovering a genetic link to homosexuality. A two-year investigation by the US Office of Research Integrity drew a blank. See Jocelyn Kaiser, "No Misconduct in 'Gay Gene' Study," *Science*, Vol. 275 (1997), p. 1251. In 1998, Hamer and Peter Copeland published *Living with Our Genes* (Doubleday). Here they argued "that many of the differences between individual personality styles are the result of differences in genes.... You have about as much choice in some aspects of your personality as you do in the shape of your nose or the size of your feet." Despite the refutation of his Xq28 study, Hamer continued to believe that "genes are the single most important factor that distinguishes one person from another." Indeed, Hamer seems defiant. He believes that the "evidence is compelling that there is some gene or genes at Xq28 related to male sexual orientation."

43. Scott M. Hammond et al., "Post-Transcriptional Gene Silencing by Double Stranded RNA," *Nature Reviews Genetics*, Vol. 2 (2001), pp. 110–119.

44. Michael T. McManus and Philip A. Sharp, "Gene Silencing in Mammals by Small Interfering RNAs," *Nature Reviews Genetics*, Vol. 3 (2002), pp. 737–747.

45. Erwei Song et al., "RNA Interference Targeting Fas Protects Mice from Fulminant Hepatitis," *Nature Medicine* (Advanced Online Publication, February 10, 2003), pp. 1–5.

## NOTE TO CHAPTER 14
## PROTECTING THE BREAST

1. Johns Hopkins University Press, 2002.

## NOTES TO CHAPTER 15
## THE FINAL CUT

1. Nalini Ambady et al., "Surgeons' Tone of Voice: A Clue to Malpractice History," *Surgery*, Vol. 132 (2002), pp. 5–9.

2. *Blood and Guts* (Norton, 2003). Porter died in March 2002.

3. Metropolitan Books, 2002.

4. J. Paul Leigh et al., "Physician Career Satisfaction Across Specialties," *Archives of Internal Medicine*, Vol. 162 (2002), pp. 1577–1584.

5. "Our Heritage and Our Future," *Journal of Thoracic and Cardiovascular Surgery*, Vol. 124 (2002), pp. 649–654.

6. "Surgery...Is It an Impairing Profession?," *Journal of the American College of Surgeons*, Vol. 194 (2002), pp. 352–366.

7. "The Fivefold Root of an Ethics of Surgery," *Bioethics*, Vol. 16 (2002), pp. 183–201.

8. Selami Dogan et al., "Totally Endoscopic Coronary Artery Bypass Grafting on Cardiopulmonary Bypass with Robotically Enhanced Telemanipulation," *Journal of Thoracic and Cardiovascular Surgery*, Vol. 123 (2002), pp. 1125–1131.

9. Richard Horton, "Surgical Research or Comic Opera: Questions, but Few Answers," *The Lancet*, Vol. 347 (1996), pp. 984–985.

10. R. C. G. Russell, "Surgical Research," *The Lancet*, Vol. 347 (1996), p. 1480.

11. H. Obertop and C. J. H. Van de Velde, "One Hundred Years of Surgical Science Behind the Dikes," *British Journal of Surgery*, Vol. 89 (2002), pp. 673–675.

12. R. H. Stables et al., "Coronary Artery Bypass Surgery versus Percutaneous Coronary Intervention with Stent Implantation in Patients with Multivessel Coronary Artery Disease," *The Lancet*, Vol. 360 (2002), pp. 965–970.

13. Ronald K. Tompkins et al., "Internationalization of General Surgical Journals," *Archives of Surgery*, Vol. 136 (2001), pp. 1342–1345.

14. Mohit Bhandari et al., "The Quality of Reporting of Randomised Trials in the *Journal of Bone and Joint Surgery* from 1998 through 2000," *Journal of Bone and Joint Surgery*, Vol. 84-A (2002), pp. 388–396.

15. Peter McCulloch et al., "Randomised Trials in Surgery: Problems and Possible Solutions," *British Medical Journal*, Vol. 324 (2002), pp. 1448–1451.

16. Michael J. Mack and Francis G. Duhaylongsod, "Through the Open Door! Where Has This Ride Taken Us?," *Journal of Thoracic and Cardiovascular Surgery*, Vol. 124 (2002), pp. 655–659.

17. Sorway W. Chan et al., "Technical Development and a Team Approach Leads to an Improved Outcome," *Australia and New Zealand Journal of Surgery*, Vol. 72 (2002), pp. 523–527.

18. Bruce E. Keogh and Robin Kingsman, "National Adult Cardiac Surgical Database Report 2000–2001" (Dendrite Clinical Systems, 2002).

19. Anders Franco-Cereceda et al., "Partial Left Ventriculotomy for Dilated Cardiomyopathy: Is This an Alternative to Transplantation?," *Journal of Thoracic and Cardiovascular Surgery*, Vol. 121 (2001), pp. 879–893.

20. "A Bypass for the Institutional Review Board: Reflections on the Cleveland Clinic Study of the Batista Operation," *Journal of Thoracic and Cardiovascular Surgery*, Vol. 121 (2001), pp. 837–839.

21. *The Puzzle People: Memoirs of a Transplant Surgeon* (University of Pittsburgh Press, 1992).

22. Angelique M. Reitsma and Jonathan D. Moreno, "Ethical Regulations for Innovative Surgery: The Last Frontier?," *Journal of the American College of Physicians*, Vol. 194 (2002), pp. 792–801.

## NOTES TO CHAPTER 16
## IN THE DANGER ZONE

1. University of California Press, 2000.

2. Murray conveys this drama by repeatedly using war metaphors. The trauma service is "battle-ready"; despite considerable efforts, his team had "not won the war"; the ICU gets "bombed" with new admissions; a treatment plan is a "full-bore attack"; and antibiotics are "broad firepower" or "big guns." These commonly used images do give a sense of the sometimes desperate atmosphere of an ICU. They also show, perhaps, the swashbuckling approach doctors take to this most acute of medical specialties.

3. New Directions, 1984.

4. Both Harcourt Brace, 1996. A new selection of Selzer's medical essays, including two new pieces, has recently been published (*The Doctor Stories*, Picador, 1998). The book contains Selzer's own account of his literary development as a doctor.

5. University of California Press, 1999.

6. Kathryn Montgomery Hunter, *Doctors' Stories: The Narrative Structure of Medical Knowledge* (Princeton University Press, 1991); and *Narrative-Based Medicine*, edited by Trisha Greenhalgh and Brian Hurwitz (BMJ Books, 1998). The journal *Literature and Medicine*, published semiannually, aims to report original research in the medical humanities.

7. *Textbook of Respiratory Medicine* (W. B. Saunders, 1994). Intriguingly, Murray's literary interests are apparent in this treatise. Murray's wife is the writer Diane Johnson, and she, together with Judy Nadel, wrote in a foreword that the work of textbook authors "had much similarity to a work of fiction," since "their idea was of course to bring order and reassurance to the turbulent field of pulmonary medicine, rather as a novelist attempts to bring meaningful order to the chaotic events of reality." I doubt that any fearsome three-thousand-page, two-volume medical textbook has ever received such a generous introduction.

8. "Deconstructing the Black Box Known as the Intensive Care Unit," *Critical Care Medicine*, Vol. 26 (1998), pp. 1300–1301.

9. A breach in the scientistic approach to medical futility was perhaps best expressed in a report from the American Medical Association last year. See "Medical Futility in End-of-Life Care," *JAMA*, Vol. 281 (1999), pp. 937–941.

10. "On the Fear of Death," in *Selected Writings* (Penguin, 1982).

11. And not only doctors. In a recent study, two thirds of sampled US medical students supported legalization of physician-assisted suicide and over half said that "they might be willing to assist a patient by writing a lethal prescription." See Richard S. Mangus et al., "Medical Students' Attitudes Toward Physician-Assisted Suicide," *JAMA*, Vol. 282 (1999), pp. 2080–2081.

12. Linda Ganzini et al., "Physicians' Experiences with the Oregon Death with Dignity Act," *New England Journal of Medicine*, Vol. 342 (2000), pp. 557–563.

13. Ronald Dworkin has been the most persuasive critic of those of us who might cling to these distinctions. See Ronald Dworkin et al., "Assisted

Suicide: The Philosophers' Brief," *The New York Review*, March 27, 1997, pp. 41–47.

14. Thomas J. Prendergast et al., "A National Survey of End-of-Life Care for Critically Ill Patients," *American Journal of Respiratory and Critical Care Medicine*, Vol. 158 (1998), pp. 1163–1167.

15. Murray and Nadel's textbook is an unusual exception, since they include a chapter on "Ethics and Withdrawal of Life Support."

16. Marion Danis et al., "Incorporating Palliative Care into Critical Care Education: Principles, Challenges, and Opportunities," *Critical Care Medicine*, Vol. 27 (1999), pp. 2005– 2013.

17. Peter A. Singer et al., "Quality End-of-Life Care: Patients' Perspectives," *JAMA*, Vol. 281 (1999), pp. 163–168.

18. Johanna H. Groenewoud et al., "Clinical Problems with the Performance of Euthanasia and Physician-Assisted Suicide in the Netherlands," *New England Journal of Medicine*, Vol. 342 (2000), pp. 551–556.

19. See Katrina Hedberg et al., "Five Years of Legal Physician-Assisted Suicide in Oregon," *New England Journal of Medicine*, Vol. 348 (2003), pp. 961–964.

20. Ganzini et al., "Physicians' Experiences with the Oregon Death with Dignity Act."

21. Mangus et al., "Medical Students' Attitudes Toward Physician-Assisted Suicide."

22. "Existential Issues in Palliative Care," *Journal of Palliative Care*, Vol. 16 (2000), pp. 20–24.

## NOTES TO CHAPTER 17
## THE HEALTH OF PEOPLES

1. www.tanzania.go.tz/vision.htm.

2. www.tanzania.go.tz/.

3. National Sentinel Surveillance System, Working Paper No. 2: "Poverty Reduction Strategy Indicators Produced Using NSS/AMMP Data for 1998–2000" (November 2001).

4. National Sentinel Surveillance System, Working Paper No. 4: "Setting Priorities in Health Care: Use of Diverse Information Perspectives at the District Level in Tanzania" (October 2002).

5. *National Mortality Burden Estimates for 2001* (Ministry of Health, United Republic of Tanzania, 2002).

6. "Health Systems: Improving Performance," *World Health Report 2000* (Geneva: World Health Organization, 2000).

7. Editorial, "Why Rank Countries by Health Performance," *The Lancet*, Vol. 357 (2001), p. 1633.

8. B.M. Kleczkowski, M.I. Roemer, and A. Van Der Werff, "National Health Systems and Their Reorientation Towards Health for All," Public Health Papers, No. 77 (Geneva: World Health Organization, 1984).

9. M.I. Roemer, *National Health Systems of the World*, Vols. One and Two (Oxford University Press, 1991).

10. R.H. Elling defined five types of health systems (and nation-state) from the perspective of labor organization, from capitalist to socialist. See his "Theory and Method for the Cross-national Study of Health Systems," *International Journal of Health Services*, Vol. 24 (1994), pp. 285–309. M. Terris divided the world's systems of medical care into those with national health services, national health insurance schemes, and market-oriented systems. See his "The Three World Systems of Medical Care: Trends and Prospects," *American Journal of Public Health*, Vol. 68 (1978), pp. 1125–1131.

11. "A Framework for the Study of National Health Systems," *Inquiry*, Vol. 12 (2 suppl.) (1975), pp. 10–24.

12. G. Yamey, "Interview with Gro Brundtland," *British Medical Journal*, Vol. 325 (2002), pp. 1355–1361.

13. V. Navarro, "Assessment of the *World Health Report 2000*," *The Lancet*, Vol. 356 (2000), pp. 1598–1601; C. Almeida, P. Braveman, M.R. Gold, et al., "Methodological Concerns and Recommendations on Policy Consequences of the *World Health Report 2000*," *The Lancet*, Vol. 357 (2001), pp. 1692–1697; P. Braveman, B. Starfield, and M.J. Geiger, "*World Health Report 2000*: How It Removes Equity from the Agenda for Public Health Monitoring and Policy," *British Medical Journal*, Vol. 323 (2001), pp. 678–681.

14. R.P. Shaw, "*World Health Report 2000* 'Financial Fairness Indicator': Useful Compass or Crystal Ball?," *International Journal of Health Services*, Vol. 32 (2002), pp. 195–203.

15. "Reflections on and Alternatives to WHO's Fairness of Financial Contribution Index," *Health Economics*, Vol. 11 (2002), pp. 103–115.

16. N. Daniels, J. Bryant, R.A. Castano, O.G. Dantes, K.S. Khan, and S. Pannarunothai, *Bulletin of the World Health Organization*, Vol. 78 (2000),

pp. 740–750.

17. R.L. Caplan, D.W. Light, and N. Daniels, "Benchmarks of Fairness: A Moral Framework for Assessing Equity," *International Journal of Health Services*, Vol. 29 (1999), pp. 853–869.

18. Michael Howard, *The Invention of Peace: Reflections on War and International Order* (Yale University Press, 2000).

19. V. Navarro and L. Shi, "The Political Context of Social Inequalities and Health," *Social Science and Medicine*, Vol. 52 (2001), pp. 481–491.

20. J. Frenk and O. Gomez-Dantes, "Globalisation and the Challenges to Health Systems," *British Medical Journal*, Vol. 325 (2002), pp. 95–97.

21. "A Framework for Assessing the Performance of Health Systems," *Bulletin of the World Health Organization*, Vol. 78 (2000), pp. 717–731.

22. R.B. Saltman and O. Ferroussier-Davis, "The Concept of Stewardship in Health Policy," *Bulletin of the World Health Organization*, Vol. 78 (2000), pp. 732–739.

23. *The Law of Peoples* (Harvard University Press, 1999).

24. R. Watson, "'Big Bang' to Reunite Europe in 25-State Nation," *The Times*, December 12, 2002, p. 20.

25. R.I. Spiers, "The United States Was Admired and Respected," *International Herald Tribune*, December 13, 2002, p. 8.

26. Harvard University Press, 1971.

27. "The Law of Peoples," in *Collected Papers*, edited by Samuel Freeman (Harvard University Press, 1999), pp. 529–564.

28. "Principles of Justice as a Basis for Conceptualising a Health Care System," *International Journal of Health Services*, Vol. 7 (1977), pp. 707–719.

29. Rawls, "Distributive Justice: Some Addenda," in *Collected Papers*, pp. 529–564.

30. G. Walt and L. Gilson, "Reforming the Health Sector in Developing Countries: The Central Role of Policy Analysis," *Health Policy Planning*, Vol. 9 (1994), pp. 353–370.

31. *The Changing Politics of Foreign Policy* (London: Palgrave, 2003).

32. United Nations Development Program, 2002.

33. K. Buse and G. Walt, "Aid Coordination for Health Sector Reform: A Conceptual Framework for Analysis and Assessment," *Health Policy*, Vol. 38 (1996), pp. 173–187.

34. G. Walt, E. Pavignani, L. Gilson, and K. Buse, "Health Sector Development: From Aid Coordination to Resource Management," *Health Policy*

*Planning*, Vol. 14 (1999), pp. 207–218.

35. "Aid Donors Should Get Their Act Together," *International Herald Tribune*, February 24, 2003, p. 10.

36. "When Stinginess Costs Plenty," *International Herald Tribune*, February 25, 2003, p. 8.

37. R. N. Haass, "The Goal Becomes Muslim Democracy," *International Herald Tribune*, December 11, 2002, p. 4.

38. J. Dwyer, E. Pearce, K. McPherson, et al., "The Ideal Health Minister," *Journal of Epidemiology and Community Health*, Vol. 56 (2002), pp. 888–895.

39. R. Horton, "North and South: Bridging the Information Gap," *The Lancet*, Vol. 355 (2000), pp. 2231–2236.

40. J. C. Moskop, for example, has reviewed how Rawlsian ideas of political justice could be applied to the notion of health as a human right. See his "Rawlsian Justice and a Human Right to Health Care," *Journal of Medical Philosophy*, Vol. 8 (1983), pp. 329–338.

41. Oxford University Press, 1999.

42. *Macroeconomics and Health: Investing in Health for Economic Development* (Geneva: World Health Organization, 2001). The views of the commission have been endorsed by many close observers of global health. For example, David Bloom and David Canning have written that "the importance of political support, organizational reform, and an approach that is dictated by end-users and results rather than professional providers and inputs—these are lessons that we have learned." See "The Health and Poverty of Nations: From Theory to Practice," *Journal of Human Development*, Vol. 4 (2003), pp. 47–71.

43. *Human Development Report 2002: Deepening Democracy in a Fragmented World* (Oxford University Press, 2002).

## NOTES TO CHAPTER 18
## TAKING DIGNITY SERIOUSLY

1. *World Health Report 2000: Health Systems: Improving Performance* (Geneva: World Health Organization, 2000).

2. Oxford University Press, 2000.

3. *Development as Freedom* (Oxford University Press, 1999).

4. S. Pearlstein, "World Bank's Quest: New Ideas to Help the Poor,"

*International Herald Tribune*, September 14, 2001, p. 17.

5. *World Development Report 2000/2001: Attacking Poverty* (Oxford University Press, 2000).

6. Andrew Haines et al., "Joining Together to Combat Poverty," *British Medical Journal*, Vol. 320 (2000), pp. 1–2.

7. *Selected Works* (Oxford University Press, 1997).

8. Richard C. Dales, "A Medieval View of Human Dignity," *Journal of the History of Ideas*, October–December 1997, pp. 557–572.

9. Pico della Mirandola, *On the Dignity of Man* (Hackett, 1998). Theological notions of dignity have continued to evolve, often more robustly than their secular variants. See *In Defense of Human Dignity*, edited by Robert Kraynak and Glenn Tinder (University of Notre Dame Press, 2003).

10. Oxford University Press, 1998.

11. *Maxims* (Penguin, 1959).

12. "Of the Dignity or Meanness of Human Nature," in *Selected Essays* (Oxford University Press, 1998).

13. *Political Writings* (Oxford University Press, 1994).

14. *Grounding for the Metaphysics of Morals* (Hackett, 1993), and *The Metaphysics of Morals* (Cambridge University Press, 1996).

15. Jonathan Mann was fifty-one when he died. He was the first director, in 1986, of the World Health Organization's Special Programme on AIDS. He resigned that position in 1990, in protest at WHO's lack of commitment to HIV/AIDS, and created the François-Xavier Bagnoud Center for Health and Human Rights. There, he was professor of health and human rights, as well as professor of epidemiology and international health at the Harvard School of Public Health. Mann later became dean of the Allegheny University School of Public Health in Philadelphia.

16. Jonathan Mann et al., "Health and Human Rights," *Health and Human Rights*, Vol. 1 (1994), pp. 7–23.

17. "Dignity and Health: The UDHR's Revolutionary First Article," *Health and Human Rights*, Vol. 3 (1998), pp. 31–38.

18. There are some examples of progress beyond Mann's conceptualization of dignity. For example, Steven Malby, in the setting of the cloning debate, has tried to develop a model of human dignity based on "existing scientific and legal literature" with the aim of creating "a tool for the international community to analyse biotechnological practices." Malby's model has four levels based upon three "strands." The three strands include agency and

autonomy (the capacity for individual thought and action), value and restraint (the inherent dignity of all human beings, which limits autonomous action), and collectivity and culture (the dignity of groups, reflecting their particular ways of life). These three strands exist in a permanent tension with one another. Malby goes on to construct four levels in a working model of dignity. Level one is the underlying basis of the three strands, as identified above. The second level concerns the parameters of that underlying basis—for example, for agency and autonomy, "dignity is violated when an individual experiences a rights-based violation." Level three balances subjective (the *effects* of an action on the person or group) with objective (the *reasons* behind an action) perspectives on dignity. And finally, level four identifies violations and responsibilities—e.g., denial of autonomy for the first strand, degrading of the individual for the second strand, and observance of social norms for the third. See Steven Malby, "Human Dignity and Human Reproductive Cloning," *Health and Human Rights*, Vol. 6 (2002), pp. 103–135. Frances Fukuyama has also offered an eclectic view of dignity—moral choice, reason, language, sociability, sentience, emotions, consciousness—in his survey of the consequences of the biotechnology revolution. See his *Our Posthuman Future* (Farrar, Straus and Giroux, 2002).

19. Carolynne Shinn has also approached dignity from a violation perspective, concluding that "its antonym is surely stigma." See "The Right to the Highest Attainable Standard of Health," *Health and Human Rights*, Vol. 4 (1998), pp. 115–133.

20. Few writers have tried to work out a theory of dignity in the context of death. One exception is Darryl Pullman. See "Dying with Dignity and the Death of Dignity," *Health Law Journal*, Vol. 4 (1996), pp. 197–219. Another approach involved asking dying patients to rate their sense of dignity on a seven-point scale: from zero (no sense of lost dignity) to six (extreme sense of lost dignity). The scale emphasized feelings of degradation, shame, and embarrassment. Loss of dignity also seemed to be related to requests for euthanasia. See Harvey M. Chochinov et al., "Dignity in the Terminally Ill," *The Lancet*, Vol. 360 (2002), pp. 2026–2030.

21. E. Diczfalusy, "In Search of Human Dignity," *International Journal of Obstetrics and Gynecology*, Vol. 59 (1997), pp. 195–206. He constructs "nine pillars of human dignity," which, like the World Bank's approach to poverty, tries to conflate a great deal into a single idea.

22. "Towards Further Clarification of the Concept of 'Dignity,'" *Journal*

*of Advanced Nursing*, Vol. 24 (1996), pp. 924–931; A. Soderberg et al., "Dignity in Situations of Ethical Difficulty in Intensive Care," *Intensive and Critical Care Nursing*, Vol. 13 (1997), pp. 135–144; and L. Shotton and D. Seedhouse, "Practical Dignity in Caring," *Nursing Ethics*, Vol. 5 (1998), pp. 246–255.

23. H. Bosma et al., "Low Job Control and Risk of Coronary Heart Disease in Whitehall II Study," *British Medical Journal*, Vol. 314 (1997), pp. 558–565.

24. "Dignity-Conserving Care—a New Model for Palliative Care," *JAMA*, Vol. 287 (May 1, 2002), pp. 2253–2260.

25. Social capital takes up three pages in the World Bank's 335-page 2000/2001 report.

26. I. Kawachi et al., "Social Capital, Income Inequality, and Mortality," *American Journal of Public Health*, Vol. 87 (1997), pp. 1491–1498; and B. P. Kennedy et al., "Social Capital, Income Inequality, and Firearm Violent Crime," *Social Science and Medicine*, Vol. 47 (1998), pp. 7–17.

27. "The Myth of Development," in *Critical Development Theory*, edited by R. Munck and D. O'Hearn (London: Zed, 1999).

28. To be fair, Sen does mention the importance of "social support in expanding people's freedom." And his exploration of "human capital" extends beyond a narrow definition that dwells on economic productive power. But neither of these ideas is fully worked out.

## NOTE TO A NOTE ON ORIGINS

1. See David Wootton, "The Hard Look Back," *The Times Literary Supplement*, March 14, 2003, pp. 8–10.

# INDEX

– dignity (p. xiii) – what relⁿ to science?

– ch. 1 – whole questⁿ of evaluating error in med as a feature of the system, not individ^l responsy

– significance of further scientific advances (pp. 14 f)? – cf meaning of Canguilhem's humanistic pathology (p. 23)

---

– emerging infections – due to "sociocultural traits" (p. 74) → call for research in social & biological, surveillance etc (81-82) – reductionist science no answer (83)

– esp poverty (p. 130)

– war also – but medicine as site for reconcilⁿ & collaborⁿ (154)

– "infrastructure of care"

---

– issue of publicⁿ procedures – Wakefield on MMR – Pusztai on GM foods – Duesberg on HIV

– more generally, key issue of balancing scientific, political, public & commercial interest